Managing Healthcare Information Systems with Web-Enabled Technologies

Lauren B. Eder
Rider University

IDEA GROUP PUBLISHING
Hershey USA • London UK

Senior Editor:	Mehdi Khosrowpour
Managing Editor:	Jan Travers
Copy Editor:	Maria Boyer
Typesetter:	Tamara Gillis
Cover Design:	Connie Peltz
Printed at:	BookCrafters

Published in the United States of America by
  Idea Group Publishing
  1331 E. Chocolate Avenue
  Hershey PA 17033-1117
  Tel: 717-533-8845
  Fax: 717-533-8661
  E-mail: cust@idea-group.com
  Web site: http://www.idea-group.com

and in the United Kingdom by
  Idea Group Publishing
  3 Henrietta Street
  Covent Garden
  London WC2E 8LU
  Tel: 171-240 0856
  Fax: 171-379 0609
  Web site: http://www.eurospan.co.uk

Library of Congress Cataloging-in-Publication Data

Eder, Lauren B., 1960-
   Managing healthcare information systems with Web-enabled technologies / Lauren B. Eder.
     p. cm.
   Includes bibliographic references and index.
   ISBN 1-878289-65-9 (pbk.)
     1. Health services administration--Computer networks. 2. Medical care--Computer networks. 3. Medicine--Computer networks. 4. Browsers (Computer programs) 5. World Wide Web. I. Title.

RA971.23 .E34 2000
362.1'0285--dc21   99-088700

British Cataloguing in Publication Data
A Cataloguing in Publication record for this book is available from the British Library.

NEW from Idea Group Publishing

Excellent additions to your library!

**Receive the Idea Group Publishing catalog with descriptions of these books by
calling, toll free 1/800-345-4332
or visit the IGP Web site at: http://www.idea-group.com!**

Managing Healthcare Information Systems with Web-Enabled Technologies

Table of Contents

Preface

In recent years, healthcare organizations worldwide have undergone major reorganizations and adjustments to meet the demands of improved health service accessibility and quality as well as lowered costs. In addition, the use of information technology to process health data continues to grow, and much of the critical information needed by healthcare administrators, providers and other users is being stored digitally in a variety of formats, often at multiple locations. As a result, an open network architecture to support data access and integration from a multitude of internal and external sources has become essential.

A major trend in healthcare computing involves the use of Web-enabled technologies to address the complex information-processing requirements that are emerging in this transforming industry. Web-enabled technologies refer to information systems that utilize standard Web browser utilities as a front-end to combinations of existing software applications with other information sources. These systems generally reside on an organization's intranet and may be connected to the Internet, providing heterogeneous connectivity for all authorized systems and users.

Web-enabled systems can provide strategic advantages for healthcare organizations. For example, the transparent streamlining of organizational processes with existing transaction processing systems can significantly reduce overhead costs while improving the delivery of health services. Secondly, Web-based interorganizational systems can lead to the establishment of more efficient and effective relationships with affiliated healthcare organizations. Finally, using a standardized Web browser provides a universal user interface for disparate systems and applications that can be accessed globally.

Web-enabled technologies are being integrated with many existing computer-based healthcare applications. Examples of successful implementations include expanded access to computer-based patient records and improved access to large data warehouses. Additionally, Web technologies are being utilized to enhance the effectiveness of telemedicine applications in rural and underdeveloped areas. There are some areas for concern, however, as Web-enabled technologies 'open the door' for greater accessibility of health data. Issues such as information privacy and adherence to information standards are just some of important challenges being faced by many organizations.

This book presents a selection of research and case studies from academics and practitioners around the world that are paving the way for the emergence of Web-enabled healthcare information systems. Their chapters focus on the critical management decision-making areas that are being realized by both healthcare and computer information systems professionals as these systems evolve. They address many of the current technological, organizational, and ethical concerns associated with the use of Web-enabled technologies to access and integrate health information.

Readers of this book will find that the chapters provide a global perspective of Web technology use in healthcare that is truly multidisciplinary. Research from several bodies of literature, including management information systems, medical informatics, computer science, clinical medicine, and organizational science are represented in this collection of highly informative readings. Together, the contributions provide experiences and insights that are both practical and theoretical in nature.

The book is divided into four general themes. First the issues surrounding Web-based interorganizational communications in healthcare are addressed from multiple perspectives. Transformations in legacy relationships are discussed, as are existing technological challenges and potential benefits for stakeholders. Second, the transition to become a Web-enabled healthcare organization is explored from both a technology-oriented and an organizational viewpoint. Strategies, proposed models, and 'lessons learned' are presented and evaluated. Web-based clinical applications are illustrated in the third section. Proposed system architectures as well as potential implications for researchers and practitioners are explored. In the final section, the Internet and the World Wide Web are considered enablers for empowering health practitioners and their patients. Several examples demonstrate how the Web-based interface to health information is having a profound impact on physicians and patients alike.

In closing, I wish to thank all of the authors for their insights and excellent contributions to this book. I also want to extend my gratitude to all of the people that assisted me in the reviewing process. In addition, this book would not have been possible without the ongoing professional support from Mehdi Khosropour and Jan Travers at Idea Group Publishing. Last, but not least, I want to thank my husband Scott and my children, Brooke and Marc, for their love and their support throughout this (and every other) project.

Lauren B. Eder, Ph.D.
Lawrenceville, New Jersey, U.S.A.
October 1999

Section I: Web-Enabling Interorganizational Communications in Healthcare

This section contains four chapters that examine the use of Web-enabled technologies across organizational boundaries. The potential impact and the potential barriers associated with the implementation of these systems are explored. The chapters represent several disciplinary perspectives, including management information systems, computer science, marketing, and economics. Each chapter proposes a unique framework for understanding the issues involved with implementing shared access to health information over a standardized Web-based interface. Together they encompass many of the critical technological, organizational, and behavioral factors associated with the impending transformation of legacy relationships in the healthcare industry today.

Forslund and Kilman discuss the technical issues associated with the evolution of globally standardized electronic health records. Specifically, they analyze the role of standards in the development of electronic health records and the current barriers impacting the growth and diffusion of globally accessible Web-based health records. Furthermore, they propose ways in which these obstacles can be overcome. Forslund and Kilman focus on some of the major projects currently under development by the Object Management Group (OMG), a non-profit consortium founded to provide an open and interoperable distributed object architecture. In their discussion, the need for standardized globally accessible health records is demonstrated, as are the benefits that can be realized with a universally accepted standard.

Hackney and McBride describe how a Web-based communication system throughout the UK can provide the foundation for a major social and cultural transformation of the UK healthcare delivery system. The authors begin with the evolution of the UK National Health Service (NHS). They discuss the importance of determining stakeholder expectations and benefits as a precursor to a successful national healthcare communications system. Hackney and McBride propose that while a sound technological infrastructure is important, it will not be sufficient in the successful deployment of a national electronic healthcare delivery system. The nature of the stakeholders must be carefully considered. Hackney and McBride develop a detailed framework for understanding the role of stakeholders, and the benefits that can derived from a national Web-based healthcare delivery system when stakeholder interests, reservations, and expectations are addressed early.

Johnson, Kumar, Ramaprasad, and Reddy propose that as a result of the rapid diffusion of Web technology and Internet access, the relationships between players in the healthcare industry will change significantly. Centering on the physician-patient relationship, the authors broadly consider the impact of Web-enabled technologies on four key players in the healthcare industry—physicians, patients, pharmaceutical firms, and insurance firms. They suggest that relationships that have traditionally been dyadic in nature, such as the physician-patient relationship or pharmaceutical firm-physician relationship, will be transformed because information technology is changing the communication path characteristics among the players. The authors propose a model in which the information exchanges among the four players become integrated and more equalized. The authors present their argument from two perspectives. The impact of Web-based technologies on the four players is explored, and their influences on the physician-patient relationship are considered from both outside and inside the clinical/hospital setting.

Kirn and Heine focus on the potential advantages and barriers that can exist when linking hospitals together on an Internet-based network to share clinical medical information. They present the ARIS methodology (architecture of integrated information systems) to describe a technical approach to developing a Web-based teleradiology network. The deployment of this system among a small consortium of hospitals in rural Germany is explored. The authors discuss the existing challenges faced by the disparate hospitals and present several conceptualizations for a Web-based scenario. Potential challenges inherent to each project as well as the expected benefits are evaluated, and an outlook to the future is proposed.

Chapter I

The Impact of the Global, Extensible Electronic Health Record

David W. Forslund
Los Alamos National Laboratory

David G. Kilman
Theragraphics, Inc.

With the arrival of the "World Wide Web," we have witnessed a transition toward a truly global perspective with respect to electronic health records. In recent years, much more discussion has focused on the potential for international virtual electronic health records and what is required for them to become a reality in the world today (Kilman & Forslund, 1997). As the Internet becomes more ubiquitous and Web-enabled, we see access to electronic health records using these technologies becoming more commonplace. Even so, these Web-enabled health records still remain technologically isolated from other medical records in the distributed continuum of care; much of the standardization challenge still stands before us. We have witnessed startling technological advances, but we still face considerable obstacles to the goal of having globally standardized electronic health records.

In this chapter we describe some of the issues associated with Web-enabled health records, the role of standards in the evolution of Web-enabled health records, and some of the barriers to the development of globally accessible electronic health records. We discuss possible ways to overcome these barriers and the kinds of benefits and opportunities that global health records will help provide. The global scale perspective makes more evident the very real and potentially tragic consequences of prolonged and unnecessary delays in deploying these technologies. Therefore, in an effort to promote a fuller consciousness of health safety, the chapter concludes with a comparative look at the negative impact of impediments in the movement toward global extensible electronic health records.

BACKGROUND

The early years of health informatics were dominated by health information systems running on mainframe computers and minicomputers at large medical facilities (Collen,

1995). These involve significant expenditures to support large central data repositories. These may efficiently solve the needs of the local hospital, but they are difficult to modify, have primarily proprietary interfaces and data representations, and provide little, if any ability to extend them into new areas without major expenditures. We characterize this state of healthcare information technology as a "stovepipe" industry with relatively limited communications between facilities and little motivation to communicate. HL7 (Health Level Seven, 1999), one of the dominant standards developing organizations for health related information, has provided an important data interchange capability. However, HL7 still has interoperability limitations that result in proprietary implementations utilizing interface engines to meet the need of connecting smaller systems into the domains of the large mainframe repositories. HL7, itself, was founded in 1987 and is an ANSI (American National Standards Institute) accredited Standards Development Organization (SDO). The term Health Level Seven comes from the seventh, or application, level in the ISO (International Standards Organization) communications model for Open Systems Interconnection (OSI).

With the evolution of distributed computing technology, paved by the rapid adoption of Web technology, the need for a central system becomes less compelling. Moreover, with the advent of privacy concerns recognizing the patient's right to control his/her medical record (Shalala, 1997), the notion of a single healthcare institution maintaining the complete medical record becomes less likely. The need for data to be shared through a secure referral process and the increasing need for a longitudinal medical record to establish long-term effects of slowly evolving diseases such as Hepatitis C and HIV, not to mention management for chronic illnesses like diabetes, pushes one away from the "stovepipe" model to one in which data exchange becomes the central paradigm.

The evolution of the Web (WWW) has helped break down these "stovepipes" by making it almost trivial to publish a database on the Internet (cf. Mactaggart, 1999). For a very low cost one can use a simple "application server" to create a Web presence for a clinical repository. The low cost results in the development of thousands of medical repositories offering the capability of managing some portion of a patient's data. This includes numerous examples of Web technology being used to manage teleconsultations. However, these developments don't really provide the patient access to a longitudinal medical record that they could understand. One would have to use an Internet search engine to assemble the long-term medical record of a patient in this distributed healthcare treatment world, although this, in fact, is not practical from a security standpoint. Additionally, this approach has essentially no architectural design behind it and thus is at best an ad hoc solution to the medical record problem with unknown scalability and extensibility capabilities. So how do we resolve this problem?

STANDARDS

How should we link the Web of health records together? The easy publication of electronic health records enables an organization to make information available to patients, but it does not enable a patient to manage all of their own information possibly stored in a number of geographically dispersed clinical repositories.

The resolution of this problem involves more than simply setting up a set of data standards and providing data feeds to those interested. This might work reasonably well within a single enterprise, but is woefully inadequate when extended to a broader region. One solution to facilitate the more dynamic linkage of systems required over a wide area is to adopt some form of "middleware" technology which can abstract away the server from the client. In addition, if this middleware has the ability to support encapsulation, polymorphism, and inheritance, it can provide a data processing environment much more capable of handling the complexities of wide area integration than simply relying on standardized data models.

The premier example of this approach is the Object Management Group, a nonprofit consortium founded (OMG, 1989) to provide an open, interoperable, platform and language independent distributed object architecture. This approach has been enormously successful and has been adopted by numerous large firms around the world as the basic architecture for their complex information systems (Carlson, 1999). While this infrastructure provides a great deal of power, scalability, and interoperability, it helps little if every healthcare institution has their own object model which is uninterpretable by most other healthcare institutions. To alleviate this problem the OMG has sought to provide direct support for vertical markets, with healthcare being a significant example. The OMG healthcare taskforce, CORBAmed, (1999) was formed in 1996 to create standard object interfaces so that the OMG CORBA (Common Object Request Broker Architecture) middleware would provide full interoperability between disparate systems and organizations. This ultimate goal would result in plug-and-play objects on the CORBA software bus capable of extending across the Internet. The interface specification language called IDL (Interface Definition Language) is a language-neutral way of expressing this capability and can be used independent of the CORBA middleware. Because OMG IDL does not specify implementation details, it provides an ideal way to specify object models capable of accommodating backward compatibility with the installed base of systems in the healthcare industry. The OMG recently began to issue interface specifications for a number of

Figure 1: Schematic of a True Web of Information Not Easily Supported by Normal WWW Protocols

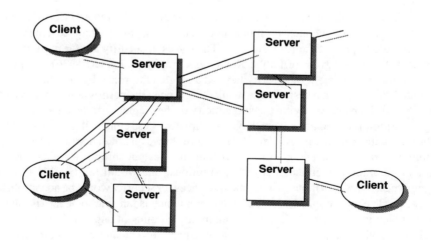

healthcare related services that can be managed with security and distributed transaction controls.

If we desire the patients eventually to have the capability or even the possibility of managing their own healthcare, a true Web of clinical information must be developed. By a "true Web" we mean a truly distributed environment, where information from multiple sites is viewable and analyzable from any point of entry, in many cases without the linkage of information even being visible. The "publish" paradigm of current Web technology does not directly support this required capability. Any viable standards must also support the ability for the content and use of the medical record to grow and evolve over time without having to replace the existing infrastructure. The CORBAmed standards provide a set of framework objects whose content can change with time and which are extensible in their capabilities.

The Person Identification Services (PIDS) specification became the first CORBAmed standard (PIDS, 1998). We view the PIDS specification as a potential key to mediating global level exchanges of health-related information (Kilman & Forslund, 1997). Interestingly, HL7 has a highly related standardization effort under development through the HL7 Master Patient Index Mediator Special Interest Group (MPISIG). The latter has the goal of harmonizing the object approach of PIDS with the message-oriented approach of HL7. Historically, both of these efforts sprang from the same series of workshops. Some organizations have participated in both efforts with the goal of keeping the two standards harmonized as much as possible. HL7 has a high interest in standards based on object models that will also assure backward compatibility with existing systems in the healthcare industry. In addition, HL7 seeks to provide a common data model that will not require healthcare institutions to use CORBA ORB technologies. Below, we describe in more detail the current challenges the HL7 MPISIG faces and the approach we recommend.

How will the Web interact with these rapidly evolving standards?

CHALLENGES

Security

To have an acceptable wide area access to their own health record information without providing access to someone who should not have access, patients require a robust security infrastructure to protect their information. The issues of security are far more than simply technical. With the advent of Public Key Cryptography (Schneier, 1996), the promise is there for the management of security beyond a single enterprise, by enabling a system of delegated trust. In such a system, one would "negotiate" the permission of access by using a certificate chain and verifying the authenticity of the elements of the chain. In this way a single institution would not have to have a complete access control list, but would manage it through authenticated roles. This does require, however, the adoption of a significant common infrastructure and common mechanism of establishing roles and permissions. Without common agreements between institutions, one would not be able to negotiate secure access. This distributed set of linked services for security would be accomplished via federation. The most common form of federation which is familiar to people is the Internet Domain Naming Service (DNS). There are multiple points of entry with caching at many levels but with a common registration mechanism so that one can obtain the relevant information from multiple locations. Utilizing federation one can provide an infrastructure to support the identification of users and their requisite permissions.

Ultimately, using public key cryptography and trusted certificate authorities, the patient should be able to control access to their distributed medical record and know with certainty who has looked at their medical record. This is possible not only in a single institution but also across multiple institutions. It would be like being able to control access to your financial transaction record across banking institutions and know who has looked at your financial record over time, much like the way you can find out who has run a credit check on you. However, we are proposing a much more organized, systematic and secure mechanism for healthcare than currently exists in the banking industry. If your medical record resides fragmented at multiple "secure" disconnected sites through the Web, it would be much more difficult for you to manage your own information. The Health Insurance Portability and Accountability Act (*cf.*, Shalala, 1997) is seeking to standardize some of this security technology to facilitate the transmission of healthcare information for reimbursement purposes.

One mechanism being developed to provide a scalable management of the permissions is the Resource Access Decision (CORBAmed RAD, 1999) interfaces being developed by the OMG. This interface enables one to express arbitrarily fine-grained access of information based on dynamic relationships between, say a patient and a physician. Based on the role of the provider, they may only be allowed to see certain pieces of a specific patient's medical record. This mechanism is designed in such a way as to be independent of the specifics of an implementation and interoperable between healthcare enterprises. This mechanism would provide a tool for restricting access to individual pieces of patient information depending on the provider's credentials, role, and location, for example. As such it sits above current security mechanisms and provides much more adaptable mechanism for satisfying authorization requests that might ordinarily be handled through Access Control Lists (ACL). Although it has just recently been adopted as a standard, such mechanisms have already been used in proprietary systems in banks and hospitals for managing access to medical records. It now is a standard and will soon be available in the commercial marketplace for many different systems.

Standardization Process

A standardized global electronic health record necessarily requires "Open" standards in order to provide sustainable and extensible systems available at low cost. This includes coordination between some of the healthcare information standards bodies and careful management of the standards process. Global level standardization requires large-scale consensus coupled with a very high quality modeling effort. The quality of the model itself becomes the critical factor since it drives the consensus, stability and sustainability of the standard. A well-designed model will accurately mirror the real world while also providing a high level of adaptability, making it easily extensible.

By mirroring the real world, a high quality model will have a higher degree of stability; it will require changes only as the real world changes and changes only to those aspects of the model that reflect the parts of the real world that change. Changes should not propagate throughout the model, entailing enormous expenditures to adapt to the changes. Models based on the idiosyncrasies of existing systems, rather than on observed features in the real world, will ultimately require higher levels of maintenance due to the dynamic character of systems compared to the relatively stable character of the real world. Because all human healthcare around the world deals with the health of real-world humans who all share a common real-world DNA heritage, we can hope to reach consensus on a common model capable of abstracting the relationships between the objects of healthcare at the global level.

The early versions of the HL7 Reference Information Model (RIM) provide illustrations of an approach to object modeling based more on the idiosyncrasies of existing systems. This does not imply that the HL7 RIM does not have the capability of evolving into a more robust model. Neither should it surprise us to discover a consensus building effort based on a model influenced heavily by the constraints of backward compatibility with existing systems. After all, most of the organizations involved in the HL7 standardization process have an installed base of systems they have an interest in preserving as much as possible. In contrast, the OMG CORBAmed modeling effort has the luxury of a relatively clean slate with respect to existing systems. While seeking to accommodate HL7 and other existing standards, the organizations involved in the OMG process have more limited interest in preserving at least some aspects of existing systems.

For example, the HL7 RIM has object-oriented hierarchies and relationships, but does not include object-oriented behaviors, often referred to as methods. This "oversight," as compared to the OMG CORBAmed models, stems from the fact that most HL7 modelers anticipate using some form of message-passing communications to implement the model. Existing HL7 systems all use message passing and we discover the influence on the model of the idiosyncrasies of the existing systems. In fact, the HL7 Modeling & Methodology Committee has produced a Message Development Framework document that details the official formal process of moving from model to message implementation.

The HL7 modeling effort makes perfect sense within the context of the HL7 perspective on systems, but does it make sense from the perspective of a global-level modeling effort for healthcare? Keep in mind that some areas of the world have much less investment or no investment in an installed base of electronic health record systems. Knowledgeable healthcare informatics professionals in developing countries will likely see that they have more in common with the "clean slate" of the OMG than they do with the backward compatibility issues of HL7. After witnessing the Y2K debacle, they will also understand the importance of a sound theory of modeling influenced by the need to accommodate changes without suffering the heavy expenses of ramifying system modifications. Any approach to modeling in healthcare that lacks the extensibility required to accommodate new technologies betrays the interests of developing regions of the world and effectively constrains their freedom to select to use the newer technologies.

Therefore, we face the challenge of arriving at an approach to modeling that will accommodate all concerns. Recent work of the HL7 MPISIG seeks to do just that. In an effort to harmonize with the OMG PIDS specification, the MPISIG has developed some use case scenario examples that it has already begun to advocate at HL7 technical meetings. These use cases include a message-passing approach as well as object methods. The MPISIG has also decided to use the OMG PIDS specification as the base specification to work from since it covers more of the landscape for MPI mediation than the existing set of HL7 messages. This does not imply an inevitable incompatibility with current HL7 messages. In fact, HL7 has a "clean slate" when it comes to object methods, which makes harmonizing with PIDS relatively straightforward. The existing set of HL7 messages becomes one means of implementing the OMG PIDS specification.

Since the OMG IDL for PIDS exists as an implementation-independent specification, providing a PIDS harmonization by developing an HL7 modeling effort for implementing

PIDS serves well as an example approach that will accommodate all concerns. In fact, it helps to disambiguate the set of HL7 messages related to MPI mediation and leads to a stronger consensus on those aspects of the healthcare modeling efforts related to identifying persons receiving healthcare. By harmonizing in this way between the HL7 standards and the OMG standards, we have some hope of evolving a single object model capable of having global consensus.

Additionally, we see the electronic medical record as an evolving, rapidly changing system. The object modeling enables one to isolate various components and construct a medical record system from a set of these components that can change over time. The CORBAmed healthcare task force is attempting to define some of these large-scale components (CORBAmed Roadmap, 1999). An institution then can build its health information system from a set of best-of-breed components from multiple vendors that may be replaced over time as technology and requirements change. This approach has recently been adopted as part of the Government Computerized Patient Record Framework Project (GCPR, 1999). It has established the following goals: (1) Create a collaborative membership to appropriately share clinical information via a standards-based, comprehensive, lifelong medical record. (2) Where no standards exist, the partnership will seek to advance the development, establishment, and adherence to standards.

Another factor which could assist the adoption of sufficient global standards to achieve a "globally extensible health record" is the open source movement (OpenSource, 1999). It has resulted in the highly acclaimed Linux operating system and is assisting in the adoption of common solutions to problems, which helps to promote the standards necessary to support this global concept for medical records.

One of the barriers to the achievement of integration on a wide scale is the disparate naming conventions and standards that exist both within countries and between countries. To address this terminology problem, the OMG has recently adopted a Terminology Query Service (CORBAmed LQS, 1998) which provides a mechanism to ask what terms in one namespace correspond to in other namespaces and what they mean. This can support the National Library of Medicine's Unified Medical Language System (NLM UMLS, 1999), for example, which is providing knowledge sources and lexical programs to assist in managing healthcare and related information. Related efforts in linking relevant information in healthcare are in Problem Knowledge Couplers (PKC, 1999), which seek to couple the uniqueness of the patient's situation to the body of relevant medical knowledge during the initial stages of diagnosis and management. Efforts are also underway to standardize the interface (CORBAmed HDIF, 1999) to systems such as the knowledge coupler to assist the provider to make appropriate healthcare decisions. Without the standardization of terminology and access mechanisms, this too, will be difficult.

In the long run, political and sociological barriers may be the hardest to overcome. The difficulty of meeting all the demands of security, connectivity, and information standards may be limited by various special interest groups and agendas unrelated to quality of care. However, the rapid adoption of Internet technologies may help to reduce the parochialisms that would otherwise impede new technology adoption. An example is the impact of the facsimile machine in stimulating the rapid changes in the governmental systems of Eastern Europe in the late 1980s.

BENEFITS AND OPPORTUNITIES

More advanced standards will help to raise the level of sophistication for decision support systems. These standards will also accommodate techniques for assisting healthcare practitioners to draw from data distributed across the continuum of care. The next generation of distributed decision support systems will bring together a diverse set of computational resources to help more quickly resolve difficult health problems. Distributed decision support might also lead to earlier detection of emerging infectious diseases by helping to more quickly analyze a real-time population base of clinical information. Collaborative decision support technology should also blend naturally into the telemedicine consulting sessions and help to supplant the "traditional" telemedicine video conferencing technology by enabling ad hoc, real-time consults between providers utilizing information-rich data sources.

Concerns about the rise of naturally occurring infectious diseases has led to apprehensions about our ability to respond to those diseases in a timely manner. An improvement in the global infrastructure could go a long way to reducing or at least detecting these threats early, and thus potentially saving thousands if not millions of lives. Surveillance of health trends also could reduce the threat of bio-terrorism by supporting the early identification of the potential sources of these threats and thus lowering their probability. Efforts to accomplish this are underway through the Centers for Disease Control and Prevention working with local and state public health organizations (CDC, 1999).

Patient empowerment over their healthcare history is an important opportunity of Web-enabled healthcare. But, as mentioned above, it requires more organization that currently exists on the Web to enable patients to comprehend and organize their information. There must be a considerable level of "coherence" in the medical record in order for the patient to be able to understand the information in the record. At the present time, the healthcare provider can be challenged to understand the entire longitudinal healthcare record, let alone the patient. By enabling the patient to better understand their longitudinal healthcare record and have convenient, secure access to it, the patient can participate much more completely in the management of their health, a process that could have significant impact on the cost and quality of healthcare in this nation.

How do we minimize the dichotomy between the "haves" and "have-nots?" We expect that the declining costs of networked computers around the world together with the expansion of the software base will eventually enable "poorer" countries to have access to resources not much worse than those of highly developed countries. This rapid change in technology will also enable third-world areas to leapfrog some of the more developed countries by skipping several generations of technological development. We are attempting to assist in this process by testing some of this advanced technology in technologically "poor" areas of the United States through grants from the National Telecommunications and Information Administration and making our prototype software available on the Web (Forslund, 1999).

Investment in public health fuels general industrial productivity and lowers healthcare costs. As Gro Harlem Brundtland, WHO Director General, recently put it (Brundtland, 1999), "Improving health in poor countries leads to increased gross domestic product per capita. In richer countries it reduces overall costs to society. From often being seen as an unproductive consumer of public funds, health is now being seen as a central element of productivity itself." The expansion of the Internet and the Web into healthcare, if done wisely, has the potential of improving the condition of society in several ways.

Healthcare information technologies will impact other industries in ways similar to the impact space technologies has on other industries. Industries outside of healthcare can reuse system components developed originally for healthcare. We anticipate many business opportunities to continue to increase in an era of high technological change. We contend that wise investments that consider the quality of healthcare a higher priority than short-term profitability will flourish and have high financial success in the long-term.

Another example of this approach is being recognized in new public-private partnerships involving shared health information. One excellent documented example has been provided by the Massachusetts Health Data Consortium (Stone, et al, 1998). They indicate how these public-private demands have stimulated the need to reorganize previously proprietary health information systems. Among their significant conclusions two salient points involve designing an interoperable network, modeled on the Internet and private intranets, using national electronic data standards to ensure interconnectivity among proprietary data systems at each point of care and emphasis on ad-hoc data release rather than centralized data pooling. The approach we are recommending is exactly that: emphasizing interoperability and a distributed architecture.

The National Committee for Quality Assurance (NCQA, 1999) recently published a report which supports this concept of a unifying Health Information Framework emphasizing standard data formats and linkages between records, while protecting security and confidentiality of the data.

IMPACT OF DELAYS

In moments of disaster, people race against time to prevent the loss of life or to help relieve suffering. For example, following a catastrophic earthquake, people work together and waste little time digging through the rubble while looking for survivors. Indeed, people often act heroically during such moments of crisis. Whether it's an earthquake, an avalanche, a flood, a storm or whatever natural disaster threatens people, we witness large numbers of people launching into action on very short notice and with a minimum amount of delay.

In 1918, the so-called "Doomsday Flu," taught us how our global civilization can interact over a short amount of time in ways that can have tragic consequences. Within a matter of months, between twenty and thirty million people (many of them healthy young adults) died in a worldwide pandemic. That's more people dead than the total number of people who died as a result the tragic Holocaust during World War II. Before its eradication, the Smallpox virus resulted in the death of 500 million people in this century (*Albuquerque Journal*, 1999).

The danger of a similar pandemic happening again remains with us today. Having a globally standardized health record has the potential to help minimize or even prevent pandemics like the Doomsday Flu. By providing a linked electronic repository of anonymous clinical information in real time, it should be possible to detect unusual healthcare events, determine their potential origins and thus respond quickly to either natural or man-made biothreats. In addition, using this large repository of data, new information could be gained as to the effective treatment and management of diseases around the world. More work needs to be done to establish the value of such a system to establish its efficacy in adding to the knowledge base of the treatment and management of disease. This could include the linking together of disparate databases including environmental, weather and health-related information (RAMBO, 1999). The potential impact on the global health of people on the planet warrants an increased commitment to the deployment of this technology. We also believe that this can be done at a reasonable cost as Web technology becomes more ubiquitous worldwide. The neglect of the adoption and deployment of the technology could result in major negative consequences for the human race.

CONCLUSIONS

We concur with others that the ubiquitous connectivity and access of the World Wide Web provides an important infrastructure for the distribution and management of healthcare information. However, a coherent software architecture is crucial for the evolution of the virtual medical record. This architecture should facilitate the use of arbitrary computer platforms and languages, and specify the type of information and access and storage methodologies. This includes the discovery of the type of information managed by a system (metadata), as well as the publication of information in an understandable way for other systems to utilize. Such an approach is necessary for the medical record to be of value to both the patient and to large scale detection of population-based health threats. We urge the evolution of the use of the World Wide Web in healthcare to include the adoption and extension of standardized interfaces and data models for exchange of information between servers around the world. This includes the adoption of a standard security infrastructure and nomenclature to preserve the integrity, privacy and confidentiality of an individual's medical record. The World Wide Web may be an excellent presentation and distribution mechanism, but by itself, it should not be thought of as the organizing architecture behind health information.

Pilot projects exist in an effort to stimulate the evolution of this global approach to the medical record. Such a pilot has been undertaken in New Mexico to demonstrate the power of the virtual medical record (Forslund, 1999). Many others are underway including the Government Computerized Patient Record project (GCPR, 1999), with additional impetus coming from the Open Source software efforts (OpenSource, 1999).

REFERENCES

Albuquerque Journal (1999). "Virus samples to be retained," May 25, 1999, A3.
Brundtland, G.H. (1999). Better Health Stokes Productivity. *International Herald Tribune.*
Carlson, D.S. (1999). Manageable Information system Development, *Component Strategies, May 1999, 58-70.*
Collen, M.F. (1995). *A History of Medical Informatics in the United States 1950-1990.* Indianapolis, IN: Hartman Publishing, 183-187.
CORBAmed (1999). retrieved May 25, 1999 from the World Wide Web: http://www.omg.org/corbamed.
CORBAmed HDIF (1999). Retrieved September 3, 199 from the World Wide Web, http://www.omg.org/corbamed/docs/98-03-30.pdf .
CORBAmed LQS (1999). Retrieved Sept 3, 1999 from the World Wide Web: CORBAmed RAD (1999), Resource Access Decision: http://www.omg.org/docs/corbamed/99-04-

04.pdf

CORBAmed Roadmap (1999): http://www.omg.org/corbamed/Roadmap/roadmap.htm

Forslund, 1999. The TeleMed Project, retrieved May 25, 1999 from the World Wide Web: http://www.acl.lanl.gov/TeleMed

GCPR (1999), Government Computerized Patient Records, retrieved May 25, 1999 from the World Wide Web: http://www.gcpr.gov

Health Level Seven (1999). Retrieved May 25, 1999 from the World Wide Web: http://www.hl7.org

Kilman, D. G., & Forslund D.W. (1997). An International Collaboratory Based on Virtual Patient Records. *Communications of the ACM,* 40, 110-117.

Mactaggart,M. (1999). "Web-Enhanced Databases Made Easy", *Component Strategies,* May, p. 62. SIGS Publications.

NCQA (1999) "Enhancing Performance Measurement, NCQA's Road Map for a Health Information Framework", Eric C. Schneider, Virginia Riehl, Sonja Courte-Wienecke, David M. Eddy, and Cary Sennet, *Journal of the American Medical Association,* September 22/29, 282(12).

NLM UMLS (1999). The Unified Medical Language System, retrieved September 3, 1999 from the World Wide Web, http://www.nlm.nih.gov/research/umls

OMG (1989). The Object Management Group, retrieved May 25, 1999 from the World Wide Web http://www.omg.org

OpenSource (1999). Information on the open source effort can be read about at http://www.opensource.org and for healthcare at: http://www.openhealth.com

PIDS (1998). Person Identification Service, retrieved May 25, 1999 from the World Wide Web: http://www.omg.org/cgi-bin/doc?formal/99-03-05.

PKC (1999). Problem Knowledge Couplers, PKC Corporation, retrieved September 3, 1999 from the World Wide Web, http://www.pkc.com

RAMBO (1999). Research Association of Medical and Biological Organizations, retrieved May 25, 1999 from the World Wide Web: http://www.acl.lanl.gov/RAMBO.

Schneier, Bruce (1996). *Applied Cryptography, 2nd Edition,* New York: John Wiley & Sons.

Shalala, Donna (1997). Confidentiality of Individually-Identifiable Health Information. Retrieved May 25, 1999 from the World Wide Web: http://aspe.os.dhhs.gov/admnsimp/pvrec0.htm

Stone, et al. (1998). "Comprehensive Health Data Systems Spanning the Public-Private Divide: The Massachusetts Experience", E. M. Stone, M. H. Bailit, M. S. Greenberg, G. R. Jones, *American Journal of Preventive Medicine,* 14(38), 40-45.

Chapter II

UK Primary Healthcare Groups: Stakeholders, Technology and Benefits

Ray Hackney
Manchester Metropolitan University

Neil McBride
DeMontfort University

INTRODUCTION

The UK Information Management Strategy (NHS, 1998) for the period to 2005 envisages the implementation of a Nationwide private network which will support clinical and administrative functions throughout the National Health Service (NHS). Using Web-based technologies, a wide variety of applications will enable rapid communication between professionals. Secondary, acute services and primary care services will be linked in a way that has not been previously possible. Communications concerning hospital appointment booking, referrals, discharges from hospitals, radiology results and laboratory test requests will all be mediated by the NHSnet, producing faster, more accurate communication and increased integration of services. Electronic patient records (EPRs) will be transmitted between general practitioners (GPs) and hospitals, prescription requests will be transmitted to pharmacists, even patients will be able to access information concerning conditions and treatment and communicate with health professionals from their homes. In effect we are observing the potential for technology-enabled change as 'information powers the NHS' (Nicholls, 1995).

The UK information management strategy provides the foundations for radical changes in healthcare philosophy: shifting the focus of activity to primary care, increasing patient responsibility and involvement in the healthcare process and increasing the information available to healthcare professionals and patients. Thus, an agenda for social and cultural change within healthcare delivery is to be driven by the availability of technical infrastructure (Lenaghan, 1998). It would be naive to consider that the availability of the technology will naturally lead to its acceptance as a communication media or to the required organizational and cultural change. The management of a Web-enabled infrastructure and its Web-based information systems is as much about the management of its social construction as its physical construction. Stakeholders within the health service will have individual perceptions and expectations of the technology which through discussion and interaction within groups will determine the social construction placed upon the technology and ultimately the benefits incurred by its use. This social construction will be significantly affected by the context within which the technology is implemented. Contextual issues may include the attitude of stakeholders and stakeholder groups to the technology, economic drivers which influence the availability of the technology, and previous implementations of information and communication technology.

If the implementation of a Web-based communication system throughout the UK NHS is to be successful, the needs of stakeholders and the types of application possible should be matched to produce benefits. The management and delivery of benefits requires an understanding of stakeholders' interests and the implementation of applications appropriate to those interests. This chapter considers the following questions: Who are the stakeholders involved in a Web-based information infrastructure? What applications are possible? How do we match applications to stakeholders to achieve benefits? In each of these areas a research agenda is developed, Firstly we provide and overview of the technology which will enable a new approach to healthcare communications in the UK.

BACKGROUND

Since its inception in 1948 the National Health Service (NHS) has attempted to provide care to all regardless of their ability to pay. It is one of the largest employers in Europe with over 1 million employees in the UK. It has undergone significant government generated reforms over the years where, most recently, change has been implemented to make the NHS more accountable and competitive (Gillies, 1998). The election of a Labour government in 1997 has led to another recent and significant reform. The White Paper 'The New NHS, Modern Dependable' (DoH, 1997) outlines these changes for the integration of services through GPs and the abolition of so called 'fund holding'. Under the new proposals GPs may control up to 90% of hospital budgets as health authorities lose their purchasing role (Deam, 1997). The NHS is a distributed organization. Services are distributed clinically and geographically. Patient services may be distributed between GPs surgeries, hospitals, community clinics, specialist services, hospices and so on. Support services such as laboratories, central administration, research, education and supplies are similarly widely distributed. This distribution results in a large amount of paper-based communication, redundant and repeated data, long waiting times and general disruption in the patient service. A computer-mediated network enables virtual organizations to be created in which allegiance, relationships and shared goals are established and maintained through electronic communication. Computer Mediated Communication (CMC) offers significant opportunities for the establishment of networks of communication within the health sector in which geographically dispersed workers—GPs, consultants, specialists, pharmacists, nurses and social workers—may be involved in the care of the same patient. An alternative future can be envisaged involving a completely networked health service in which information flows freely, resulting in a more efficient system in which quality data promotes the formation of virtual networks of clinical expertise for the benefit of patients (Hackney et al., 1997). The NHSnet is intended to provide the means of establishing integrated communications within the health service.

The NHSnet is essentially an Intranet for the UK health service. As such it uses the concepts, software and technology, which are familiar through the Internet, to create an information environment internal to the NHS. It is described as a secure national network developed exclusively for the NHS (IMG, 1997). The network is serviced by two connection providers, British Telecom (BT) and Cable and Wireless Communications, each of which provides Wide Area Network (WAN) services. BT runs the core WAN services, while BT and Cable and Wireless compete for local WAN provision. Connections are provided to national applications including the Prescription Pricing Authority, NHS Supplies, and the Nationwide Clearing Service. The latter provides a central sorting point for statutory data forwarded from healthcare providers for use by government departments. A messaging service provides a link from the NHSnet to a mobile communications network serviced by RACAL. E-mail and firewalls (a secure Internet gateway) provide links to the Internet through JANET (the UK universities network) and superJANET, as shown in Figure 1.

Organizations within the health service register to connect to NHSnet. Costs include some initial capital outlay for networking equipment, servers and connection. Following connection, services are paid for as they are used. Connection involves the signing of a 'Code of Connection' which specifies adherence to the NHS security policy (IMG, 1995) as well other requirements including the appointment of one named security officer, the removal of any connection to JANET and the Internet and appropriate password authentication. An earlier edition of 'Establishing NHSnet' (IMG, 1996) highlights NHSWeb and NHSweb directory. This will include what is essentially and internal search engine which will enable users to locate information and services. Here knowledge bases, training materials and reference books will be located. It is intended that the search engine will enable searching on perspectives: 'the user perspective—as GP, clinician, manager etc. the organization perspective—information from or about the NHS Executive, NHS Trusts, Health Authorities, charities etc. the geographic perspective—structured by counties (sic)

Figure 1: NHSnet Underlying Infrastructure

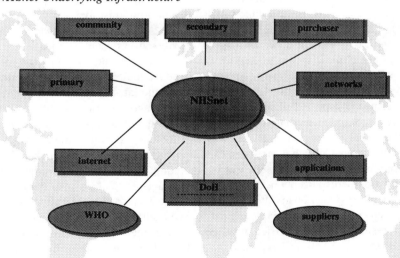

of the UK and other geographical groupings such as the English regions' (IMG, 1996). The NHSnet went 'live' in April 1997. By August 1997, 451 organizations had connected via BT, 29 using X25 rather than Internet Protocol (IP). Seventy-eight organizations had connected via Mercury. Initially, 171 GP practices from a potentially 10,000 GPs connected to NHSNet. However, incentives to join the NHSNet, including access to hospitals for appointment, results and discharge details, have increased the desirability of NHSNet connection. The fact that the NHSNet is now a central plank of the UK NHS Information Management strategy increases the likelihood of all GPs being connected by 2002.

The main thrust of this chapter concerns the question of how benefits are obtained from such a technology as the NHSNet. Some previous applications of information technology in the UK NHS have been criticized because the technology was imposed on the organization without considering the viewpoint of potential users, what the benefits would be and how they would be obtained. This may be described as a failure in the social construction of the technology, a failure to understand the user's perception of the technology and then to alter that perception or to alter the technology to suit that perception. There must be a focus on the stakeholders and the interpretation that they put on the technology. Attention must be given to the types of application and their potential for meeting user needs. There must also be a management commitment to delivering benefits. The following sections consider each of these issues.

STAKEHOLDERS IN THE NHSnet

In order to optimize the effectiveness of the NHSNet, we must understand the stakeholders who will potentially make use of it. We must identify and predict the social and cultural forces that will influence how the NHSNet is used and will determine whether it is taken-up and becomes embedded in the culture and processes of the health service or whether it is ignored. The concepts of Actor-Network Theory (ANT) provide a good basis for studying the social construction of technology. Actor-Network Theory (ACT) is an approach to structuring and explaining the links between society and technology. It offers explanations of how technology becomes acceptable and is taken up by groups in society. It suggests how technology is socially constructed. For example, How do mobile phones become widely used, Why does MS-Windows dominate the PC market? How is Linux becoming popular? Why does the same information system fail in one organization and succeed in another? How do case mix systems get established in hospitals? (Bloomfield et al, 1992) How are EDI networks and standards established? (Monteiro and Hanseth, 1996). ANT provides a fined-grained approach to analyzing the mechanism by which social action shapes technology and technology shapes social action. The primary focus is on stakeholders (actors) and how they are involved in the shaping of technology.

Actors are both human and non-human stakeholders who pursue interests that may encourage or constrain technology (Monteiro and Hanseth, 1996; Walsham, 1997). Many actors make up a network of interests, which becomes stable as they are aligned to the technology. This alignment is achieved through the translation of interests and the enrolment of actors into the network. Translating involves showing how an actor's nonaligned interests may become aligned. Skills, practices, organizational arrangements and contracts may all be part of the process of alignment. Alignment is established in inscriptions, which give a particular viewpoint precedence. For example, business processes may be established through managerial rhetoric, contracts, historical context, and so on. These business processes are then the basis for software which acts as an inscription of the organizational process, which becomes more fixed and indeed may become irreversible. It may be impossible to go back to a point where there were alternative possibilities. Another example would be standards, which once established become inscriptions for particular viewpoints within an actor-network. Networks spread, people become locked-in to the network which reinforces its spread. Once established and spread, the standards become irreversible. It is impossible to go back and start again. The standards inscribe the use of the network. They may be so deeply embedded in the system that they become black-boxes whose use is accepted without questioning how it works, or whether it represents the best way to do things.

Stakeholders can be defined as 'any human or non-human organization unit that can affect as well as be affected by a human or non-human organization unit's policies' (Vidgen and McMaster, 1995). The identification of stakeholders in NHSNet, and the study of their interests, concerns and attitudes to the NHSNet is of importance in researching CMC in the health sector. Stakeholders have different expectations and perceptions. They also have different reasons for wanting to be involved in the NHSNet. Furthermore each stakeholder will have multiple perspectives. Stakeholder analysis is valuable in helping us to understand these interests and therefore take them into account. Stakeholder's interests can be viewed from three perspectives. Firstly stakeholders have rational interests. They take a logical view of a phenomenon and consider its objective value. Secondly they have organizational interests, depending on their social position within an organization and their social agenda. Thirdly, they have individual interests, related to their status, career progression and job security, for example. The use of the NHSNet in NHS trusts will expand only as hospitals develop new systems which require links to the NHSNet. Old systems may remain outside the influence of the NHSNet, and there may be no connection with or influence on the host of disparate and unconnected specialist systems which inhabit hospitals. Patients remain excluded from the NHSNet. This gives them neither increased choice, nor access to information, which might reduce levels of anxiety and increase their involvement with their treatment. The rigorous efforts to isolate the NHSNet from public information systems may not encourage its use.

The success of the NHSNet will be influenced by the extent to which stakeholders support and use it. Barriers and differences between groups within the NHS may be reduced by the use of the NHSNet. However, a study of networked computer use in Canadian primary care suggested that computer networks may reinforce existing barriers and subcultural divisions (Legare and Douzou, 1996). Networked computer systems were installed in 105 GP surgeries in Quebec. These systems provided links with experts on mental health and were aimed at increasing GPs' interest in mental health problems. Mental health experts could be questioned by the GPs over an e-mail link; a general clinical pharmacology databank was provided together with a bulletin board on mental health issues. Professionals already involved in mental health issues made use of the network. Those with less interest rejected the mental health specialists consultation network and made use of the drug databank without reference to mental health problems, reinforcing their traditional practice approach, which concentrated on drug treatment of conditions and ignored therapy or alternative treatments. Thus the system had no effect in increasing mental health awareness. Since there were no champions of the technology who would enroll other, the system remained unused in the way it was intended.

Furthermore, the clinical and economic interests of the GPs were not aligned with the information system, and there was no natural catalyst to encourage use of the system in a way which would promote cultural change. The clear lesson is that the information system by itself will not promote cultural change. This illustrates the need to understand the stakeholders' interests and to align the Web-based health information systems with them. More research is needed into how stakeholders view the NHSNet and how they may consider using it. Also the nature of stakeholder relationships and the perceptions each group holds of other groups is an important area for investigation. Individual studies on particular stakeholders' groups, their relationship with other groups and the social and political factors which would influence attitudes toward and usage of the NHSNet should be encouraged.

Figure 2 considers the roles and interests for selected stakeholders who may have an interest in the NHSNet. The interests described are somewhat speculative. Whether the

Figure 2: Stakeholders in the NHSnet

Stakeholder	Role	Rational	Organizational	Individual
GPs	Provide primary care	Save costs of mail.(+) Provide access to clinical information.(+)	Increase power over providers through provision of information on provider performance (+)	Increase amount of time used in non-patient care activities (-) Enable moneys to be recovered quicker (+)
NHSTrusts	Provide acute care	Save mail costs (+) Increase efficiency of booking(+) Reduce non-attendance (+)	Increase control over communications (+)	Increase power of IM department (-).
Health Authorities	Purchase health-care for given geographical area	Obtain more data about demographic trends (+)	Increase control over GPs (+)	Increase quality control centres reputation (+)
Network Suppliers	Provide net-work services	Increase efficiency of communication in the health service (+)	Create a locked-in, long-term, stable market for services (+)	Compete success-fully and dominate healthcare market (+)
Outsourcers	Provide IT services	Enable better data quality and faster, more efficient services for clients (+)	Increase networking skills in order to be in a position to bid for further work.(+)	Create network of IT functions Strengthen hold on healthcare market (+)
Information Management Group	Provide over-all IS/IT policy	Reduce paper-based communications in the NHS, increase quality of data (+)	Strengthen power base of IMG (+) Increase control over IT within NHS organisations (+)	Correct tarnished reputation of IMG (+).
Patients	Consumers of services	Get more information and reduce uncertainty about what treatments are to be carried out (+)		
Self-help groups	Provide help and support to people with specific conditions	Produce strengthen-ed networks so that faster support can be provided (+)	Increase lobbying power and ability to influence GPs, consultants, etc. (+)	

interest is seen as positive or negative by the stakeholder is indicated by (+) or (-) respectively. Such a grid could result from a rigorous stakeholder research program.

GPs AS STAKEHOLDERS IN THE NHSnet

The key focus of the use of the NHSNet and the development of electronic patient records is on primary care. General practitioners, as important stakeholders, have a view of the NHSNet which will influence its use. The role of the GP within the community is pivotal to the delivery of healthcare within society. GPs reflect society's expectations of medicine and also influence those expectations. Their role extends beyond physical healthcare to the provision of advice which was once derived from within the extended family. The individualization of society, and the replacement of natural caring networks with state provision, has increased the public expectation of what the GP can provide and has resulted in an increased pressure on their time and resources. An increased focus by the media on medicine and medical matters has expanded the amount of information available to the public concerning hospitals and treatments. Some patients have begun to use this information to make more demands of their GPs. More informed patients may have greater expectations of their GPs and may expect more information from them. The notion of trust and the autonomy of the GP has been diminished. There has been a reduction of the knowledge gap.

GPs have also been subjected to significant administrative change. These changes have been aimed at allowing patients and GPs a greater choice of consultant and hospital in referrals. Information on hospital costs, waiting lists, consultants' interests and quality may be required to enable informed decisions on referrals. GPs' power has potentially increased since hospitals depend upon their patient referrals, and GPs have more freedom, in theory at least, to choose hospitals. However, GPs still refer patients primarily to local hospitals that they know. Also relationships between GPs and the consultant to whom they refer patients have become less strong over the years with the increasing workload of the GPs. There was a time when the GP would accompany the patient to the consultants and discuss the problem with the consultant. This would strengthen the GP-patient relationship and result in the informal education of the GP through discussions with the consultant. This close triangle of relationships has been lost. It could be suggested the NHSNet offers a chance to restore it as follows:

a) GPs are required to produce more information, both administrative and clinical. The growing popularity of evidence-based medicine may work in increasing information flow into the GPs practice and the flow of clinical information out. Pharmaceutical companies are seeking closer links with GPs and exploring possibilities of electronic communication in order to gather results for clinical tests.

b) GPs have a core role in the community. They provide the pivotal link between the individual in his or her home and the massive organizational structures represented by hospitals and acute services, social security and even work where illness and health issues are concerned. They are also key providers and distributors of information on a grand scale within the community. As such they are key players in the successful use of the NHSNet.

c) GPs are significant users of IT. Over 90% of GPs have computers in their surgeries, over half of those in their consulting rooms. In 1996, more than 8% of GPs were considered to be running a paperless office (Purves, 1996). However, a majority remain dependent on paper-based systems. The proliferation of computers within GP practices has been piecemeal. Hundreds of suppliers have provided a range of systems of varying quality. These have been unable to share information. Different rules for reimbursement of GPs for computer systems have been in place across the UK and attempts to link GPs has been of limited success, with unrealistic targets not being met (Jones, 1996).

It could be envisaged that access to the NHSNet from within the GPs surgery could provide instant call-up of a wide range of medical information for the use of both the GP and the patient. E-mail communications between GPs and patients could also occur in some cases. Links between GP surgeries could change the nature of consultations. GPs might employ primary care health workers who would answer patient's queries, provide reassurance—which is often all that is required—and become a virtual network of health information and family support. An electronic expansion of health care could pay dividends in preventative measures, resulting in significant savings of the GPs time. This in itself raises issues concerning the nature of the GP/ patient relationship and the extent to which patients may be willing to trust health workers other than the GP. Here, then, cultural change is occurring in an environment in which information technology is also being introduced, thus raising research questions about the interrelationship between the two and the influence of IT on culture and culture in the acceptance of IT.

Thus, in studying GPs as a stakeholder group, a number of research questions may be formulated, as noted in Table 1.

Table 1: GP Stakeholder Research

- How will increased communication and knowledge availability affect the GP/ patient relationship?
- Will the connection between hospitals and GPs' surgeries result in increased communication between GPs and consultants and a more rapid dissemination of clinical information and medical progress?
- Will electronic communication favour a particular group of patients who are affluent and educated?
- How will the use of electronic communications affect referral practice?
- What is the effect of the GPs' view of technology? Will the effective use of the NHSNet be limited to those practices where there is a GP who is a technical hobbyist?
- Does the networking of a GP practice change the nature of working relationships within the surgery?
- To what extent is it possible to replace face-to-face interactions between patients and GPs with electronic links?
- Can the NHSNet be expected to catalyse the formation of virtual networks of GPs, pharmacists, optometrists, dentists and other services within primary care?
- How does the level of computer expertise of the GP affect use of the NHSNet?
- What are the drivers for NHSNet usage by GPs?
- What are the attitudes of GPs and patients to communicating using e-mail?
- What links and contacts might develop between GPs and Internet-based special interest groups?
- What ethical worries do GPs have concerning NHSNet?

These questions centre on a main question: Will the use of the NHSNet within a GPs surgery change the behaviour, attitudes and activities of the GPs and modify the relationship between the GP and the patient? While the expectation is that the use of the NHSNet could revolutionize primary care, there appears to be little evidence for this as yet. The consideration of GPs as stakeholders raises issues about the political and social impact of the NHSNet. Knowledge availability on the NHSNet may have a significant impact on how GPs investigate conditions. However, it could be suggested that the demands of external groups —patients, pharmaceutical companies, pressure groups and special interest groups—will put significant pressure on GPs who may be acting as gatekeepers to a network of information from which the public is excluded. NHSNet security policy excludes contact with external networks and consequently involves the exclusion of large stakeholder groupings. However, attempts to exclude patients from health information sources may be fruitless. Patients can obtain health information from the Internet and arrive at surgery knowing more about a condition than the GPs does, but not having the professional expertise to sift the information and identify what is valid.

THE USES OF THE NHSnet

The NHSNet offers a platform for a wide variety of applications within the NHS. Communications between GPs and consultants can be established. Results may be transmitted directly to the GPs. Dialogue may be conducted with the consultant concerning a patient's condition. GPs may be able to obtain information on hospitals, services and standards of care through the NHSNet in order to make the best decisions on patient referrals. Electronic journals may provide the latest information for GPs, selected by relevance to the GPs interests. Special interest groups may be set up, using electronic mail to exchange information and ideas concerning specific conditions. Health warnings and health scares may be transmitted to all GPs to inform them ahead of the media. The network is a secure national system developed exclusively for the NHS. It is composed of a number of services that will support a number of communication needs of the organizations involved. It embraces voice and data over a wide area network of providers. With greater access to the NHSNet, or the use of the NHSNet, patients could be able to set up self-help networks to share experiences and information concerning specific conditions. Consultations may take place over e-mail and information provided in order to close the knowledge gap between GPs and patients. Information provided through CMC may reduce worry, enable patients to be better informed, and even reduce the number of non-attendances at clinics.

The NHSNet may aid the remote viewing of conditions by specialists at large hospitals who can provide advice remotely. Expertise and information on rare cases can be distributed through CMC. Remote tutorials may allow the sharing of information from centres of excellence. Patients may be discharged earlier and their condition monitored from home using CMC to transmit necessary clinical data. Virtual GP practices could be established over wide geographical areas. Existing services may be extended and their efficiency improved, and new services developed. Each service will require its own research agenda. Technical and social issues will have to be addressed. The use of the NHSNet will require a balanced approach in which different ways of using it are equally promoted in order to promote the widest possible stakeholder involvement.

Angehrn (1997) has proposed a useful framework for determining the strategic applications of the Internet for multinational enterprises. The so-called ICDT model reflects the variety of opportunities afforded by the Web to create 'space' for organizations or individuals to adopt 'alternative channels for exchanging information, communicating, distributing different types of products or services'. The Angehrn model is identified through the notion of 'virtual space' for Information, Communication, Distribution and Transaction (ICDT) activities. These virtual; spaces address visibility, interaction, delivery and trading respectively. These characteristics of the ICDT model are aimed at reflecting the nature of the external environment for the organization (markets and resources) and its internal processes for analyzing existing contexts. In addition, the ICDT model (Angehrn, 1997) provides a reasonable approach for designing a balanced NHSNet strategy in which a range of uses is considered. Figure 3 illustrates the ICDT model that considers uses of a network under the heading of information, communication, distribution and transaction.

The virtual information space provides channels for hospitals to display information about themselves for internal and external consumption. This information may include details of waiting lists, information about specialties and other economic and practical information about the hospitals. Access to scientific journals and the latest clinical information can be provided. Such an information network may promote evidence-based medicine. Researchers will need to ask whether the presence of the NHSNet alters the way GPs obtain their clinical information, and what factors influence the decision they make. The NHSNet could host important decision support systems which may alter decision-making activities.

The virtual communication space provides new channels for relationship-building. Dialogues concerning clinical and management decisions can take place. Opinions can be polled and ideas developed. Closer relationships between GPs and consultants may be

Figure 3: Outline ICDT Model of NHSNet

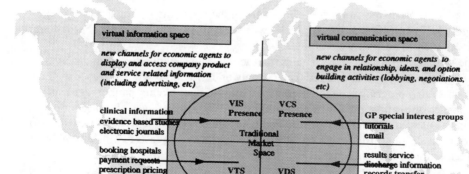

established. Researchers need to ask: Do existing relationships change as a result of the NHSnet? Are new relationships formed? What is the effect of the NHSnet on the development of attitudes and responses to comments from the Department of Health, for example. The virtual distribution space provides a new channel for the distribution of services within the NHS. Results services can provide much faster responses to GPs, providing instant test results from machine to GPs' surgery. Consultation between GPs and consultants are facilitated. Mobile links with ambulances may allow clinical assessments to be carried out on the spot. It is important that the NHSnet allows the promotion of appropriate medical support. For example, it may not be necessary to have highly qualified emergency teams attending minor incidents if mobile communications provide the assurance of the availability of specialist intervention if it is needed. It is noteworthy that the consumer of services, the patient, is excluded from the NHSnet. The possibility of providing computer-based counseling services and of using electronic communication to deal with the minor ailments and psychological problems that take up so much of the GPs' time would provide an efficient means of getting appropriate care to patients in an efficient manner. Researchers need to address the social issues around the use of CMC in distributing medical services and providing medical advice.

The concept of a Hospital at Home could be supported through the NHSnet. Patients are released from hospital at an earlier date if home facilities are suitable and clinical monitoring can continue. Biochemical and physiological monitoring takes place using CMC and removes the need for the patient to remain in the hospital. Given the right home conditions, the advantages are considerable in terms of faster recovery in a relaxing environment over which the patient has more control, and the reduced risk of infections. Furthermore, the use of CMC may enable the promotion of home births that have significant advantages over hospital births. Both technical and social issues need researching. What are the technical and data requirements for Hospital at Home? How does remote monitoring affect clinical decision making? What factors inhibit remote monitoring? Systems for remote monitoring of many patients at home, managed in a form that could be considered to be a virtual hospital already exist in the U.S. The problem is not one of establishing the technology base, but of establishing the social base. Research is needed as to what constitutes appropriate technology for home use in the UK. This will differ according to patient groups. The CMC needs of the elderly will differ significantly from those with long-term illness such as post-viral syndrome.

The virtual transaction space enables transactions between purchasers and providers to be executed quickly. It is envisaged that a variety of transactions will take place over the NHSnet, including ordering and requisitioning, item of service claims, patient registrations and exchanges of contract minimum datasets (IMG,1994). Here issues of transaction cost reduction and data quality need to be examined. The availability of the NHSnet may support applications in all four virtual spaces. Current IMG literature suggests a primary emphasis on the transaction space. We consider that effective use of the NHSnet to deliver improved services to patients requires a balanced use of all four virtual spaces. Research needs to address the use of the information, communication and distribution spaces as well as the transaction space.

The possibility of services which do not duplicate existing services using the NHSnet, but develop as new services which harness the distinctive properties of the NHSnet, need to be identified by researchers and examined for feasibility.

THE BENEFITS OF THE NHSnet

Research into the appropriate uses of the NHSNet using a framework such as ICDT needs to be matched to an understanding of stakeholders and their tasks, interests and attitudes. The Actor Network Theory suggests that the enrollment of users on to a new technology, i.e. their effective and enthusiastic use of an information, depends on there being a match between their interests and the interests of the system. Benefits will arise where the stakeholder's interest matches the proposed applications, and where new applications are championed by individuals or groups who can successfully enrol others and align their interests with the technology. In determining the benefits, analyses that consider cost savings without examining stakeholder interests may not predict the outcome of computer-mediated communication (CMC) within healthcare systems.

A study in the Netherlands (Ribbers, 1995) suggested that possible benefits of CMC included lower message cost, higher quality data and data transfer, greater social cohesion and more information available for the patient. The IMG identifies benefits in efficiency, effectiveness, working practices and delivery of patient care (IMG, 1997). The networking strategy identifies cost savings benefits through competitive procurements, reduced local networking costs and reductions in stationary and delivery costs. Benefits from cost savings need to be approached cautiously. The Netherlands study found no cost savings, although that provided the basis of the case for the implementation of the CMC pilot. It was particularly costly for GPs to link up. Systems were seen as non-user-friendly, terminals were expensive and the message set was limited. The study noted the key role of GPs in successful CMC. There is clearly a need for research to identify success factors associated with CMC in healthcare. The Netherlands study found that the primary benefit of the local CMC was in improved data quality. Similar benefits can be expected from the NHSnet. Timely and better quality information can be provided to GPs, including up-to-date, accurate results. IMG identifies other data quality improvements in administrative statistics, better collections of data and more reliable analysis. It suggests that better cashflow will follow. Efficiency benefits are also cited, including avoiding re-keying of data, reduction in paper and reduction in time looking for omitted data.

Several points can be made. Firstly, the benefits focus on administration and the flow of administrative tasks. The focus is on the transactions, rather than the activities generating the transactions. It is as if the transaction is the treatment, rather than an artifact resulting from the treatment. Researchers should question this administrative, transaction focus. There is little in the benefits cited to suggest clinical benefits to the patient. This may be a result of the exclusion of the patient from the system. The system of administrative messages and transactions runs virtually in the absence of the patient who is external to the system and merely modeled in the system. Secondly, there is the assumption that administrative benefits such as single entry point for data, reduced time opening, forwarding and filing information and reduction in telephone inquiries naturally occur as a result of the installation of CMC systems. We would suggest that this is not the case. Such administrative activities are generated from social interactions. They are a result of social activities and interpretations of events and actions by the stakeholders. The expectation of the delivery of efficiency benefits results from the adherence by technologists to a machine view of the organization (see McBride et al., 1997). Efficiency benefits are often not realized and do not represent the real benefits of the system (McBride and Fidler, 1994). Research is required to identify the benefits of the NHSnet, to look for factors that might inhibit or promote those benefits and to develop case studies that illustrate how the benefits may be obtained. This research should start with stakeholder analysis.

FUTURE TRENDS

The future of computer-mediated communications in the health service lies in networked systems which bring together geographically separated and disparate professional groups (Ahmed and Berlin, 1997). These applications will be characterized by their variety. Applications will be tailored to stakeholders interests. This variety will be built in some standard foundations. Standards for networking, communications, data representation, electronic patients records, and communication with patients will ensure the integrity of the networked communication system. While management effort will be required to establish and maintain those standards, the real management challenge lies in managing stakeholders interests in order to ensure that effective use is made of the technology. This means that issues such as enrolment, alignment and inscription are critical. The management of Web-based systems over a distributed network is as much about the management of the social construction of the technology as it is about the management of the physical technology. Such management requires an understanding of the stakeholders, through stakeholder analysis and an analysis of the potential of the technology based on frameworks such as ICDT.

Stakeholders have the key role in the development of any Web-enabled environment. It is their social, political and cultural views that will determine the direction of the NHSnet. While economic and technical drivers may have an important effect on the use of the NHSnet, the most important drivers are arguably the social drivers (McBride, 1996).

Figure 4: Research Agenda for CMC within the NHSnet

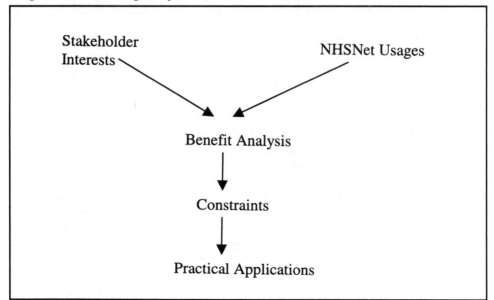

Stakeholders will place a social interpretation on the NHSnet. Interested groups will seek to influence and enroll others to their particular view. Powerful agencies will seek to enforce use through their control of resources; for example, authorities can demand submission of payment requests over the NHSnet. It is therefore important that we understand the network of alliances and explore the social and political issues that will determine the social construction of the NHSnet.

It is important that this becomes a focus for research. Figure 4 identifies relationships between the research areas outlined in this chapter. The study of stakeholders and applications leads to an analysis of possible benefits. The achievement of these benefits may be limited by constraints such as available resources and skills. However, we would suggest that, if practical applications are to emerge, a matching of possible applications with stakeholders is necessary.

CONCLUSION

The NHSnet will have significant implications throughout healthcare in the UK although there is some evidence of the 'negative' aspects of the systems (Klerker and Zetraues, 1998). There has also been much discussion on technical and security issues and the paucity of research on the social implications. For example, the Government White Paper on Primary Care (DoH, 1996) suggests alternative forms of contracting, the ability to employ doctors or alternative workers within practices in contract relationships other than partnerships; and an increased role for the community pharmacy as a first port of call for minor ailments, a source of counselling on the use of medicines and a source of health promotion. Such changed approaches could result in virtual networks of primary healthcare if appropriately supported by the NHSnet. These changing social structures and social roles need to receive the attention of researchers.

How healthcare expectations will be affected by the NHSnet and whether culture and politics within the NHS will inhibit or promote its use is a matter for urgent research. Unless we examine the nature of the NHSnet, and its social and political influence in a holistic way and do not restrict ourselves to technical and economic issues, we will find that its potential is not achieved. A system which may provide new and improved ways for delivering clinical care and promoting community health may be reduced to a glorified transaction processing system, with little benefit for the patient and an increased transaction workload for medical staff. It is up to researchers to point the way to effective CMCs for the healthcare sector in the 21st century.

This chapter has identified two important issues that managers need to consider. The nature of the stakeholders must be examined. If we do not understand the stakeholders' interests, expectations and reservations concerning Web-based applications, the success of the implementation of applications may be compromised. Indeed, technical solutions imposed on unwilling and disinterested users is a recipe for failure. Users must have an interest in the application, be enrolled onto its use and inscribe their own meaning. Secondly, the potential uses of the Web-based technologies must be explored in a manner that is comprehensive and creative. The ICDT framework provides a comprehensive framework that considers information delivery, stakeholder communications, service delivery and transactions. It is up to the manager to provide the creative input, considering applications which do not duplicate existing administrative or clinical function, but which exploit the distinctive nature of the technology to provide new services.

However, both these aspects must be grounded in a focus on benefits. The delivery of the technology is insufficient. The Web-based technology must deliver tangible benefits to all stakeholders in terms of cost savings, improved patient care, improved patient satisfaction and the integration of patient services. The management of the NHSNet, as one example of Web-based technology in the health service must be synonymous with the management of benefits. It is in this area that the major challenge lies.

REFERENCES

Ahmed, M. A. and Berlin, A. (1997). Information technology in general practice: current use and views on future development, *Journal of Informatics in Primary Care*

Angehrn, A. (1997). Designing mature Internet business strategies: The ICDT model. *European Management Journal 15*(4) 361-369.

Bloomfield, B.P; Coombs,R.; Cooper,D.J. and Rea,D. (1992). Machines and manoeuvres: responsibility accounting and the construction of hospital information systems. *Accounting, Management and Information Technologies. 2*, 197-219.

Deam, M. (1997). End of sharp-elbowed internal market for NHS, *The Lancet, 350* (9094), 1829

DoH (1996). *Choice and Opportunity. Primary Care : The Future*. The Stationary Office, London. UK

DoH (1997). *The new NHS, modern, dependable*, The Stationary Office, London, UK.

Gillies, A. (1998). Computers and the NHS: an analysis of their contribution to the past, present and future delivery of the National Health Service, *Journal of Information Technology, 13*, 219-229.

Hackney, R A; Dhillon G & McBride, N K (1997). Primary Care Information Technology within the NHS: the concept of markets and hierarchies on systems exploitation, *International Journal of Public Sector Management*, 10(4 & 5), 388-395

House of Lords Select Committee on Science and Technology (1996). *Information Society: Agenda for Action in the UK*. 23rd July 1996, HMSO, London

IMG (1994). A Strategy for NHS-wide networking. IMG Ref E5155.

IMG (1995). Data Networking Security Policy IMG Ref. E5221.

IMG (1996). Establishing NHSnet. IMG Ref C3167.

IMG (1997). Establishing NHSnet. IMG Ref H8019.

Jones, D. (1996). The National Information Management and Technology (IM&T) Strategy and its impact upon Primary Care. *Proceedings of the 2nd International Symposium on Health Information Management Research,* University of Sheffield.

Legare, J and Douzou, S (1996). Who needs information systems in the health care sector and who will use them? An experiment. *Information Technology and People* 8(3) 28-42.

Lenaghan, J.(Ed.) (1998). *Rethinking IT and Health*, Institute for Public Policy Research, London, UK.

Klercker, T. and Zetraues, S. (1998). Dilemmas in introducing World Wide Web-based information technology in primary care: a focus group study, *Family Practitioner*, 15(3), 205-210.

McBride, N. (1996). Why Businesses are Joining the Internet: Identifying the Drivers of Global Information Systems Expansion. *Proceedings of the 4th European Conference on*

Information Systems, Vol. 1, p 171 - 181. Lisbon, Portugal.

McBride,N, Lander,R and McRobb, S. (1997. Postmodern Information Management. *Business Information Technology'97*, Manchester Metropolitan University, November 5-6, 1997.

McBride, N K and Fidler, C (1994). An Interpretive Approach to the Justification of Investment in Executive Information Systems. *Proceedings of the First European Conference on IT Investment Evaluation*. Henley-on-Thames, England. 13-14th September 1994, pp 16-26.

Monteiro,E and Hanseth,O (1996). Social shaping of information infrastructure: on being specific about the technology. In Orlikowski,W; Walsham,G; Jones, M.R and DeGross,J (Eds) *Information Technology and Changes in Organisational Work*. Chapman and Hall, London.

NHS (1998). Information for Health [WWW] Available from: http://www.imt4nhs.exec.nhs.uk/strategy/full/content [Accessed 25 March 1999]

Nicholls, I (1995). An information management and technology strategy for the NHS: getting better with information, *Centre for Health Information Management Research Conference*, University of Sheffield, UK

Purves, I.N. (1996). The paperless general practice. *British Medical Journal*. Vol 312.

Ribbers,P.M. (1995). EDI in regional healthcare - THe case of RHCNET in the Netherlands, in EDI in Europe: How it works in practice, Ed. Krcmar, H; Bjorn-Anderson,N. and O'Callaghan,R, pp259-276. John Wiley, Chichester

Vidgen, R and McMaster, T. (1995). Black Boxes,Non-Human Stakeholders and the Translation of IT Through Mediation, in *Information Technology and Changes in Organisational Work* edited by Orlikowski, W; Walsham, G, Jones, M R; and DeGross, J I Pp 250-270. Chapman and Hall, London.

Walsham, G. (1997). Actor-Network Theory and IS Research: Current status and future prospects. In Lee,A; Liebenau,J and DeGross,J (Eds). *Information systems and qualitative research* Chapman and Hall, London.

Chapter III

Technology-Based Marketing in the Healthcare Industry: Implications for Relationships Between Players in the Industry

Grace Johnson, Anand Kumar, Arkalgud Ramaprasad
and Madhusudhan Reddy
Southern Illinois University at Carbondale

The past few years have seen Web-based technology diffusing into a wide cross-section of industries, cutting across various barriers, and changing the way many companies do business. The healthcare industry, though relatively slow to adopt information technology (Eder and Darter, 1998), is no exception. Information technology is transforming the healthcare environment in ways that go beyond simple consumer health information Web sites (Hagland, 1997). Increasingly, the industry is leveraging information technology effectively to manage its business and address issues affecting patient care (Lankford, 1999).

At the heart of the healthcare industry lies the patient-physician relationship. The interaction between these two players usually occurs in a clinic/hospital setting. It is generally believed that the relationship between the patient and the physician is influenced not only by this interaction, but also by other interactions that a patient may have *inside* a clinic/hospital setting, such as interactions with nurses, staff, the registration desk, etc. However, changes brought about by information technology (a) allow players outside the clinic/hospital setting to influence the patient-physician relationship and (b) affect the way in which players and processes inside a clinic/hospital setting influence the patient-physician relationship. This chapter examines how Web technology affects the patient-physician relationship through its impact on players and processes both *outside* and *inside* a clinic/hospital setting.

The healthcare industry is complex and comprises many relationships between different players in the industry, for example, physicians, patients, pharmaceutical firms, and insurance firms. These relationships are often developed as separate dyads that are independent of each other. This has led to the healthcare industry being described as diverse and disconnected (*Business Wire*, 1999). However, information technology is changing the industry by introducing technology applications that increase and strengthen *connectivity* between the different players in the industry. The increased on-line connectivity is influencing marketing practices within the industry, which in turn are affecting the dynamics of the relationships between the different players in the industry.

In this chapter, we focus on the impact of Web-based technology on marketing practices within the healthcare industry and its impact on the relationships between the major players in the industry. In particular, we focus on the relationship between the patient and his/her physician. The first part of the chapter examines the dynamics of this relationship in the context of exchanges and interactions that patients and physicians have with the pharmaceutical and insurance companies, i.e., players outside the clinic/hospital setting. We present a simple conceptual model that shows how relationships in the industry have evolved as a result of technologically driven marketing practices. In the second part of the chapter, we examine how Web technology affects the way in which players and processes inside the clinic/hospital setting influence the patient-physician relationship. Specifically, we explore how Web technology streamlines administration within a clinic/hospital, increases patient education about their illness, enhances communication between patients and physicians and leads to an overall improvement in the quality of patient care. We balance our discussion of the virtues of Web technology by briefly discussing thorny legal and public policy issues that have been raised by the use of this technology in the healthcare industry.

CONCEPTUAL MODEL DEPICTING INFORMATION FLOW

The traditional flow of information between three important players in the healthcare industry has been *sequential* as shown in Figure 1.

The exchange that typically takes place between the pharmaceutical company, physician, and the patient can be depicted as sets of *informational exchanges* or *transactions*. Pharmaceutical companies communicate directly with physicians to promote their products to them while physicians interact with the company representatives to learn more about their products. The information flow is two-way: from the company to the physician, and from the physician to the company.

The physician and the patient also form a dyad where exchange of information takes place. Interestingly, in this dyad, it is very likely that the amount of relevant information that is exchanged between the two parties is asymmetric. This asymmetry arises from differences in motivation and knowledge structure between the two parties. The patient comes to the doctor because he/she needs information on his/her condition or ailment and describes his/ her symptoms. The physician combines this *external* information from the patient with

Figure 1: Model of Traditional Communication Flow between Primary Players in the Healthcare Industry.

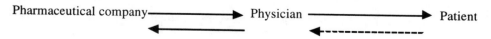

an *internal* source of information, his/her prior knowledge and experience, to make a diagnosis. Once a diagnosis is made, a decision for the best possible treatment for the patient has to be made. The physician does not have the time or the motivation to engage in a detailed discussion of suitable alternatives with the patient. Instead, the physician decides which drug would be the most suitable for the patient and conveys only what he/she thinks is "relevant" information to the patient. The result of this decision process results in a prescription that the patient will use to obtain the specified product from the pharmacy.

It is interesting to note that the patient, the actual *consumer* of the product, who also pays for it, is more or less a recipient of the one-way flow of information (Mechanic, 1998) calls such a physician-patient relationship a *paternalistic* relationship). Patients usually do not and cannot participate in the communication process as equal partners as they have limited knowledge abou medicines and treatments. However, pharmaceutical firms, the sellers of the prescribed drugs, need to promote their products, but under the model shown in Figure 1, these firms did not directly interact with the end consumer, the patient. Instead, they relied completely on a *push* strategy to increase sales of their products. That is, they would try to convince physicians to prescribe their products and then hope that a large enough number of prescriptions would be generated by patients purchasing their prescribed drugs.

As depicted in Figure 1, there was no direct interaction between all three parties; the three parties performed as two separate sets of *dyads* or pairwise relationships (Hall, 1996). Also, as shown in Figure 1, flow of information from the patient to the physician was tentative and minimal. It was confined to a recounting of the signs or symptoms he/she was experiencing. The flow from the physician to the patient would account for the major portion of this interaction, because of the knowledge, expertise, experience, and perceived power imbalance between the two parties.

It would be quite natural to expect this perceived "power" imbalance because patients only visit a physician when they have a problem and insufficient information to solve it by themselves. ("Power" is defined as the capacity of one party to influence the behavior of another). The marketing and social psychology literature have identified various sources of power (Eyuboglu and Atac, 1991; French and Raven, 1959). According to this literature, the physician's medical expertise gives him/her *expert* power, which is based on medical knowledge. Another kind of power is *information* power (the physician has information that is relevant to the patient but the patient does not have that information). The different power

Figure 2: Model of Current Communication Flows Between Selected Members of the Healthcare Industry

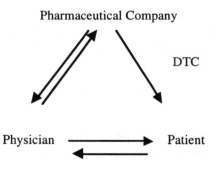

bases in Figure 1 all favor the physician.

With the advent of the relatively new phenomenon known as direct-to-consumer advertising (DTCA) of prescription drugs, the flow of information changed quite dramatically, as shown in Figure 2.

Figure 2 shows a new link connecting the three parties; it shows an arrow from the pharmaceutical company to the patient, representing information flow between the two for the first time. This has had some impact on the physician-patient relationship; a solid line has replaced the dotted arrow of Figure 1. The reason for this is explained below.

DTCA came about partly due to relaxation in regulations relating to prescription drug advertising, and partly because of increasing competitive pressures within the pharmaceutical industry. As more and more brands and categories of drugs proliferated in the market, companies found it increasingly difficult to communicate messages about their products to the physician, the important influencer in the purchase. Since the 1980s, this factor, together with concern about losing market share particularly to generic drugs, led to a new direction of promotional activity, this time targeted at the consumer. Advances in information technology also made it possible for marketers to think in terms of targeted marketing where firms would send marketing communications directly to an individual through direct mail campaigns. Beginning in the Eighties, but much more prominently in the early Nineties, several companies began to utilize various forms of direct-to-consumer advertising. In 1983, the FDA imposed a moratorium on this strategy, and then lifted it in 1985 (Food and Drug Administration, 1985). In August 1997, the FDA further relaxed regulations governing DTC marketing of prescription drugs on television and radio by issuing exploratory guidelines that permitted marketers to run commercials naming the prescription product, the condition it is used to treat, and some side effects. This resulted in a virtual explosion of spending on such advertisements. Figures rose from $55 million in 1991 to $516 million in 1996 to over $1.3 billion in 1998, and are projected to reach $6 billion by 2005 (*Business Wire*, Nov 19, 1998).

The introduction of DTCA coincided with the explosion of information availability via electronic media such as the Internet. The hitherto passive patient became an active *consumer* of information. It is estimated that there are at least 10,000 World Wide Web sites devoted to healthcare, with information on everything from innumerable medical conditions, to individual advice, second opinions, support groups, and actual diagnoses ("Practicing Medicine on the Net," 1997). Consumers obtain information from these Web sites and initiate dialogues with their physicians on the basis of this newly obtained knowledge (Kaplan, 1998). DTCA prompts patients to initiate dialogues with their physicians, asking questions about specific brands of drugs. By adopting DTCA, pharmaceutical firms were explicitly incorporating a *pull* strategy in their marketing plans. Firms tried to push their products to the physicians so that physicians would prescribe these products *and at the same time*, tried to get patients to ask their physicians for these products, thus creating a demand (pull) for these products.

The net effect of patients getting additional information from various sources including direct-to-consumer advertising has been that many patients are now motivated to learn more about medical conditions and treatment options, and to consult their physicians more (Holmer, 1999). These patients may be called "empowered patients," as they are empowered with greater levels of information relevant to their situation. Such patients can and often will query the physician about the prescribed treatment and also about alternatives that may not have been mentioned by the physician initially. Figure 2 captures this change in the physician-patient relationship by having a solid line showing the exchange between the patient and the physician. Many physicians might perceive the empowered patient to be a threat to their authority. But, as has been pointed out by some commentators, the patient has been empowered with *information*, not prescribing authority (Holmer, 1999). The physician's information power base is weakened in the Figure 2 scenario compared to that in Figure 1. However, his/her expert power base remains the same, because the power to write prescriptions still rests with the physician. Once the dialogue has been started, the physician's role always takes precedence. With adequate cooperation from the physician, communication flows can be continuous, sustained, and enhancing to the relationship.

The separate *dyads* of Figure 1 have merged to some extent to form a single *triad*, but it must be noted that the information flow is not perfectly symmetric and balanced in the triad. A greater balance and symmetry of information exchange is seen in what we call the third phase of our conceptual model.

The third phase is (and will be) characterized by extensive diffusion and use of on-line technology in the healthcare industry. This phase is currently in its infancy. What is described here is our envisioning of the very near future. Web technology can enable hitherto disperse players in the industry to forge stronger communication links, enabling a high degree of *connectivity*. Instead of separate pairs of dyads or triads, we can increasingly observe the formation of *networks* of relationships characterized by increased levels of collaboration. The improved collaboration efforts are focused on the patient, now perceived as a *consumer* of healthcare.

Figure 3 shows our conceptualization of the communication flows between four key

Figure 3: Diamond Model of Technology-Enabled On-line Interconnectivity

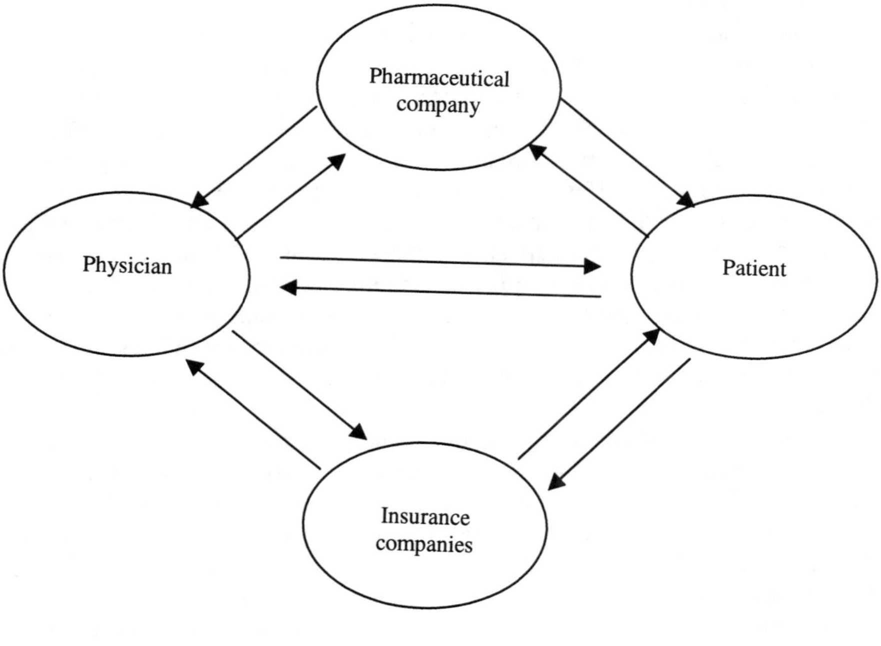

players in the health care industry enabled by on-line connectivity. Under the new model, the patient-physician relationship is an ongoing one supported by online communication such as e-mail whereas previously, the relationship was a series of discrete interactions. There is also a greater perceived equality in the exchange of information between physician and patient, enabled by continuous patient education with Web resources. Our model also suggests relationships between other players in the healthcare industry and thus allows us to explore the impact of technology on the healthcare industry as a whole.

Insurance Companies and Connectivity

Insurance companies can be connected online to both patients and physicians. Insurance companies can be connected electronically to physicians' offices for rapid, efficient claims processing that could potentially cut down costs, time, and paperwork. Actual transfer of money can also be done electronically (*Star Tribune,* Oct. 1998). In addition to expediting payments, the claims process can be entirely transparent to the patient over the Web so that he/she can observe whether the company has processed a particular bill. Patients can correspond with the companies by e-mail, so that communications such as filing a complaint can be responded to very quickly.

Currently, most insurers have Web sites and use them for some or all of the following services: descriptions of the plans they offer, but not the prices for each plan; lists of doctors affiliated with their plan; and basic preventive health information, such as timetables of children's immunizations.

Spurred by the new connectivity, some insurance companies have progressed much more than others have. For example, Aetna has included a health encyclopedia that it has jointly developed with Johns Hopkins University (http://www.aetnaushc.com). Kaiser also offers an online encyclopedia at its members-only site (http://www.kponline.com). Other innovative services include:

- On-line health assessments that identify patients' biggest health risk and provide links to follow-up information;
- On-line advice from nurses and pharmacists, who will respond by e-mail within 24 hours;
- On-line discussion groups on topics ranging from HIV to parenting, some moderated by doctors.
- Appointment making online.

Kaiser officials envision a "virtual medical center" that will cater to a wide range of patient needs. All these developments show how technology can be used in the healthcare industry to improve the patient-insurance company relationship. Given the present debate in the United States over Patients' Bill of Rights, insurance companies should welcome the opportunity provided by technology to enhance their relationship with their clients, the patients.

The implications of technological advances for insurance companies are that they are going to be much more closely involved with their customers. In terms of business practices, this will mean that patients will come to expect a lot more information and many more services from them. As patients get more informed about various illnesses, they will have more questions for the insurance and pharmaceutical firms. To ensure that insurance companies provide accurate responses that are likely to satisfy their customers, they may have to be in closer contact with physicians and pharmaceutical firms, not just in terms of being connected electronically, but also in terms of exchange of information. For example, if information provided by an insurance company is contradicted by a patient's physician or a pharmaceutical firm, it is likely to erode the credibility of the insurance firm.

The Diamond model in Figure 3 also suggests implications for marketers in the healthcare industry that are a result of the patient-insurance company-physician-pharmaceutical company relationships. We illustrate the marketing implications of the aforementioned relationships by considering the following scenario. A patient may see an advertisement for a particular drug on the television or in a magazine. While this may prompt the patient to ask his/her physician about this drug (which is the goal of current DTC advertising by pharmaceutical firms), it may also prompt the patient to ask his/her insurance company whether that particular drug was covered by their policy. Many patients will not want to ask their physician about a drug that is not covered by their policy. These patients will first contact their insurance company and if they find that the drug is covered by their policy, then they are likely to ask their physician about this drug. If the advertised drug is cheaper than the drug presently being prescribed by the physician, the insurance companies are likely to put some pressure on the physician to change his/her prescribing habits. Any such action on the part of an insurance provider represents a threat for a pharmaceutical firm whose drug is presently being prescribed and an opportunity for another firm whose drug is not being prescribed. The physician may also be forced to seek more information from a pharmaceutical firm about a drug, especially if he/she has limited knowledge about it. Though the above scenario was based on the patient – insurance company – physician – pharmaceutical firm relationship, it serves as an illustration of how any relationship shown in the Diamond model in Figure 3 can either directly or indirectly influence marketing practices in the healthcare industry.

Pharmaceutical Firms and Connectivity

Pharmaceutical companies can continue to communicate with consumers directly through advertisements (and also through on-line communications using e-mail and relevant discussion groups). However, instead of the burden of responding to patients' queries being placed fully on physicians, companies can support queries interactively through their Web sites. Doctors and other qualified company personnel can be available online to help assess individuals' suitability for the advertised drugs. Patients can also have access to all the research related to the drugs through links. In order not to alienate physicians in this process, the companies can be available online to talk to doctors also. They can respond to their questions and requests for samples, and can support physicians with updates on the latest research findings and progression of clinical trials.

In fact, in many instances, pharmaceutical firms may find that the increased levels of connectivity can enable them to offset and complement their sales representatives' efforts at detailing the physician. For example, a physician may not give much time to the sales representative of a pharmaceutical firm selling drug A. The physician may regularly be prescribing drug B and ignoring the efforts of the drug A salesperson. However, inquiries from the patient and/or the insurance company may lead the physician to seek information about the drug. At this point, the pharmaceutical company gets an opportunity to persuade the physician about the merits of its drug and can possibly persuade the physician to give its sales representative a few minutes of his/her time. Thus, increased connectivity can be a useful tool for pharmaceutical firms if it is used in a strategic manner to complement their existing marketing practices.

The greatest help that pharmaceutical companies can offer patients and physicians through the enhanced connectivity brought about by technology is in the area of *patient compliance*. Poor patient compliance is one of the biggest problems encountered by physicians, as it directly affects the successful outcomes of the prescribed treatment. Pharmaceutical companies can directly tackle this problem through on-line connectivity and database technology. They can do this by establishing connections with patients and supporting them through the duration of the therapy, something that physicians just do not have the time or resources to do. For example, AllerDays is a new comprehensive wellness program for patients on Hoechst Marion Roussel's Allegra. It is operated by McKesson Corporation through its database-driven Patient Care Enhancing Program. The program enables manufacturers such as Hoechst, in cooperation with retail pharmacies, to enhance patient understanding of their conditions and adhere to their prescribed drug regimen. The program has seen excellent response and significantly increased compliance rates (*Business Wire,* Sept. 1998). It can easily be envisioned how these compliance rates can be further enhanced with on-line support.

IMPLICATIONS FOR DYADIC AND NETWORK RELATIONSHIPS

It is relevant and important for the different players in the industry to understand the impact of the enhanced relationship between members of any one dyad on other dyads in the health care industry. We believe that proactive firms will attempt to understand the implications of these changes being brought about by information technology and be prepared to not only deal with the consequences, but also plan on ways to leverage these changes to their advantage.

Clearly, patients who have a high level of connectivity with the pharmaceutical and insurance companies, and who make use of the above listed services being offered by these firms, will have a very different knowledge structure about their health than patients who do not make use of these services. It is important for physicians to anticipate and be aware of the changes in their patients' knowledge structures, because such changes will lead to changes in the patients' expectations of information to be received from the physician. Physicians who are unprepared for these changes are likely to respond to all patients in the way they have dealt with them in the past. This may lead to many patients feeling dissatisfied with the amount of information they receive or the level of detail provided to them by the physicians. Prior research in marketing has shown that satisfaction with information has a major effect on overall satisfaction with a product or service (Spreng et al., 1997). Thus, physicians who do not understand the implications of increased connectivity in the different dyads in the health care industry are likely to be faced with problems related to patient satisfaction. Though we have used physicians as an example in the scenario described above, the necessity of understanding the impact of technology and increased connectivity between players in the healthcare industry is equally critical for every player in the industry.

The rest of this chapter examines how information technology influences the patient-physician relationship in a hospital setting and discusses other important issues that are raised by the new connectivity.

WEB TECHNOLOGY IN THE CLINIC/ HOSPITAL SETTING

Streamlining Administration and Enhancing Communication

Marketers know the importance of overall customer experience with a firm in influencing a customer's loyalty to that firm and his/ her desire to talk favorably about that firm to others. In the literature on marketing orientation, it is pointed out that in market oriented firms, marketing is not viewed as the sole responsibility of the marketing department. There is a company-wide focus on marketing as every department realizes that it can influence customers directly or indirectly. Highly market-oriented firms are typically characterized by better levels of inter-departmental coordination than firms that are less market oriented (Kohli and Jaworski, 1990). These findings from the marketing literature are equally applicable in a hospital/clinic setting where patients' overall experience is determined not only by the interaction with the physician but also by their interactions with various other employees such as the nurses. Information technology can now make it possible for hospitals/clinics to coordinate their various activities much better than before and enhance the overall patient care experience provided by these institutions.

A recent survey conducted by editors of *Hospitals and Health Networks* and Deloitte Consulting queried 277 health organizations nationwide on their use of online technology and classified respondents into "most wired" organizations and "less wired" depending on the extent of usage of this technology (Solovy and Serb, 1999). In this survey, the hundred most wired health organizations offered a variety of patient services online. These included (in decreasing order of availability) preregistration (73%), physician referral, support groups, nurse advice, reviewing test results, reporting self-tests, appointment scheduling, claims query, and prescription renewal (4%). Similarly, services offered to doctors and nurses using the Internet were access to patient data (29%), viewing radiology results, viewing lab results, viewing pathology results, decision support, lab order entry, pathology order entry (12%), pharmacy order entry (12%), and radiology order entry (12%). The following types of patient data were available online, for access by authorized medical personnel — clinical results, current medical record, medical history, nurses' notes, and patient demographics. Sixty-one to eighty percent of the most wired organizations had this type of information available online compared to 21 to 40 percent of less wired organizations.

The above functions are primarily those that use technology to streamline clinical and administrative operations, and are the very basic improvements to organizational efficiency and effectiveness that online technology can bring about. We look beyond these, and explore the possible greater contributions that Internet and intranet technology can make, to improving the *quality of care* that the consumer, the patient, receives.

At their core, Intranet and Internet technologies are a mechanism for improving communication and connectivity. Improving formal and informal communication channels has been one of the most appreciated contributions made by this technology. For example, many physicians are increasingly using e-mail to communicate with their patients. Kansas University Medical Center has found that patients find the convenience and comfort of e-mailing their physicians far outweigh their confidentiality concerns (Hagland, 1997). E-mail interactions can enable a physician to make a more considered response to patient inquiries than on the phone, at his/her own leisure. This can also be time efficient for physicians constantly under time pressure.

E-mail and related services are also used by physicians to enhance their communication and connectivity with other physicians. This might not affect the patient directly, but in the long run, is likely to enable higher quality of care rendered to the patient. These higher levels of patient care would be a result of sharing of information, knowledge, and experience. Physicians are also joining on-line news groups and listservs to obtain clinical consultations with large groups of colleagues or specialists (Pinkowish, 1999).

Patient and Provider Education in Disease Management

Patient education has been an issue widely discussed as exemplifying the impact of the Information Age on health care. Forty percent of people surfing the Web use it to get health care information (Solovy and Serb, 1999). A number of health care organizations give their patients online access to information about their chronic conditions, ranging from AIDS to diabetes to substance abuse (Solovy and Serb, 1999).

Many physicians have had the experience of a patient bringing a printout from a medical Web site to their office. If the information obtained is from a reputable source such as the Mayo Clinic Web site, the only negative aspect might be that the patient does not understand the material. If the information is incorrect or misleading, there is potential for plenty of damage to the patient personally, and also to the patient-physician relationship. There is evidence of numerous unscrupulous sellers wanting to sell medications, devices, and services on the Internet (Pinkowish, 1999). Apart from Web sites, patients may also obtain virtually unlimited information from the thousands of discussion groups that supply medical advice, information and support. These on-line groups have been described as being "double-edged swords," as the potential for *misinformation* is as high as that for education.

In discussing patient education, it is important to differentiate between the *informed* patient and the *knowledgeable* patient. The difference between the two is the mere possession of information on the part of the informed patient and the possession of knowledge by the latter. The patient possessing information is largely unequipped to put that information to any use because of his/her lack of technical knowledge or expertise. Ideally, the physician can help the patient process the information he/she brings into the interaction, place the processed information in the context that is most relevant for the patient, and point out ways in which the knowledge so generated can be applied to best benefit him/her. Doctors have the medical judgment to filter and explain information from the Internet and help patients interpret it with appropriate skepticism (Sandrick, 1998). Researchers have pointed out that a dialogue between patient and physician that is open, nontechnical, compassionate, and receptive to questions can, in most cases, bring about meaningful patient comprehension and can serve a valuable therapeutic purpose at the same time (Greenfield et al., 1985).

Some physicians have pointed out that as long as potential misinformation is an issue, it would be in the patients' and the physicians' best interest for the doctor to point out suitable Web sites where the patient can be assured of reliable information. This would suggest that doctors and/or clinics would be expected to be aware of relevant medical Web sites and patients may expect the doctors to give their evaluation of the content at different sites. This would be a new role for many physicians who are unprepared for the rapid changes affecting the industry. On the other hand, physicians who anticipate such patient expectations may promptly guide the patient to sites such as Healthfinder (http://www.healthfinder.org), which was developed by the U.S. Department of Health and Human Services, and is designed to contain links only to high-quality health information (Pinkowish, 1999).

Many organizations have exploited Web resources to benefit physicians in their education and continuing education. This education can have two purposes: to update their professional employees on technology, and encourage them to use the Web as an online library. Physicians, as a group, lag behind other scientific and technical professionals in their facility with computers (Pinkowish, 1997). Though all information available online is also available in print, the advantage with using on-line resources is the ease of access and substantial savings in time.

Group Health Cooperative, a Seattle-based HMO, has made this technology part of the core of its operations, and has received national recognition for its success with disease management. Its Clinical Roadmaps disease management program is entirely supported by an extensive on-line library. Doctors have access to a wealth of practice knowledge on some of the most common chronic diseases they work with every day (Hagland, 1997). The advantage is that doctors can stay up-to-date in their knowledge and thus contribute directly to the quality of service offered to their patients. To support physician education, an increasing number of medical textbooks are available online. MD Consult is a very comprehensive source for on-line textbook access, with links to nearly 40 full texts online. These electronic textbooks have the tremendous advantage of being updated on a regular basis. In addition, nearly all the major, peer-reviewed medical and scientific journals have an on-line presence (Pinkowish, 1997).

In addition to influencing the quality of care provided, shared knowledge can facilitate collaborative patient/physician decision making (also called participative decision making). When patients are more *involved* in their own care and *understand* the treatment being offered them, their *compliance* with the treatment is likely to improve significantly. This will directly impact the effectiveness of the outcome of the interaction, both for the physician, whose performance is being implicitly evaluated by this measure, and for the patient who needs to comply in order to see progress.

Physicians work under dynamic and difficult conditions in trying to provide the best care for their patients (*Business Wire*, 1999). Web technology can make easily available all the information they need for quick and effective decision making, allowing them to focus on what is really important—patient care.

Legal and Public Policy Issues

There are some prickly legal and public policy issues that accompany the tremendous opportunities presented to the healthcare industry by information technology. We discuss some issues that are a consequence of the industry's attempt to leverage information technology to manage its business.

The first legal issue that arises from the use of communications over the Internet pertains to the security of documents transmitted in this manner. E-mail may not be secure and breaches of patient confidentiality are possible. Attorneys particularly warn that forwarding, printing, and copying e-mail messages from or to patients be done with a great deal of caution. Some go so far as to recommend obtaining informed consent before using e-mail (Pinkowish, 1999). The legal issues are far from clear or resolved. A recent editorial in *JAMA* discussed how lawyers have yet to reach a consensus on whether encryption of e-mail messages is needed to preserve attorney-client privilege (Spielberg, 1998). Some organizations have preempted any potential problems by incorporating e-mail messages into the formal patient medical records maintained. In such cases, doctors routinely copy all communications to the medical records section, where they are printed out. When a patient comes in, the doctor requests that he/she go through the printed message and sign it in order to validate it (Hagland, 1997).

A second legal and public policy issue that is raised by the industry adopting technological applications pertains to licensing physicians to practice medicine (Keltner, 1998). Under the present laws, anybody who practices medicine has to be licensed by the state in which he/she intends to practice. However, the Web makes it possible for a person sitting in one state to advise patients sitting in another state, another country, or even another continent. It is unclear how we as a society should deal with this development. Should we have laws that govern physicians practicing over the Internet? If we do need laws, should the states make these laws (just as states give licenses) or should it be national-level legislation, or should it be an international standard?

Public policy efforts are aimed at protecting the public from individuals who might be unqualified to render medical diagnoses and opinions. While that argument would suggest that there is a need to have some kind of licensing requirement for those who practice medicine (or give medical advice) over the Internet, the same argument would then raise some more questions about some common practices seen on the Internet today. The questions that are raised pertain to the accuracy of medical information provided on the Web. Patients can get information by clicking through hyperlinks from one site to another, i.e., an insurance company's Web site may have information about coverage for diabetes treatments and then one can click on a hyperlink to go to a site giving medical information about diabetes. If the patient comes across and uses inaccurate information which harms him/her, then who should be held responsible for the damage caused — the insurance company or the site that put up the information as a free service and has no contractual relationship with the patient? If public policy aims to protect individuals from getting advice from unqualified sources, should it matter whether the source is a live person or a Web site that has the aura of medical authority. How far can public policy go with legislation on these issues? At present, most companies that provide hyperlinks to sites containing medical information tend to provide prominent disclaimers that clearly state they are not responsible for any damages that may result from the use of information contained at these sites (Keltner, 1998). Should public policymakers intervene or is it appropriate for insurance or pharmaceutical firms to put a disclaimer and not worry about the accuracy of the information that can be accessed from their site? These are indeed thorny issues that have the potential to slow down the rate of adoption of information technology in certain areas of the healthcare industry.

FUTURE RESEARCH

Though patient care, in general, seems to be the beneficiary of the changes being brought about by information technology, one of the most promising areas for future research is the impact of this technology on rural health care. Our discussions with information technology specialists and healthcare professionals, including physicians and managed care providers, suggest that rural healthcare is likely to be the area where information technology can make its biggest impact by radically improving the quality of patient care. For example, rural areas tend to have far fewer physicians servicing large areas. Often, physicians in rural areas travel to a different town on different days of the week to look after their patients. Information technology is now making it possible for patients in rural areas to have much better access to their physicians. The physicians, in turn, are able to better serve their patients. It is possible for them to stay in one place and coordinate activities in others. They could have their patients' test reports sent to them electronically from different places, communicate with their patients electronically, and in some cases, (as with the elderly) even monitor patient compliance. These are fascinating developments made possible by information technology and future research should address the best ways for us to harness the technology and improve the quality of patient care.

CONCLUSIONS

The impact of information technology is being felt by the healthcare industry in many different ways. At the core of the industry lies the physician-patient relationship. The average number of physician contacts per person per year has ranged between 5.3 and 6.0 during the period 1987 to 1995 in the USA. In 1987 it was 5.4 and in 1995 it was 5.8. It peaked in 1993 and 1994 at 6.0 and was the lowest in 1988 and 1989 at 5.3 (Pamuk et al, 1998). Given the above trend, or more correctly the absence of one, it is unlikely that the *number* of physician contacts per person per year will be significantly affected by the increased connectivity and interactions fostered by the emerging information technology in the healthcare industry.

However, in contrast to the constancy of the number of physician contacts, the *nature* of physician contacts has already changed significantly and is likely to change even more dramatically. As depicted in the Diamond Model of Figure 3, every physician contact involves two physically present participants—the physician and the patient—and two virtually present participants — the pharmaceutical companies and insurance companies. Although the latter two have always been "present" during a physician-patient interaction, they have lurked in the shadows. The pharmaceutical companies have acted through the physicians; the insurance companies have acted after the contact. Now, due to greater connectivity and interactions, the pharmaceutical companies are acting through the physician and the patient; the insurance companies are acting prior to, during, and after the contact.

Naturally, the new relationships among the four key players in the healthcare industry have changed and will continue to change the balance of power, especially informational power. These changes, when harnessed properly, can dramatically improve the *quality* of the physician contact. One of the major constraints in healthcare is the physician's time. It is not surprising therefore that about two-thirds of physician office visits last less than 15 minutes (Woodward, 1997). The new technologies make it possible to focus the few available minutes on the core issues concerning the physician and the patient, rather than on peripheral issues that can be addressed without the need for physical contact between the physician and the patient. The emerging connectivity makes it possible for both physicians and patients to obtain and assimilate information asynchronously online rather than synchronously on-site — in the presence of the other party. An informed patient can be an asset to a physician in diagnosing and treating his or her own disease. Such a patient is also more likely to comply with a course of treatment than an uninformed patient. The new technologies can help inform the patient prior to and following the physician contact and thereby reserve the contact time for processing the information.

In concluding, one must acknowledge the possibility of adverse effects as well. An uninformed patient may be benign and an informed patient an asset, but a misinformed patient may be a liability. Such a patient can diminish the quality of the physician contact. The very technology that makes it possible to inform a patient also makes it possible to misinform him/ her. There are many Web sites that provide information of questionable credibility. Either out of ignorance or out of desperation many patients may be drawn to these sites. The physician is then compelled to correct the misinformation during his or her contact with the patient. One can minimize such dysfunction if the pharmaceutical companies, insurance companies, and hospitals ensure the availability of certified, credible information and the physicians point their patient to such information.

REFERENCES

Business Wire (1998), "Boston Area Doctors Use the Internet to Share Medical Data for Faster Diagnosis," (June 15), New York.

Business Wire (1998), "McKesson's Patient-Direct Program Generates 9.2% Response Rate for "AllerDays" Wellness Program; Informed Patients Adhere to Drug Regimens for Better Outcomes," (Sep. 1), New York.

Business Wire (1998), "Physicians' Online to Help Doctors Create Web Presence, Obtain Prescription Samples Via Internet," (Sep. 18), New York.

Business Wire (1999), "CyBear to Partner with Sun Microsystems to Develop Healthcare Internet," (Feb. 1), New York.

Business Wire (1999), "Data General and HealthGate Alliance Brings Critical Information to Patients," (Feb. 22), New York.

Business Wire (Nov 18, 1998), "$5 Million Online marketing program landed by Mediconsult.com: One of the largest Direct-to-Consumer Web Marketing Programs," New York: Business Wire.

Ditto, Steve and Briggs Pile (1998), "Marketing on the Internet," *Healthcare Executive*, Sep/Oct., 54-55.

Eder, Lauren and Marvin E. Darter (1998), "Physicians in Cyberspace," *Communications of the ACM*, 41(3), 52-54.

Eyuboglu, Nermin, and Osman A. Atac (1991), Informational Power: A Means for Increased Control in Channels of Distribution, *Psychology and Marketing*, Fall, 197-213.

Food and Drug Administration (1985), "Direct-to-consumer advertising of prescription drugs: withdrawal of moratorium," *Federal Register*, (September 9), 50:36677-36678.

French, John R.P., and Bertram Raven (1959), *The Bases of Social Power in Studies in Social Power*, ed. Dorwin Cartwright, Ann Arbor, MI: University of Michigan, 612-613.

Greenfield, S., S. Kaplan, & J.E. Ware, Jr. (1985), "Expanding patient involvement in care: Effects on patient outcomes," *Annals of Internal Medicine*, 102(4), 520-528.

Hagland, Mark (1997), "How "WebCare" is Changing Health Care Delivery, Hit by Hit," *Health Management Technology*, (March), 22-26.

Hall, Richard H. (1996), *Organizations- Structures, Processes, and Outcomes*, (6th ed.), Englewood Cliffs, NJ: Prentice-Hall.

Holmer, Alan F. (1999), "Direct-to-consumer prescription drug advertising builds bridges between patients and physicians," *Journal of the American Medical Association*, 281, 4 (Jan 27), 380-382.

Kaplan, Debbie (1998), "Working with the Internet—and your Patients," *Patient Care*, 32(4), 4.

Keltner, Kristin B. (1998), "Networked Health Information: Assuring Quality Control on the Internet," *Federal Communications Law Journal*, 50(2), 417-439.

Kohli, Ajay K. and Bernard J. Jaworski (1990), "Market Orientation: The Construct, Research Propositions, and Managerial Implications," *Journal of Marketing*, 54 (April), 1-18.

Lankford, Dawn (1997), "Health Care Moves into Cyberspace," *Wichita Business Journal*, (Jan. 3), 1.

Mechanic, David (1998), "Public Trust and Initiatives for New Health Care Partnerships," *The Milbank Quarterly*, 76(2), 281-302.

Medical Economics (1997), "Practicing Medicine on the Net," 74, 23, 64(3).

Pamuk E, Makuc D, Heck K, Reuben C, Lochner K (1998), "Socioeconomic Status and Health Chartbook," Health, United States 1998, Hyattsville, Maryland: National Center for Health Statistics.

Pinkowish, Mary Desmond (1997), "The Physician's Guide to the Internet," *Patient Care*, 31, 3, 26-53.

Pinkowish, Mary Desmond (1999), "The Internet in Medicine: An Update," *Patient Care*, 33, 1, 30-54.

Prelter, Robert (1998), "Vendors expand Web sites from Marketing to Transactions, Data Management, Communications," *Employee Benefit Plan Review*, 52(12), 30-34.

Solovy, Alden and Chris Serb (1999), "Health Care's Most Wired," *Hospitals and Health Networks*, 73, 2, 43-51.

Spielberg, A.R. (1998), "On Call and Online: Sociohistorical, Legal, and Ethical Implications of Email for the Patient-Physician Relationship," *Journal of the American Medical Association*, 280, 1353-1359.

Spreng, Richard A., Scott B. MacKenzie, and Richard W. Olshavsky (1996), "A Reexamination of the Determinants of Consumer Satisfaction," *Journal of Marketing*, 60 (July), 3, 15-34.

Star Tribune (1998), "How Internet Could Change Patient Care," (Oct. 1), Minneapolis, Minnesota.

Woodwell, David A. (1997) *National Ambulatory Medical Care Survey: 1995 Summary*, U.S. Department of Health and Human Services, Centers for Disease Control and Prevention, National Center for Health Statistics.

Chapter IV

Teleradiology: IT-Based Co-operation and Networking in Public Health

Stefan Kirn and Christian Heine
Technical University of Ilenau
Institute of Information Systems

In most countries of the world, public health is an important indicator for the prosperity of a society. However, due to increasing deficits in public households, more and more conflicts arise between new medical approaches and traditional medicine, between technology-centered and human-centered care, and between increasing demands of patients (societies) and limited, sometimes even decreasing healthcare budgets.

In this context, telecommunication-based medicine (telemedicine for short) provides for economies of scale, for sharing of investments, for speeding up clinical and healthcare business processes, for bridging geographical distances and, last but not least, for fundamentally re-designing, and innovating diagnostic, administrative, therapeutic and nursing processes (Hammer, 1993; Berger, 1997).

Telemedicine-networks can only be established and operated efficiently
- if all relevant information and objects are in digital form (providing for a dematerialization of healthcare processes!)
- if high-speed networks are available with acceptable bandwidth,
- if the telemedicine-software can be integrated with the administrative and clinical systems of healthcare institutions, and
- if the clinical and administrative processes of healthcare institutions are adapted to the challenges of telemedicine.

Up to now, it is quite usual to support administrative processes (such as billing), patient management, education, research or procurement by telematics. In contrast, telematics in diagnostics and therapy is still at its very beginning in most countries. First examples are emerging in telepathology, in teledermatology, and in telerobotics for surgical operations. The most emergent field in telemedicine, however, is teleradiology. Probably the most important reason is that information, objects, and thus most processes in radiology can be dematerialized much more easily than in other clinical fields.

Regarding the points mentioned above, and with particular respect to the requirements of teleradiology, the current state can be characterized as follows:

- There is an increasing availability of digital modalities in hospitals. Thus, digital representations of images will be standard in the near future.
- The Internet provides a public infrastructure for telecommunication. Increasing bandwith provide for a much better reliability than in the past. Recent achievements in communication security (e.g., electronic signatures, virtual private networks, tunneling) facilitate the development of telemedicine applications (Müller, 1999).
- Expenses for telecommunication (dollar per unit) are decreasing rapidly due to technical innovations, extensive worldwide competition, cost reduction in hardware, etc.

However, there are also open problems, in particular in software management / software technology, in the future development of standards (HL7, Dicom), and, finally, in the organizational systems/management structures typically found in public health organizations.

Information systems in healthcare are not at all open systems. For example, the architectures of most systems do not meet the state of the art in software technology. Modularization, object orientation, component technology, open interfaces and the like are still not common today. Even the commitment to standards such as HL7 or Dicom that are really important for teleradiology cannot be taken for granted. This is quite an important difference to up-to-date information systems in industry and manufacturing.

Problems in management include that the IT departments of most public health institutions are not very experienced in large software projects, and in running/maintaining inter-hospital computer networks. On the side of software companies, there are bottlenecks in manpower (Y2K problem, Euro, fairly not enough programmers/IT experts on the market) and in competence (in particular, system integration, operation/maintenance of large inter-organizational computer networks, telematics, IT support along the healthcare value chain).

A particular technological risk relates to the further development of the standards HL7 (representation/transmission of textual and numerical information) and Dicom 3.0 (representation/transmission of images). The definitions of both standards are not consolidated yet. Problems may arise due to the rapid success of the new Internet standard XML (eXtended Markup Language). XML provides quite a natural way to structure and access documents composed of text, images, audio and video sequences. The historical reasons behind the distinction into these two standards have therefore become obsolete already. Thus, an upcoming integration of HL7 and Dicom may be expected (HL7, 1999). Healthcare institutions then could apply to XML for ease exchange of information between disparate software applications. This, in turn, will impact the architectures and the functionality of future hospital information systems (HIS) as well as of dedicated radiology information systems (RIS).

On the organizational side, problems of change management are important. They result from the specific organizational cultures in healthcare, from shortcomings in process management, and also from inefficient management structures in public health institutions. This may cause risks and difficulties (i.e., cost-raisers) if technology-driven change management aims to adapt a healthcare institution to a new organizational situation.

Contribution

The chapter describes the potential benefits and the challenges small hospitals are faced with if they aim to establish and run a teleradiology network supporting their every-day processes in radiology. The next section introduces the technical approach and the methodology being used throughout the project. Then, the initial situation of the hospitals involved, the benefits expected from teleradiology and an overview of those conceptualizations of the teleradiology network that have been suggested are covered. Three of them are described and evaluated in more detail. The final section summarizes the results and gives the outlook of future work.

TECHNICAL APPROACH, METHODOLOGY

The technical approach we have applied to refers to ARIS (= architecture of integrated information systems). ARIS provides a methodology and a set of tools for developing information models. An information model of a hospital is an abstract description of the relevant activities, information objects and information flows in a real-world hospital. A telemedicine information model is thus an adequate basis for designing, implementing, and maintaining a telematics-based inter-clinical software system. A detailed description of ARIS is available in Scheer (1998).

On the one hand, ARIS provides an integrated modeling framework including expanded event-driven process chains (eEPC's) for business process representations, function trees for representing business functions in enterprises, organizational charts for representing the organizational structure of a firm, and entity-relationship models (ERMs) for data modeling. These four modeling concepts stand for different, however interdependent perspectives of the modeling task. In ARIS, these modeling concepts refer to each other in such a way that any changes of the information model, e.g., a modification of the organizational chart, can easily be mapped to the data model, to the process chains, etc.

On the other hand, ARIS also provides an approved software design process model in that it distinguishes five stages of software development (see Figure 1):

- *Application problem:* still outside of the methodology
- *Requirements specification:* First ARIS stage of modeling. Contains pre-formal, semantic model of the requirements of a business application. On this level, ERMs and EPCs are used to represent particular information systems requirements.
- *Information system (IS) concept:* Second stage of ARIS modeling. Contains detailed formal descriptions of the conceptual data model (database design), and of the software architecture on the overall systems level.
- *Implementation description:* Third level of ARIS modeling. Contains the physical data model (database design) and formal specification of the detailed software architecture (level of modules).
- *Implementation:* Outside of ARIS, addresses the physical implementation of the system.

Figure 1: ARIS Methodology

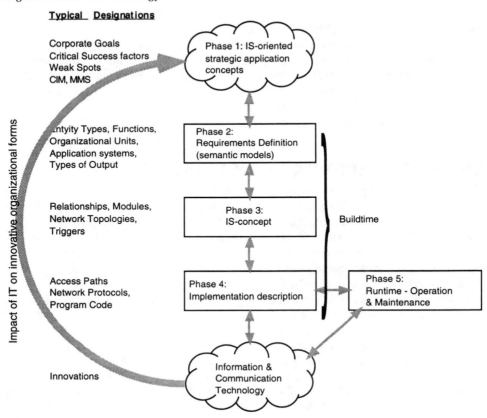

Typical Designations

Corporate Goals
Critical Success factors
Weak Spots
CIM, MMS

Phase 1: IS-oriented strategic application concepts

Entyity Types, Functions, Organizational Units, Application systems, Types of Output

Phase 2: Requirements Definition (semantic models)

Relationships, Modules, Network Topologies, Triggers

Phase 3: IS-concept

Buildtime

Access Paths Network Protocols, Program Code

Phase 4: Implementation description

Phase 5: Runtime - Operation & Maintenance

Impact of IT on innovative organizational forms

Innovations

Information & Communication Technology

DESCRIPTION OF PROJECT

Background

Thuringia is a German state with a square dimension of 18.400 km^2 and about 2.5 million inhabitants living mostly in small towns (< 100.000 inhabitants). Currently, there are about 45 hospitals, 35 of them are too small (< 300 beds) for further reductions in size (at current level of technology). However, recent forecasts say that the demand for healthcare services in Thuringia will further decrease by about 15% in the next five years. It is expected that this will cause sincere economic problems for at least 50% of the hospitals in the region. The public authorities currently owning those hospitals will probably not be able to cover the resulting burden of debt. Two possible solutions are currently under consideration: (1) Further decrease the minimum firm size required for survival through organizational networking, outsourcing/insourcing, and telematics; (2) Sell distressed healthcare institutions to a privately owned hospital chain.

In this context, three small Thuringian hospitals formed a consortium in order to evaluate whether telematics can help them survive under these uncomfortable constraints at least in the interim. They thus decided to investigate the risks and the strategic contribution of a teleradiology network to their competitiveness in the regional healthcare market.

Benefits Expected

Telemedicine in general is supposed to provide for economies of scale, for sharing of financial investments between hospitals, for efficient cooperation among clinical experts, and for providing small hospitals with access to up-to-date, university-level diagnostic competence (there is only one university hospital in Thuringia).

In this context, teleradiology is supposed to provide for the following advantages:

- *Standardization:* Concerns technical equipment, software systems, diagnostic and administrative processes in the radiology departments involved. Also leads to detailed documentation of processes, etc. and improves the quality standards in radiology across the members of the network.
- *Radiological competence:* A teleradiology network provides for specialization, and, thus for better radiological competence available to each node in the network.
- *IT competence:* Due to the increasing number of digital modalities, teleradiology will soon enter the local routine processes in hospitals. However, it may prove difficult to build up and keep the necessary IT competence available. Thus, a teleradiology network will also support specialization in IT.
- *Availability:* Enlistment periods for radiologists can be much better coordinated across a teleradiology network. This is especially important at night and during weekends.
- *Second opinion:* It is sometimes necessary to call for a second opinion, e.g., in case of strokes, in neurosurgery, etc.
- *sharing of digital archives:* Digital archives are an expensive resource. They require specialized IT competence, dedicated building infrastructures, etc. Expectation: significant economies of scale through decrease of fix costs per hospital and of unit costs per stored radiological image.
- *Procurement:* A teleradiology network may have a much better position in radiology-related procurement than a single hospital on its own.

Conceptualizations of Different Types of Networks in Teleradiology

Teleradiology can run in very different forms. Examples are the operation of a telearchive, different approaches to teleconsultation, telecommunication-based exchange of radiological expertise, telecooperation of radiologists in diagnosis and therapy, but also telerobotic-like control of the operations of a remote modality (e.g., movements, taking pictures, etc.). This made it necessary to limit the scope of the study to four concrete teleradiology scenarios:

Scenario 1: Joint operation of a centralized picture archive, where each remote user (radiology department) can only access its own database partition. In this scenario, there are no local picture archiving systems (PACS).

Scenario 2: Joint operation of a centralized picture archive, where each remote user only accesses its own database partition. In addition to Scenario 1, each radiology department runs and maintains a local PACS for caching purposes.

Scenario 3: Teleconsultation with access to local software systems (in particular, RIS and HIS [hospital information system]) and local PACS.

Scenario 4: Teleconsultation with access to local RIS/HIS and to a jointly operated, centralized PACS. This approach integrates Scenarios 2 and 3.

There is a partial order defined on these scenarios: 1 —> 2, 1 —> 3, {2 and 3} —> 4.

For each of these scenarios, a detailed analysis of its particular risks and promises has been undertaken. Based upon empirical research, detailed evaluations of the functional, organizational and information processing settings in each hospital have been performed.

On this basis, the feasibility, the risks, and the potential advantages of setting up and operating the teleradiology network under consideration have been determined. The investigations also addressed the readiness of software providers to actively support the prospective teleradiology network.

The following general results have been achieved:

- Expected benefits (listed above) can be achieved.
- The economic feasibility depends upon the cost for software (including. project management) and for data transmission over a telecommunication network. An important promise is that currently the cost of telecommunication is decreasing very rapidly.
- The organizational and functional structures and the processes within each involved radiology department do not provide any sincere innovation barriers. It may, however, be necessary to establish a coordination unit supporting the adaptation of local structures and processes to the requirements of a teleradiology network.
- Similar points apply to the coordination of tasks, responsibilities, and processes across the different information systems departments of each network member.
- The benefits of standardization may not so easily be achieved. Basically every member of the network wants to stay independent in its local hardware/software choices (e.g., RIS, HIS, PACS) from the network.
- The most important precondition, but probably also the highest barrier for an efficient operation of the teleradiology network, is thus the integration of different radiology information and picture archiving systems. Up to now, these systems are proprietary legacy systems. They are not at all on the current state of software technology. That makes it difficult to add necessary functions and to adapt parts of the internal architectures, data models, and data flows. It thus cannot be taken for granted that the relevant software providers really will support such a project.
- A bit surprisingly, the relevant standards HL7 and DICOM3 are not consolidated yet. Due to the rapid emergence of the Internet, and to the overwhelming success of the just recently developed information representation language XML (eXtended Markup Language) an impact on further definitions of these standards must be expected.

SELECTED SCENARIOS

Centralized archive, exclusive database partitions for each network member, and local picture archiving systems for the purpose of caching (Scenario 2):

Each member of the network (hospital) runs its own radiology information and picture archiving systems under local control. The primary objective behind this scenario is economies of scale by a common archiving system for long time storage of radiological data (pictures).

Figure 2 illustrates a possible realization of this scenario. This scenario involves a

Figure 2: Telearchive with local PACS for caching at each network node

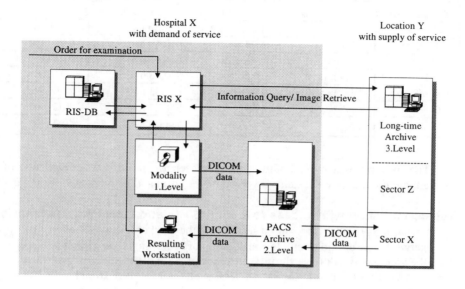

storage hierarchy with three levels. On the first level, there is a storage at each modality. On the second level, the local PACS provide for a short-term storage of pictures. The local PACS serve as a buffer or prefetching memory with a pre-calculated capacity (e.g., up to one month). On the third level, the telearchive provides long-term storage capacities.

Organization and size of the local archives depend on technical and economic factors. Figure 4 provides an example.

The costs of telecommunications depend on the capacity of the local PACS (in days of caching), on the volume of the data transmitted per archiving operation, and on the bandwith available. The following figure presents an example for a data transmission calculation.

Figure 3: Calculation for a local PACS (example)

- average examinations of patients per day	150 patients/day
- average size of radiological data per examination	15 MB/examination
- average accesses to the central archive	150 accesses/day
- average size of loaded radiological data per examination	15 MB/examination
- amount of created radiological data per day	2,2 GB/day
- amount of loaded radiological data per day	2,2 GB/day
- daily backup-volume per night to the central archive	2,2 GB/day
- amount of created radiological data per month	65 GB/month
- amount of loaded radiological data per month	65 GB/month
- amount of archived radiological data per month	130 GB/month
- Size of the RAID System (Level 1)	260 GB

Figure 4: Data transmission calculations (example)

Time required for data transmission depending on amount of data and bandwith				
	64 kbit/s	128 kbit/s	2Mbit/s	34 Mbit/s
100 kByte	12,5 sec	6,25 sec	0,4 sec.	0,024 sec
1 Mbyte	128 sec	64 sec	4,1 sec	0,24 sec
10 Mbyte	21,3 min	10,66 min	0,68 min	2,41 sec
100 Mbyte	213,3 min	106,6 min	6,83 min	24,01 sec
1 Gbyte	35,5 h	17,7 h	68,3 min	4,02 min
10 Gbyte	355,5 h	177,7 h	11,3 h	40,2 min

The only necessary precondition for this scenario is DICOM-compliance of the different picture archiving systems involved on the local and network-wide storage level.

Teleconsultation with access to local RIS/HIS and local PACS (scenario 3)

Scenario 3 provides all required services on the level of teleconsultations. Examples:
- network consultation: remote consultation of a radiologist providing his services for the whole network (e.g., during weekends or at night)
- be on call: remote radiologist transfers results, for instance from home
- expert consultation: remote radiologist provides a "second opinion"
- transport consultation: remote specialized radiologist decides whether a patient can be / needs to be transported to a specialized clinic (e.g., case of neurosurgery)
- emergency consultation: remote radiologist needs to be accessed / consulted as fast as possible.

The data transmission capacities in this scenario are not as high as in the telearchive scenario. At present, there exists only some interest for teleconsultation in computer tomography (CT) and magneto resonance tomography (MRT). The bandwith needed depends primarily on the required transmission speed.

Thus, when setting up a teleconsultation network, the maximum acceptable transmission times for the different consultation scenarios needs to be determined first.

The following figure shows exemplary data transmission times for CT- and MRT-studies.

Figure 5: Data transmission for CT- and MRT-studies (values based on theoretical bandwith)

Time required for data transmission for CT- and MRT-studies with different bandwiths		
Bandwith	CT-Study (approx.15 Mbyte)	MRT-Study (approx.60 Mbyte)
64 kbit/s	32 min.	128 min.
128 kbit/s	16 min.	64 min.
768 kbit/s	2,7 min.	10,7 min.
2Mbit/s	1 min.	4 min.
34 Mbit/s	3,5 sec.	14 sec.

Teleconsultation with Access to Local RIS/HIS and to a Central PACS (Scenario 4)

The scenarios outlined above assume a proprietary telecommunication infrastructure where security requirements are not such important. It is, however, absolutely necessary to also consider teleradiology across public networks, e.g., the internet. In this case, it is absolutely necessary to meet the relevant security constraints as they have been laid down in the respective national and international legal regulations.

A teleradiology system that meets these requirements is available with CHILI. CHILI has been developed by the Steinbeis-Transferzentrum Medical Informatics (TZMI), Heidelberg, and is available on the market since 1997. The particular strength of CHILI is its well-developed security system. This meets the strong data privacy requirements of the German Data Privacy Law (Bundesdatenschutzgesetz BDSG) and also the technical aspects of data security, which have been defined by the Commission of the European Community in its IT Security Manual. This makes CHILI quite appropriate for any teleradiology cooperation accessing the internet.

The following figure gives a description of a CHILI-based architecture as a possible solution to the requirements specified in scenario 4.

CHILI does also include a WWW concept. This provides tools for secure transmission of medical data on WWW basis, e.g., all information is being transmitted on basis of SSL (Secure Socket Layer) applying to the HTTPS-protocol. Every PC equipped with an internet browser can thus be used to directly access the CHILI database.

The implementation of billing mechanisms on basis of HL7 and XML is the next step to real internet-based teleradiology. Currently, there are only solutions on the market that support a small selection of those processes running in the daily routine of a radiology department.

Figure 6: Teleconsultation architecture based on CHILI

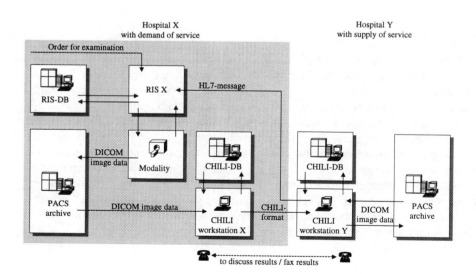

Figure 7: Architecture of viewing components and plug-ins [ENGELMANN (WWW)]

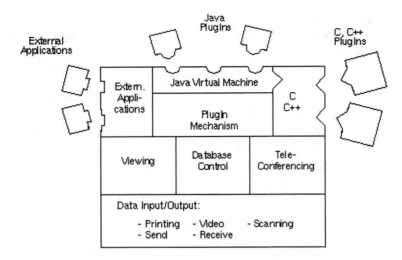

Another interesting advantage of CHILI is its plug-in concept. Software developers can thus easily add new functionality to the system. In doing so they are free in the choice of programming language and interface toolkits (e.g., C, C++, Tcl/Tk). The following figure shows the architecture of viewing components and plug-ins.

In the perspective of true, open internet-based teleradiology, also some shortcomings of the CHILI system need to be reported. At the moment, there is no solution available for billing teleradiology services (e.g., consultations). Further issues relate to an integration of CHILI with the information systems of other hospitals, health assurances, etc. Thee are still a lot of interfaces to be developed. Another important point is that, up to now, CHILI does not support the HL7 standard yet.

SUMMARY

The research in this project has shown, that teleradiology can provide hospitals with a decrease in their costs in radiology while at the same time their competence in diagnostic, and therapy quality increases. Teleradiology has thus a clear potential to contribute a significant competitive advantage to small and medium-sized hospitals.

On the other hand, the research undertaken has also shown several risks and other important innovation barriers. The risks are mainly related to the proprietary nature of current hospital information systems, and to the missing competence of most RIS/HIS-supplying software companies in inter-organizational networks, and telecommunication. The most important barrier, however, seems to be that the strategic impact of teleradiology (and telemedicine in general) has not been recognized yet broadly (at least in Germany). This is in a hard contrast to the situation industry, where networking, telecommunications, division of labor also between competing enterprises is very common today.

REFERENCES

Adler, R.M. (1995) Emerging Standards for Component Software. *IEEE Computer*, March, 68-77.

ACR (WWW). (1998). American College of Radiology: Radiology: an Inside Look. http://www.acr.org.

Berger, Roland (1999).Telematik im Gesundheitswesen: Perspektiven der Telemedizin in Deutschland. München http://www.rolandberger.com (only in German).

Callon, J. D. (1996). *Competitive Advantage through Information Technology*. McGraw-Hill International Editions, New York.

Cash Jr., J.I.; Eccles, R.G.; Nohria, N.; Nolan, R.L. (1994). *Building the Information-Age Organization: Structure, Control, and Information Technologies*. 3rd ed. Richard D. Irwin Inc..

Engelmann, Uwe et al. (1998). A Three-Generation Model for Teleradiology. In : IEEEb(Hrsg.): *Transactions on Information Technology in Biomedicine, 2(1)*, 20-25.

Engelmann, Uwe (1999). Das CHILI-Plug-in-Konzept: Funktionale Offenheit in einer radiologischen Workstation. (only in German) http://mbi.dkfz- heidelberg.de/mbi/TR/Papers/P5-98.html.

Gogan, J.L. & Guinan, P.J. (1999). Fletcher Allen Health Care's Telemedicine Initiative. *Journal of Information Technology Cases and Applications*, 1(1), 41-72.

Hammer, M. & Champy, J. (1993). *Reengineering the Corporation: A Manifesto for Business Revolution*. New York: Harper Collins.

HL7: HL7-DICOM IMSIG (1997). http://dumccs.mc.duke.edu/standards/HL7/sigs/image-management/HTML/goals.html.

HL7 (1999). HL7 version 2.3 draft standard, http://www.mcis.duke.edu/ standards/HL7/pubs/version2.3/html/hl7web.zip. Download: 20.08.1999.

Jarke, M. & Kethers, S.(1999). Regionale Kooperationskompetenz: Probleme und Modellierungstechniken. In: *Wirtschaftsinformatik* 41/4, 316-325, (only in German).

Johnson, C.R., MacLeod, R.S. & Matheson, M.A. (1993). Computational Medicine: Bioelectric Field Problems. *IEEE Computer*, October 1993, 59-67.

Kidd, P.T. (1994). *Agile Manufacturing: Forging New Frontiers*. Addison-Wesley, Wokingham/GB.

Kirn, St. & O'Hare, G. (eds.) (1997). Cooperative Knowledge Processing: The Key Technology for Intelligent Organizations. *Springer Series on Computer Supported Cooperative Work*. Springer London.

Müller, G. & Rannenberg, K. (eds.) (1999). *Multilateral Security in Communications — Technology, Infrastructure, Economy*. Addison-Wesley, München.

Rosemann, M. (1998). Managing the Complexity of Multiperspective Information Models using the Guidelines of Modelling. In: *Proceedings of the 3rd Australian Conference on Requirements Engineering*. Ed.: D. Fowler, L. Dawson, Geelong, 26./27, 101-118.

Rosemann, M.; Becker, J. & v. Uthmann, C. (1999). Guidelines of Business Process Modeling. In: W. v. d. Aalst; J. Desel; A. Oberweis (eds.): *Business Process Management: Models, Techniques and Empirical Studies*.

Scheer, A.-W. (1998). *Business Process Frameworks*. 2nd ed. Springer, Berlin.

Schnepf, J.A.; Du, D.H.C.; Ritenoux, E.R. & Fahrmann, A.J. (1995). Building Future Medical Educaion Enviroments over ATM Networks. *Communications of the ACM*, 38, (2), 54-69.

Smither, R.S. (1994). *The Psychology of Work and Human Performance*. Harper Collins College Publishers, New York.

Section II: Web Enabling the Health Organization

This section is aimed at providing readers with an understanding of some of the principal concerns within healthcare organizations as they begin implementing Web-enabled information systems. The common theme among these chapters is the focus on the transition process. We begin with an overview of the transformations affecting clinical healthcare delivery, and then present three case studies depicting the transition process of several healthcare organizations that are moving their legacy information systems applications to a Web-based environment. Each of the three cases presented in this section provides detailed assessments of the strategies used, including expected benefits, lessons learned, and directions for further research and development.

Turner begins by discussing the historical development of telemedicine and proposes that evolving Web-based telemedicine applications are leading to the creation of virtual organizations for the provision of healthcare services. Healthcare organizations that are transitioning to a virtual mode of delivery are being faced with a new set of challenges including provider licensing, liabilities, and reimbursements. Turner suggests that new patterns of healthcare delivery will continue to emerge as Web-based technology forces the change of existing processes. As changes occur at the interorganizational level (as introduced in Section I by Johnson et al.), managers also need to be aware of the intraorganizational changes that are likely to occur. Management should understand how telemedicine fits within their organization's current mission, procedures, and policies. Identifying and planning for key change areas, such as social, cultural, and technological factors within the organization, will lay the foundation for a smoother transition.

In their case study, Lehmann and Wee describe the process reengineering efforts of a New Zealand hospital that is transitioning to become an electronic community for its organizational members. The authors focus specifically on the objectives of the patient admission process at a suburban Auckland hospital. The previous manual system is evaluated and the newly developed Web-based system is explained in detail. The system architecture is defined as well as the impact of the system on members of the hospital community, particularly the medical practitioners. Beginning with the expected benefits, Lehmann and Wee precisely describe the migration process and the lessons learned, providing both researchers and practitioners with a solid understanding of one hospital's experiences. They conclude with the hospital's future plans for the expansion of their system.

Korpela, Mykkanen, Rasanen, Ruonamaa, and Sormunen focus on the migration process associated with transforming proprietary legacy systems to open Web-enabled systems. Many hospitals around the world still operate within the dumb terminal/mainframe context for information processing. The authors describe the problems inherent to this architecture in light of both current user requirements and the technology that is available today. They present a well-defined migration strategy that focuses on preserving existing IT investments while transitioning first to a client/server and finally towards an object oriented, Web-based network computing environment. The authors base their discussion around a migration strategy that was deployed for a specific legacy system in Finland. In doing so, they provide a detailed analysis of the project's migration objectives and the tools used to accomplish those objectives. They extend their discussion by demonstrating the applicability of their migration approach to both American and Nigerian health organizations. Korpela, Mykkanen, Rasanen, Ruonamaa, and Sormunen provide a useful framework for practitioners and researchers that are involved with the transition from legacy systems to a Web-enabled environment.

In the third case study, Kohli and Ziege focus on the re-design of the cost accounting process within the context of a large, multi-location health organization. Specifically, they describe the Web-enabled intranet infrastructure that was developed to support the cost management operations throughout the Holy Cross Health System in Indiana. The authors begin with a descriptive overview of the cost management process. They describe the selection process for the IT that was ultimately deployed, emphasizing the importance of communicating with the end users. The authors also discuss the decision to internally develop the cost accounting application, and provide an assessment of the pros and cons. Kohli and Ziege's conclusions suggest that more than the technology, a clear understanding of organizational processes is the most critical aspect in the design and the development of a Web-enabled cost management application.

Chapter V

Telemedicine: Generating the Virtual Office Visit

Jeanine W. Turner
Georgetown University

Telemedicine is redefining the boundaries of the doctor and patient encounter. No longer do the doctor and patient need to be in the same room. No longer does the doctor have to visually see the patient to develop a diagnosis. New telecommunications infrastructures have created the possibility for a virtual office visit, outside of the constraints of time and space. This radical change in physical boundaries creates a profound transformation of the doctor and patient relationship, the organizational cultures of the healthcare institutions involved, and the administration, management, and reimbursement of services. Debakey (1995) argued that telemedicine, or the use of telecommunications technologies within the field of healthcare, has the potential for having a greater impact on the future of medicine than any other modality. Although the term telemedicine can include a wide variety of applications and technologies, including database management, distance education, and electronic patient records, this chapter will focus the application of telemedicine on delivery of remote electronic clinical consultations. This chapter will discuss telemedicine's historical development, the transformation of the clinical environment from an external, internal, and individual perspective, and future trends.

TELEMEDICINE'S HISTORICAL DEVELOPMENT

The intersection of communication technology and medicine is not new. In 1877, 21 local doctors built one of the first telephone exchanges to allow easier communication with the local drugstore (Starr, 1982). However, more recent characterizations of "telemedicine" date back over the past three decades. Lovett and Bashshur (1979) divided the development of telemedicine into three stages. The first stage was characterized by pioneering efforts exploring use of telecommunications modalities in the delivery of care across distance with few public or private resources to support them.

The second stage, between 1965 and 1973, was marked by deliberate efforts towards research and development and received short-term federal support. The third stage began in 1973, continuing through 1979, and for the first time, involved evaluation by interdisciplinary teams with social scientists and specialists in medical care organization, planning, and delivery. During this time, the knowledge gained from the space program and the public telecommunications efforts cooperated to form STARPAHC (Space Technology Applied to Rural Papago Advanced Health Care). STARPAHC was a $3.3 million project that used expertise gained from the space program and applied it to the problem of delivering medical care to the Papago Indian reservation. This effort was an exemplary program that integrated designers, users, care providers, and evaluators in determining the system's objectives, design, criteria for performance, and responsibility for its operation (Lovett & Bashshur, 1979).

Regardless of their success, the majority of the programs started prior to 1986 have not survived due to the lack of federal funding based on the inability to justify the programs on a cost-benefit basis (Perednia & Allen, 1995). Although the data from these early efforts are limited, early reviews and evaluations indicate that the technology that was used was reasonably effective in transmitting the information needed for most clinical uses, and the majority of the patients were satisfied with their treatment (Perednia & Allen, 1995).

What might be considered the fourth stage of telemedicine is occurring in the mid to late 1990s and has several driving factors. These factors include: the strong need for clinical medicine in remote areas, the politics and economics of a managed care approach to medicine, the suppliers of telemedicine equipment and telecommunications carrying capacity (Perednia & Allen, 1995). The 1990s have also witnessed large investments in telemedicine development, with the total amount of money spent by the federal government on grants, contracts, and appropriations for telemedicine in the '90s approaching $700 million (Perednia & Grigsby, 1998). Bashshur (1995a) noted, "Unlike the early pioneering efforts of the 1970s in the development of telemedicine systems, which operated somewhat independently and in relative isolation of each other, the current generation of telemedicine systems is emerging as part of a larger social and cultural movement, embedded in the information age" (p. 81).

As attempts were made to mimic the appearance of the doctor and patient traditional encounter, the early approaches to telemedicine focused on technologies that facilitated both visual and audio cues. The doctor and patient could hear and see each other in real time, but were each in distinct locations. The first official telemedicine program review of U.S. programs conducted by Telemedicine Today in 1993 revealed 12 active telemedicine programs, all employing interactive video technology as a means of mediating doctor and patient interaction. The fourth telemedicine program review of U.S. programs revealed a total of 80 telemedicine programs across 38 states, including Washington, D.C. (Grigsby and Allen, 1997). The majority of the programs incorporated interactive television applications, while a few employed store and forward technology. During 1996 and the first four months of 1997, the survey found a total of 21,274 patient-clinical interactions taking place (Grigsby and Allen, 1997).

As the costs of interactive television have decreased with the creation of the CODEC and the improvement of telecommunications infrastructures, expensive room-based videoconferencing systems are being replaced with desktop and Web-based versions. The development and increased use of the Internet has expanded the use of telemedicine in real time, interactive videoconferencing applications to Web-based, store-and-forward applications. One specialty that has achieved success in this area is teledermatology. In May 1998, Walter Reed Army Medical Center created a Web-based system for providing primary care physicians the opportunity to consult with dermatologists regarding specific patients. A 1999 study of 224 teledermatology consults showed that 54% of the patients were able to be treated at the primary care facility, never having to make the trip to see the specialist (Welch, Pak and Poropatich, 1999). Often these specialty specific programs allow better triage capabilities for channeling patients to appropriate specialist care.

In addition to programs within medical centers, private companies are creating Web-based programs that provide real-time doctor and patient consultations. AmericasDoctor.com is a World Wide Web company headquartered in Owings Mills, Maryland, contracting with about 100 medical professionals to answer "guest" concerns. The company opened in 1998 and currently attracts approximately 3,000 people a day to its "Ask-the-Doc" feature. Brown (1999) reported that at its busiest time, as many as 20 physicians at two call centers can be answering "guest" questions. The company likes to think of itself as an extension of the "ask-a-nurse" service that provided telephone advice to concerned callers. The company characterizes itself more as a medical information provider rather than a provider of a doctor and patient relationship. It seems that as the doctor and patient encounter moves away from synchronous, video-enhanced connections, the systems supporting the encounter (like reimbursement, credentialing, licensing, and legal systems) are having difficulty defining what constitutes a doctor and patient visit. The next section will discuss the characteristics of the doctor and patient visit and the impact that new technologies are having on what constitutes that virtual office visit.

TRANSFORMATION IN THE CLINICAL ENVIRONMENT: THE NEW VIRTUAL VISIT

Telemedicine technology, in its current state, influences many levels of communication. Turner and Thomas (1999) argue that telemedicine constitutes a virtual service. Through the use of a telecommunications infrastructure, the traditional office environment is expanded in time and space to create a new service that has unique implications on the provider and patient relationship. First, it influences the relationship between the provider organization and the location receiving the consultation. This relationship can be recognized through any number of combinations of healthcare professionals — from a specialist at an academic medical center and a family practice practitioner at a rural, remote site, to a physician responding to a worried caller over a Web-based session. Secondly, telemedicine forces the creation of a virtual organization to support the development of a relationship among members. This new organization, comprised of each of the distinct sites involved in the interaction, must coordinate and manage the relationships influenced on both an intra-organizational and an inter-organizational level, as well as manage its relationship with patients. These include the creation of a vision for each individual organization and the combined virtual organization. These visions describe the way telemedicine fits within the current practice of medicine, as well as procedures and policies that will direct its use.

Thirdly, telemedicine requires new patterns of medical practice because the current technology often requires that healthcare practitioners change processes of care. These practitioners must learn to interpret information in new and different ways. Information that used to be provided within the richness of a face-to-face setting is now provided at a distance with fewer verbal and nonverbal cues to consider. And finally, on a patient to provider level, this technology is a radical departure from the way that care is currently provided to a patient. The doctor-patient relationship is being expanded to include an interaction that does not necessarily include touch. A doctor may examine a patient from thousands of miles away. In this way, telemedicine constitutes a major influence on the way that the relationship between a physician and a patient is developed and on expectations regarding this relationship.

Bashshur (1995b) delineated six essential characteristics of a telemedicine system: (1) geographic separation between provider and client or provider and provider; (2) the use of some type of telecommunications technology that facilitates the interaction and transfer of information between parties; (3) appropriate staffing to perform all necessary functions within such systems; (4) the development of an organizational structure uniquely suitable for implementing telemedicine systems; (5) the development of clinical protocols for triaging clients to appropriate diagnostic and treatment sources; and (6) the development of normative standards of behavior to replace the norms of face-to-face contact between client and provider. Of these characteristics, one refers to physical separation, one refers to the telecommunications product itself, and the rest refer to processes of communication that must support the telecommunications service. Whitten (1995) supports the importance of recognizing these processes in citing organizational problems, inadequate dissemination of information regarding telemedicine, and existing referral patterns and practices as the primary obstacles to telemedicine acceptance by physicians participating in the Kansas program. These characteristics can be understood as they relate to the external regulatory environment, the internal organizational environment, and the individual virtual environment of the doctor and patient encounter.

The External Regulatory Environment

The healthcare visit is embedded within a complex regulatory environment that is based in the assumption that doctors provide consultations with their patients face-to-face and in the same room. Most of these regulatory conditions provide challenges when moving from a traditional office visit to a virtual one. Sanders and Bashshur (1995) identified six problems facing the development and deployment of telemedicine: (1) interstate licensing and institutional credentialing of physicians; (2) legal liability and litigation; (3) individual client or patient autonomy and the right to privacy; (4) reimbursement; (5) knowledge about telemedicine; and (6) system design and infrastructure. These challenges reflect much of the research and discussion surrounding telemedicine.

Through the use of telecommunications connections, it is now technologically possible for a physician in Boston, Massachusetts, to consult with a patient in Laramie, Wyoming. It is technologically possible for a primary care physician in Orlando, Florida to receive a second opinion from a cardiology specialist in Seattle, Washington.

However, in these virtual environments, where the patient and physician are located in different physical environments but connected via a telecommunications connection, where does the consultation happen? When an interaction occurs between a primary care physician in one state and a specialist in another, where does that consultation happen? Who should be held accountable if something goes wrong? The consulting physician? The technology employed? The phone company providing the transmission service? Who should be reimbursed for the service and how? How should information transmitted be stored? To answer these questions, laws, credentialing systems, and reimbursement mechanisms from the physical world have been applied to this new virtual environment. Unfortunately, instead of recognizing the uniqueness offered by virtual space, the licensing, credentialing and reimbursement systems have refused to acknowledge this new environment. Instead, these systems have tried to force the physical world laws into virtual space. Therefore a concrete location had to be chosen for these systems to be applied. As a result, the consultation in a virtual environment occurs where the patient is located. In most states, the physician must be licensed in the state where the patient is located, regardless of the physician's location. Therefore, efficiencies and economies gained by employing a physician from a remote location are lost, because licensure and credentialing systems now force these individuals to align themselves with the physical space of the patient (Mun & Turner, 1999).

A specific example of the concerns being raised by these virtual office visits can be seen in the approach that the Ask-a-Doc system (discussed earlier) takes when referring to the people that connect to its site. The organization specifically refers to the Web callers as "guests" and not "patients." They characterize themselves as providing medical information much like a library, not diagnoses. AmericasDoctor.com emphatically states that it is not providing an on-line medical practice. However, patients may be characterizing these services differently. The "guests" go to the Web site with specific health-related questions and receive answers from qualified physicians. On some Web sites, visitors to the site pay for medical information. If legally challenged, courts will have to decide whether these Web-based services are providing information that might be received at a cocktail party or in a library, or if the services are more like traditional consultations (Brown, 1999).

Reimbursement systems have taken a very cautious approach to virtual environments as spaces for doctor and patient consultations. The Health Care Financing Administration (HCFA), which provides reimbursement for Medicare, has funded several demonstration projects to investigate telemedicine consultations, but does not yet reimburse most clinical telemedicine services. Many insurers are watching the development of HCFA's reimbursement policies to provide models of their own. Face-to-face, in-the-same-room care is still required for reimbursement of most consultation services (Perednia & Grigsby, 1998).

At this point in telemedicine's development, many of these external regulatory issues are following telemedicine deployment. As issues concerning liability are raised, the courts will continue to define the boundaries of these new virtual environments. Agencies and constituents are gradually exploring reimbursement and licensure concerns. Although these external issues create challenges for deployment, they have not prevented trials and applications of telemedicine consultations. Another area that has provided interesting challenges has been the organizational environment that supports telemedicine encounters.

The Internal Organizational Environment

In addition to the complex regulatory environment where telemedicine occurs, it is also important to consider changes to the organizational environment that supports the new doctor and patient environment that is created. The adoption and implementation of medical technology within healthcare organizations comprise complicated processes. The dual authority system within healthcare organizations creates opportunities for potential conflicts in telemedicine-related decisions. The juxtaposition of two power groups, administration and medical staff, within the same organization requires acceptance and adoption by both groups for implementation efforts to be successful (Coe, 1970). Although many decisions within the healthcare organization concern areas that are clearly demarcated as belonging to one group's authority versus the other, telemedicine applications fall into a common area where both the medical staff and the administration have valid interests. Telemedicine applications offer the opportunity to develop efficient connections between healthcare organizations so as to facilitate the creation of integrated delivery systems. Coordination of administrative details and concerns associated with the development of these relationships may use the same telecommunications infrastructure as the one developed to facilitate remote clinical care. The different uses and concerns, coupled with potentially different goals of fiscal survival versus clinical efficacy, can create challenges in the adoption and implementation of telemedicine systems. New virtual service healthcare systems must be created that span the organizational boundaries of any one healthcare organization (Turner, 1998; Turner & Peterson, 1998; Warisse, 1996).

The adoption and implementation of the innovation by the telemedicine network members requires special attention to the building of relationships and the coordination between organizations and individuals (Warisse, 1996). When distinct organizations are connected through telecommunications connections to facilitate work practices, a virtual organization is formed (Lipnack & Stamps, 1997). This new virtual organization is comprised of members of each of the distinct organizations. Each distinct organization operates within its own culture, goals, hierarchical structure, norms, rules, and procedures. The emerging virtual organization must develop its own culture, structure, norms, rules and procedures that accommodate the needs of each distinct organization involved (Turner, 1998; Warisse, 1996).

A clear example of the need for a new virtual organization to support the virtual healthcare system can be seen in the adoption and implementation of telemedicine by an academic medical center and a prison system to augment the delivery of specialty care to the state's inmate population (Warisse, 1996). Prior to telemedicine, specialists from the academic medical center would travel to a maximum-security clinic housed within a prison hospital to provide specialty consultations to inmate patients. Inmates would travel from their own institutions around the state to the prison hospital during a scheduled consultation time. After the consultations were completed, the inmates returned to their institutions and the specialists returned to the medical center.

The implementation of a videoconferencing connection between the academic medical center and the individual institutions facilitated telemedicine clinics while eliminating travel for both the specialist and the inmate. With the telemedicine clinics, the academic medical center connected directly to the individual institutions. At prearranged times, the specialist would meet with the patient and the institutional physician over video. Prior to telemedicine, the specialist never had the opportunity to meet the institutional physicians. In this way, telemedicine opened up a new avenue of communication. Each healthcare practitioner could learn from the other's experience. Eliminating inmate transportation and additional security officers saved dollars. The specialist saved time by eliminating his/her trip to the inmate clinic (Mekhjian, Warisse, Gailiun, & McCain, 1996).

However, regardless of the viability of the solution that telemedicine offered to the academic medical center and the prison system, the initial diffusion of this application was relatively slow. Many of the reasons for this gradual acceptance of telemedicine by the adopting organizations can be based in the difficulty in establishing a virtual organization (Warisse, 1996). Within the prison and medical center example, the prison system had its own unique hierarchical structure, norms, rules, and protocols for delivering healthcare to inmate patients. Similarly, the academic medical center had its own unique process, structures, norms and protocols for delivering care. Prior to telemedicine, each organization could practice the delivery of healthcare within its own boundaries. Although the organizations did collaborate on the provision of care, they did not have to incorporate one another's ways of accomplishing work within their system of care. For example, specialists would make suggestions in an inmate's chart for follow-up by the institutional physician. However, each task was accomplished individually and passed to the next organization involved. The organizations did not have to practice synchronously. The creation of a synchronous healthcare delivery system across organizational boundaries required the creation of a virtual organization (Turner, 1998; Warisse, 1996).

The virtual organization needed to create new practices and structures for facilitating work. Issues of leadership, control, incentives, and protocols needed to be worked out. Since each member of the virtual organization had first an allegiance to their own organization, it was hard to work out these leadership roles. The coordinator from the medical center was not used to accommodate the prison system's concerns, and the prison system was not used to accommodate the needs of the academic medical center.

Although this example is based in a prison telemedicine application, similar challenges to the creation of virtual organizations can arise in other telemedicine applications. The crossing of physical boundaries via telecommunications technologies requires the establishment of new virtual boundaries that facilitate the development of the new combined organization's activities. Whether these virtual boundaries connect a prison to an academic medical center, a specialist to a family practice physician, or a physician to a patient in their home, these virtual boundaries provide the context for the creation of a new doctor and patient environment for clinical encounters.

The Individual Virtual Environment

Within this regulatory and organizational complexity, the doctor and patient must come together to interact in new and different ways. The doctor at one location is stripped of the multidimensional cues offered by a face-to-face, in the same room consultation and must now rely more on the patient's verbal account and maybe the existence of a healthcare provider at the remote site who can provide additional information.

Physicians across a variety of specialties have reported success with the application of telemedicine for diagnoses (see reviews of telemedicine use in dermatology, pulmonary care, infectious diseases, oncology, ophthalmology, orthopedics, plastic surgery in Bashshur, Sanders, & Shannon(1997) and in Viegas and Dunn (1998). Perednia and Grigsby (1998) argue that conditions within each specialty can be placed along a continuum of information complexity. As conditions manifest themselves within complicated presentations the diagnoses requires more information, while less complicated presentations require less information. In this way, telemedicine offers the opportunity to diagnose the less complicated conditions while providing a triage mechanism for directing treatments and further diagnoses for more complicated conditions. Satisfaction with telemedicine from a provider's perspective has come from the ability of the virtual environment to convey the information necessary to provide an adequate diagnosis.

The discussion of telemedicine within the literature tends to focus on the capacity of technology to convey the data necessary for conducting medical consultations in various specialties (Grigsby, 1997; Perednia and Grigsby, 1998). Research emphasis has been on efficient information transfer. However, the practice of medicine is more than the transfer of information. Medical care involves human communication between the doctor and the patient. Both informational and relational aspects of communication must be addressed when understanding the communication processes involved (Cegala, McGee and McNeilis, 1996). Although providers may focus on the informational dimension, patients see the importance of the relational dimension to the provision of care as well.

Research suggests that from a patient's perspective, telemedicine has been seen as an effective way of providing care (Allen & Hayes, 1995; Mekhjian, Turner, Gailiun and McCain, 1999). However, just as in the traditional doctor and patient encounter, Mekhjian et al. (1999) found that the telemedicine interaction contained both information and relationship dimensions. These patients evaluated the ability of the consultation to transmit information, as well as provide empathic concern. The study compared two groups of telemedicine patients, one in a familiar setting with healthcare practitioners they knew, versus patients in an unfamiliar setting with healthcare practitioners with whom the patients were less familiar. Both groups were satisfied with the information exchange. However, patients in the less familiar setting were less satisfied with the relationship exchange (Mekhjian, et al., 1999). This study emphasizes the importance of examining the entire context of care.

It could be that patients would vary in their satisfaction with telemedicine depending on the severity of their condition. Although a patient may have a fairly routine type of cancer from a physician's perspective, which is amenable to the information-carrying capacity of the technology, a cancer diagnoses may not be perceived as routine from a patient's perspective. In this situation a patient may feel a context that conveys more of the relational dimension of the doctor/patient encounter is necessary. Reconciling the different perspectives of a medical diagnosis from both the patient and the physician's perspective will be important to evaluating quality and satisfaction with telemedicine in the future.

In addition, when evaluating the patient's perspective regarding telemedicine, it is important to explore the options available and the costs associated with a traditional environment versus a virtual environment. As Mekhjian et al. (1999) suggest, all things being equal, patients would probably choose a face-to-face traditional encounter over a teleconsultation. However, telecommunications solutions are usually implemented because all things are not equal (for example, barriers to access because of geographic distance or the inability to miss a day of work). Therefore, assessments of patient satisfaction in these mediated environments should include benefits gained or lost as a result of the teleconsultation instead of just comparing in-person versus not in-person.

THE FUTURE

Across the various telemedicine technologies, successful implementation and use of telemedicine applications depends on attending to the external regulatory environment, the internal organizational environment, and the individual virtual environment of the doctor and patient encounter. For example, a Web-based solution must recognize the user interface needs of the home user, the environment of the patient, as well as the patient's ability to interact with the physician and communicate his or her needs effectively. Similarly, the user interface concerns of the physician, the organizational constraints and rules within the hospital, and the ability of the physician to communicate in this new mediated environment should also be considered. As Web-based telemedicine increases in its availability and use, home care solutions will become more prevalent. Dakin (1998) notes that about seven million chronic patients receive healthcare in the home annually, with the market for these services growing at approximately 24% per year. Many companies are turning to this growing market to develop telemedicine applications.

Home health services create strong opportunities for telecommunications connections. Through a variety of telecommunications technologies, patients can be connected to their physician or nurse for monitoring and diagnoses. Goldberg (1997) argued that the changing competitive nature of the healthcare marketplace requires that organizations provide a continuum of acute, subacute, and long-term care in a variety of facilities and community-based settings, including the home. Telemedicine technologies offer an efficient method of providing home-based clinical interactions. Patients and families can be involved in the process of care in a way that they have not had the opportunity before.

CONCLUSION

In the near future, telemedicine systems may be ubiquitous, as available and easy to use as the telephone. The practice of medicine between physicians and patients may be conducted using store-and-forward, Web-based technology, such that asynchronous communication is more the norm that will dominate the provider/patient relationship. However, due to existing technology, as well as norms and expectations on the part of patients and healthcare providers, these scenarios have not been fully realized. As a result, this period in time offers an optimum opportunity to study a process by which a new communication technology is adopted and implemented within a healthcare environment to create a new form of clinical encounter. As these new communication technologies are introduced and begin to diffuse within healthcare organizations, it is critical that scholars examine the implications of the use of these technologies on the organizational and individual dimensions of the doctor and patient encounter. In doing so, a better understanding of the knowledge and skills needed by individuals, as well as by organizations, can be reached.

REFERENCES

Bashshur, R. (1995a). Health policy and telemedicine. *Telemedicine Journal,* 1(1), 81-83.

Bashshur, R. (1995b). On the definition and evaluation of telemedicine. *Telemedicine Journal,* 1(1), 19-30.

Bashshur, R., Sanders, J., & Shannon, G. (Eds.). (1997). *Telemedicine: Theory and practice.* Springfield, IL: Charles C. Thomas Publisher.

Brown, D. (1999, August 22). Log on and say 'Ahhh.' *The Washington Post.* A1, A10.

Cegala, D., McGee, D., & McNeilis, K. (1996). Components of patients and doctors perceptions of communication competence during a primary care interview. *Health Communication,* 8, 1-27.

Coe, R. (1970). *The sociology of medicine.* McGraw-Hill Book Company: New York, NY.

Dakin, D. (1998). Online: ATA home care guidelines illustrate service legitimacy and association leadership. *Telehealth Magazine,* 4(7), p. 5.

Debakey, M. (1995). Telemedicine has now come of age. *Telemedicine Journal,* 1(1), 19-30.

Goldberg, A. (1997). Tele-home healthcare on call: Trends leading to the return of the housecall. *Telemedicine Today,* 5(4), 14-15.

Grigsby, B & Allen, A. (August, 1997). Fourth annual telemedicine program review. *Telemedicine Today*, 30-38, 42.

Grigsby, J. (1997). Telemedicine in the United States. In R. Bashshur, J. Sanders, and G. Shannon (Eds.), *Telemedicine: Theory and Practice*, pp. 291-325, Springfield, Illinois: Charles C. Thomas, Publisher.

Lovett, J & Bashshur, R. (1979). Telemedicine in the USA. *Telecommunications Policy*. 3(1) 3-14.

Lipnack, J. & Stamps, J. (1997). *Virtual teams: Reaching across space, time, and organizations with technology.* New York: John Wiley & Sons, Inc.

Mekhjian, H., Warisse, J., Gailiun, M. & McCain, T. (1996). The Ohio telemedicine system for prison inmates. *Telemedicine Journal*, 2(1), 17-24.

Mekhjian, H., Turner, J. W., Gailiun, M., & McCain, T. (1999). Patient satisfaction with telemedicine in a prison environment: A matter of context. *Journal of Telemedicine and Telecare*, 5, 55-61.

Mun, S., & Turner, J.W. (1999). Telemedicine: Emerging e-Medicine. *Annual Review of Biomedical Engineering*, 1, 589-610.

Perednia, D. & Allen, A. (1995). Telemedicine technology and clinical applications. *Journal of the American Medical Association*, 273(6), 483-488.

Perednia, D. & Grigsby, J. (1998). Telephones, telemedicine, and technologically neutral coverage policy. *Telemedicine Journal*, 4(2), 145-152.

Puskin, D. (1995). Opportunities and challenges to telemedicine in rural America. *Journal of Medical Systems*, 19(1), 53-61.

Sanders, J. & Bashshur, R. (1995). Perspective: Challenges to the implementation of telemedicine. *Telemedicine Journal*. 1, 115-123.

Starr, P. (1982). *The social transformation of American medicine*. USA: Basic Books.

Turner, J.W. & Peterson, C. (1998). Organizational telecompetence: Creating the virtual organization. In S. Viegas and K. Dunn (Eds.) *Telemedicine: Practicing in the information age*, 41-48. New York: Lippincott-Raven.

Turner, J.W. (August, 1998). *The integration of new communication technologies to form virtual organizations*. Paper presented at the Pacific Medical Technology Symposium, PACMEDTek, Honolulu, Hawaii.

Turner, J.W. & Thomas, R. (1999). *Perceptions of virtual service organizations: The contribution of customer expectations to adaptive structuration theory*. Paper presented at the meeting of the National Commmunication Association, Chicago, Illinois.

Welch, M., Pak, H. & Poropatich, R. (1999). The impact of the Web-based store and forward teledermatology consult system in the national capital area. *Telemedicine Journal*, 5,1,41.

Viegas, S. & Dunn, K. (eds). (1998). *Telemedicine: Practicing in the information age*. New York: Lippincott-Raven.

Warisse, J. (1996). *Communicative implications of implementing telemedicine technology: A framework of telecompetence*. (Doctoral dissertation, The Ohio State University, 1996). (University Microfilms No. 9710670).

Chapter VI

Automating Surgical Patients' Admission: Proactive Leadership on a Shoestring

Hans Lehmann and Terence Wee
University of Auckland

The rationale for using a single case study approach is set out and put into context of current case research literature and thinking. The validity of the approach and its implications for being able to generalise from its findings are discussed.

The key point in the case is the determination of a private hospital in Auckland, New Zealand, to re-engineer its processes with information technology. Persisting in the face of apathy and even resistance by its main business partners, they achieved a viable pilot system on a minimum budget, using common, off-the-shelf software and technologies.

Starting from a modest electronic presence, the hospital's aim is to become the centrepiece of an electronic community, offering a rich set of communications and other media for the medical practitioners who use the hospital facilities. The case in this chapter is the history of the first service project, an electronic interface for surgeons to book operating facilities and to automate admission procedures. The process changes and improvements are described, as are the resolution of environmental issues such as security and patient privacy. The architecture of the system, which centres on the basic structure of an intranet, is outlined. A number of points of general import for interactive surgeon-hospital systems are developed from the case in conclusion. Pointers for further and/or follow-up research are given.

INTRODUCTION

Information technology (IT) is a difficult business function to manage in the typical New Zealand enterprise, i.e., usually a small organisation with fewer resources but usually with a broader scope then comparable enterprises in a larger economy. The difficulty often increases when information technology moves to the more critical areas of the enterprise's operation (Jackson et al., 1994). The health industry in New Zealand is undergoing a phase of accelerated change at present. A strong focus of the current change is the area of productivity improvements. Health enterprises have thus begun to embrace information technology to much greater extent than before. The relative inexperience with information technology within the industry, coupled with the new application areas the technology is used for, makes for exciting times.

Another significant factor shaping the development of information technology in the New Zealand health industry is the fact that most information technology management theories and their respective 'how-to' guides are based on a North American — and to a lesser extent, European — environment. These are characterised by larger enterprises, often with comparatively narrow scopes, operating in large markets with a wide variety of supply for technology and advice. In contrast, the small New Zealand enterprises usually rely on limited, often unstable supply and advice in a tiny market.

Therefore, the objective of this study is to take an in-depth look at how a small private hospital in Auckland, New Zealand, copes with applying information technology in the health sector, using Web-enabled technologies. The project in question is part of a larger plan. The strategic intent behind the project was one of establishing an electronic presence for most of the Hospital's dealing with its community and stakeholders (trustees, patients, medical providers and internal staff). The very first step along this route was the establishment of a 'homepage'. Apart from fulfilling a general marketing objective, it was also designed to become the focal point for an 'electronic community' of all people who use the hospital facilities. The case under analysis is the history of the first 'electronic service' project, an electronic interface for surgeons to automate admission procedures.

The chapter is structured as follows:
- A brief overview of relevant literature is outlined and justification for using a case method is given in the next section ..
- A critical assessment of the original manual admission procedure is the start of the case 'story.'
- The re-engineered process is introduced and the development of its architecture together with an evaluation of the technology options is presented.
- The experiences with the implementation are relayed.
- Finally, conclusions are drawn and lessons are outlined.

RESEARCH METHODOLOGY AND APPROACH

Most of the literature on information technology in use in the health sector is still contained in the medical literature, mainly in the sectors of community medicine or health management. A brief survey of the literature which has the development and implementation of Web-based information systems as its focus shows that a common use of web technology is in the first instance internal to health institutions. In their simplest form, such systems are predominantly used for the transmission of information (such as x-rays) over an intranet, for which Evans (1997) provides a good example. However, more sophisticated information systems strategies (such as reported by Hoyt, 1998) focus firmly on operations within the institution, too. Reports of lacklustre success with Web-centric information systems such as Infoworld (1997) seem symptomatic for the prevailing opinion that the time for using Web technologies for external linkages has not yet come to the health sector. The objective in the project reported in this paper thus seems to be from a minority of cases, where an external link was attempted — and furthermore attempted with a minimal budget.

The focus of this research was to:

- study the issues arising from the re-engineering of the interaction between medical practitioners and a hospital by introducing an automated system — in the face of negative attitudes from the practitioners;
- analyse the experiences of a small development team with limited resources as they were implementing an information system with standard, off-the-shelf technology within a minimum budget;
- derive lessons from the systems building process as it applied to such a system in the specific health industry setting of hospital/medical practitioner interaction.

Appropriateness of Single Case Research

AS Benbasat et al. (1987) noted, information systems (IS) researchers should learn and theorise from studying systems in practice as, typically, much IS research trails behind practitioners' knowledge. Case research, with its emphasis on understanding empirical data in natural settings (Eisenhardt, 1988), seems therefore an appropriate method for studying information systems issues and practice in general. Other researchers, such as Zinatelli et al. (1992) have provided valuable guidelines for the conduct of case study research.

Yin (1989) names three rationales for choosing a single case study. The first two, namely where the case in question is either *critical* (in testing a well-formulated theory) or *extreme or unique* (i.e., so rare that any single case is worth analysing) do not apply. The *revelatory* rationale (i.e., observing a previously inaccessible phenomenon), however, applies in our case. In the same vein, Benbasat et al. (1987) confirm that single cases are useful at the outset of theory generation. The main argument against single cases, namely that their findings are not generalisable, is largely answered by Lee (1989). He points out that single cases differ from multiple cases only in their degree of generalisability: none lead to instant and complete general theories. In this sense, the 'lessons' learned from our case have been formulated as postulates, with a specific view to their validity being confirmed, or otherwise, in future research.

BACKGROUND: THE MANUAL ADMISSION PROCEDURE

The Hospital in the case is a small but fully integrated acute care hospital located in the eastern suburbs of Auckland. It provides a full range of specialist services, offering medical and surgical facilities that range from an Accident and Medical Clinic (operated by over 40 local general practitioners) through to the hospital's Specialists Centre with over 25 consulting specialists. Services include radiology, laboratory, physiotherapy, pharmacy, day surgery, five operating theatres, wards and an intensive care unit. The case focuses on the way in which surgeons arrange for operating facilities and for the admission of their patients to the hospital.

The original process by which the hospital accepted patients and theatre bookings was predominantly a manual system. There were a number of ways (shown in the diagram below) in which a surgeon could admit a patient into the hospital for operations or day surgery and book Hospital facilities for this purpose. They were:

a) doctor's referral letter (by fax or mail),

b) admission form (filled out by the patient and sent in by fax or mail),

c) telephone (to the Hospital by the surgeon and *vice versa* for confirmation),

d) list printed out from the doctor's practice information systems (and subsequently mailed for faxed to the hospital).

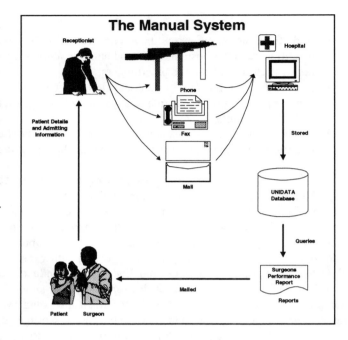

Upon receipt of admission details, any one of the three receptionists would enter the information on the forms or lists into the Hospital's existing database system. At the same time, one of the three receptionists would also manually schedule the Operating Theatre times as information is received. Admission information was usually received a week in advance.

Should the time slots chosen by the surgeons not be available, the hospital would call the surgeon to inform him or her of the unavailability and request an alternative date. Once the necessary details have been keyed into the system, the documents required by each patient for their respective surgeries are collected and put into an envelope, which contains all other patient details. After this is done, a schedule for the Operating Theatres is also printed out and filed.

One day prior to a patient's surgery, one of the staff would a check on patient details and print out the necessary patient labels. These labels were then kept in the respective patient's envelope. Also, a patient file would be opened where all the patient notes would be placed into the envelope for easy reading. After the patient has been through the surgery, their notes/details would be put back into the envelope and sent to the patient records department where they would be stored for future reference.

The admission staffs would also make phone calls to patients having surgeries on the day before just as a reminder of their appointments. Copies of the Operating Theatre schedule would also be distributed around the hospital. Surgeons who come in a half hour before their surgery time would then have a chance to see which Operating Theatre they will be in.

Currently monthly doctors' 'audit reports' are prepared from the hospital's information systems. These reports contain surgeon performance information, which the surgeon uses to do their surgical audit. This information is then sent to the surgeon through the mail.

Problems with the Manual Procedure

The manual system of admitting patients had a number of limitations. These include:
- *Risk of Errors:* Because very often handwritten information (in 'doctor's writing') is

keyed in manually by the hospital staff. Errors, which potentially can effect the lives of patients, are possible; furthermore, due to the numerous ways in which admission could be processed or received, there is the possibility of omitting some of the surgeon's admission requests. This can have adverse consequences on both the patients and the surgeons.

- *Redundant and Duplicated Effort*; details of the patient were recorded twice, once at the remote site where the surgeon fills in the Doctor's Referral Letter, and a second time when the hospital receives the admission details. This duplication of effort may have adverse effects, especially when information sent in by the surgeons is handwritten and often illegible. In addition, because of this lack of confidence in what has been recorded, thorough checks of all details were carried out on the day prior to a patient's surgery. Finally, an admitting staff at the hospital would make a phone call to remind both surgeon and patient of the following day's appointment.

- *Lack of Privacy*; because admission information pertains not only to the operating procedure, but also to dietary considerations and instructions for nursing care, the majority of staff at the Hospital use the same information represented on the 'Operating Theatre Schedule' for their respective jobs. The private and often sensitive nature of some of the information was not well protected in the manual system; the electronic admission system is designed to eliminate and/or reduce most of these shortcomings of the manual system.

A critical requirement for the hospital was a consequence of the introduction of new and unified codes to New Zealand health sector to ensure appropriate classification of patient information. This has two main aspects:

a) A correct patient's NHI (National Health Index)[1] number has to be input in the form to enable the hospital to apply for payment from the New Zealand health authorities. With the paper-based system, most surgeons simply ignored them. An Electronic Admitting System would have such checks built into the relevant form.

b) The hospital also has to adhere to a set of operations codes (the 'ICD9' codes[2]) originally set by the World Health Organisation (WHO). However, the codes do not mean much to a surgeon, who would prefer to input "artificial pacemaker rate check" while the hospital requires "O8945" as the operative procedure, not least for facilitating claiming reimbursement from health-insurers.

Another problem with the manual system is a consequence of success: As the numbers of referrals grew, managing patient admission became a labour intensive task for the Hospital. From the surgeons' point of view, the manual system worked well because for them, all that was required was at worst to fill in a form and submit it to the Hospital – most of them just had their receptionist phone the Hospital and make them fill in any forms. All other logistic issues are dealt with by the Hospital. Furthermore, the number of patients dealt with by each individual surgeon was insignificant compared to the hospital.

From the hospital's perspective, however, admitting patients soon required excessive administrative work per patient and thus became expensive in terms of labour costs. The repeated form filling and filing of patient records in time required the employment of a number of full time staff to ensure that all patients were admitted correctly.

Objectives of a Solution to the Problems

The problems of the manual admitting system described above made the automation of some or all of the admission procedures   a plausible avenue of improvement. Because of the peculiar dichotomy of motivation for the participants in the system—big problem for the hospital, no problem for the surgeons—any automation solution to would have to address a number of essential issues:

- The solution will have to make admission of a patient to the hospital easy for the surgeon — otherwise there would be no incentive to change.
- On the other hand, however, some responsibility of filling in an admission form needs to be passed to the surgeon, if the hospital is to make any savings;
- There should be no, or at least only a minimum requirement for capital information technology investment on the side of the surgeons;
- Any technology needs to be easy to use and robust to mishandling by untrained users;
- The same requirements for low cost, ease of use and low-maintenance operability apply for the information technology installation on the hospital side, too;
- Any procedure needs to be self-checking to ensure that only correct ICD9 codes and NHI identifiers are entered into the system.

An analysis of these requirements quickly reduced the options for a solution that satisfies all these constraints. Most alternative intermediate forms of communication (e.g. electronic mail), whilst not changing anything for the surgeon, also do not significantly reduce the need for control effort and checking activity at the hospital end. This meant that electronic submission through an on-line interface was identified as the preferred resolution to the problem. Input into an electronic form would eliminate legibility problems and impose a discipline with respect to completeness and integrity of the patient data entered. To assist with the problem of obtaining correct codes, an electronic admission system could have search capability that suits the needs of both the hospital and surgeons. For example, by entering a keyword in the "Operation Description" field, for example, the system could return all possible operations that include that keyword. On the other hand, by entering an ICD9 code in the "Code" field, its respective description will be shown in the "Description" field.

The on-line interface could in theory be a proprietary solution. However, the restrictions on capital investment (and common sense!) made Internet technology the most feasible option. Using an Internet environment as an on-line medium would have the following significant advantages:

- The Internet environment supports a consistent, standard and multi-user environment which is either already installed on surgeons information technology platforms or can be implemented readily and cheaply.
- An on-line system would make the services offered by the Electronic Admitting System available for 24 hours a day, 7 days a week and not, as at present, from 9:00 to 17:00, Mondays to Fridays only. This requirement, albeit not a frequent one at present, was seen as a distinct competitive advantage for the hospital.

However, two issues with an on-line system that need careful consideration are the security of access to the system and the privacy of the information contained in it. This leads to three design considerations:

- First, for user access, security facilities such as user login identification and passwords need to be provided:
- Secondly, in order to secure the transfer of information over the network connection, encryption technology would need to be used for all data transmitted.
- Finally, if the network medium used were to be the Internet, then the admission database and the other information systems used by the hospital need to be protected

from unauthorised access. This would need to be done with the use of a 'firewall', i.e. a computer situated between the hospitals computer systems and the external users, allowing only through-connections with the required and correct access rights.

However, for all these design considerations there exist a wide body of design knowledge and development experience as well as a range of readily available standard software products. For this reason, it seemed a safe assumption that any such automated, on-line system could be built within the financial constraints recognised by the hospital and the surgeons.

USER ATTITUDES TO THE WEB-BASED SYSTEM

After the hospital had decided on the automation project in principle, all affected hospital staffs were given an opportunity to contribute with suggestions as to what the system should do and how it should be. Furthermore, the existing staffs were assured that there would be no redundancies and that any excess clerical capacity would be dealt with by internal redeployment. This had a marked positive effect on staff moral and motivation – it meant that the hospital staff became positive and convinced ambassadors for the new system *vis á vis* the surgeons.

However, while the internal users had been intimately involved in the development of an automated solution, the reaction to such a system by the hospital's external customers, i.e. the surgeons, was a considerable unknown. Before the development project was started, therefore, the hospital decided to canvass the opinions of a sample of surgeons (with whom it had done business before) to assess the potential acceptance of an electronic admission system.

70 surgeons who frequently use the operating facilities at the hospital were contacted and asked to participate in a survey concerning the proposed electronic admission system. Of the 70 surgeons, 33 (47.14%) decided to participate in the survey.

The survey was carried out in semi-structured individual interviews, followed by an inventory and classification of the information technology platform available to each participant. Included questions about the current system in place for admitting a patient at the Hospital. The paragraphs below summarise what the surgeons thought about the current system and its proposed replacement. Appendix A contains more detailed results in tabular form.

The majority of surgeons perceive no problems with the current system, a few mention that there is too much paperwork to fill out, and others complain that it takes too long to get a response back from the hospital about their booking. '*Other*' responses include such issues as the admitting staff at the hospital "can't understand them sometimes when using the phone to admit a patient."

Surgeons use on average 1.7 methods of admission. Phoning the hospital is the most popular. However, this is also the most labour-intensive method for the hospital, albeit the most accurate. All other methods may require checking back, which can be cumbersome.

A further set of questions was aimed at assessing the preparedness of the surgeons to use an electronic admission system. Only about one in six surgeons would use such a system voluntarily when the still have the choice of the present, manual, admission systems. However, slightly more than half would comply with an electronic admission system if it were a requirement strongly encouraged by the hospital. However, nearly every third

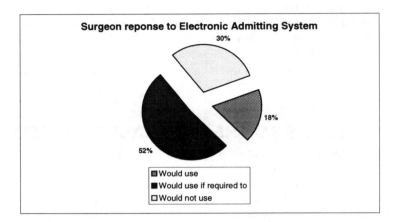

surgeon would prefer not to have to use the system at all. These findings are illustrated above.

Following up on the surgeons' resistance to the electronic admission system, it was discovered that the primary reason was a perceived need to upgrade the computer system already in place at the surgeons' practice.

While only 2 out of the 33 surgeons surveyed currently use a modem, about three quarters of surgeons' practices already have a computer system installed. Furthermore, a small minority (10%, i.e., three surgeons) of participants are currently in the process of contemplating acquisition of a computer, but still undecided, indicated that the hospital's electronic admission system might just swing their resolve to now install information systems at their practice.

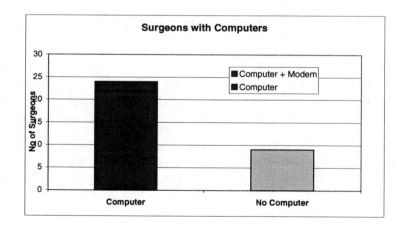

From these findings, it was concluded that there is a viable base of information technology in surgeons' practices to accommodate an electronic admission system. However, nearly one in three surgeons would have to invest in new computer hardware and software in order to use such a system. They coincide largely with the 30% of recipients who indicated that they are not willing to participate in an electronic admission system.

After careful weighing of the probabilities, the hospital felt that despite the surgeons' comfort with the current system and despite a notable level of resistance to a new electronic admission system, they would take a proactive stance and develop a prototype of an electronic admission system regardless.

An important factor for this decision was the fact that over two-thirds of the surgeons indicated that they would use such a system if they were *"forced to by the hospital"*. Although the hospital is in no position to *"force"* surgeons, current trends in the health sector in New Zealand are creating an environment where the role of information technology is becoming very rapidly a *sine qua non* for medical practitioners. Examples are:

- Payment procedures from government and quasi-government agencies are being computerised and on-line use of these systems is strongly encouraged; doctors receive a large proportion of their income through those channels;
- Medical services (laboratory analyses, radiography, etc.) are increasingly using e-mail and other electronic links to transmit information (i.e. reports and images, etc.);
- There is an accelerating trend for medical practitioners to computerise as software becomes more reliable, easier to use, cheaper, more readily available and vendors are more experienced in managing the substantial implementation projects often involved with computerising a busy medical practice.

It was felt that the hospital could point to this 'groundswell' when they set out to convince the surgeons to 'modernise' their communications with the hospital.

Furthermore, the Hospital hoped that a successful pilot among a selected few surgeons would generate enough 'peer-pressure' for the hesitant customers to follow suit at a 'second deployment phase'.

Lastly, the hospital strongly anticipated that an electronic admission system would bring significant benefits to the efficiency and subsequently the productivity of the hospital's clerical procedures. Some of those benefits would accrue even for the 'manual' admission (for such surgeons not participating in the electronic system) as the look-up facilities in the system's input function would considerably improve the speed and accuracy of data entry.

DESIGNING THE NEW ADMISSION SYSTEM

In conclusion, the hospital defined the objectives of an electronic admitting system as to overcome the following inefficiencies:

- Risk of errors
- Redundant and duplicated effort
- Lack of privacy
- Costly administrative work
- Submission of incomplete admission forms

At the same time, the automated procedures should provide the following value-added services at little or no additional costs to the surgeons:

- Extended patient admission hours
- Search engine for appropriate ICD9 and NHI codes.
- Quick and up-to-date feedback on surgeons' operation statistics at the hospital.

The Hospital furthermore learned that they could make use of a student team from the University of Auckland, who were electing this real-life systems project as a part of their last year as an information systems major. This, together with the fact that a computer to use for the prototype was already available, meant that the costs— and thus a main risk element —for the prototype could probably be kept to a minimum.

Organisation of the Development Process

The student team was to be supervised by the chief executive himself, assisted by the principal nursing officer, who took care of day-to-day liaison. The chief administration officer was involved as the main 'user representative'. The team met with this 'steering group' on an ad-hoc basis during the design phase of the project and on a more regular basis once testing and beta-implementation was undertaken. During most of the actual implementation, the chief administration officer became the main liaison person for the team.

Following decision in principle and having set up the project team, the design of the new electronic admission system could now begin in earnest.

Developing the New Process

The diagram below displays an overview of the new system for admitting a patient to the hospital.

The surgeon submits the patient details and admitting information to the receptionist. This information is then entered into the system using an electronic form. The information is then transferred over a network connection, whether it is a remote access connection or

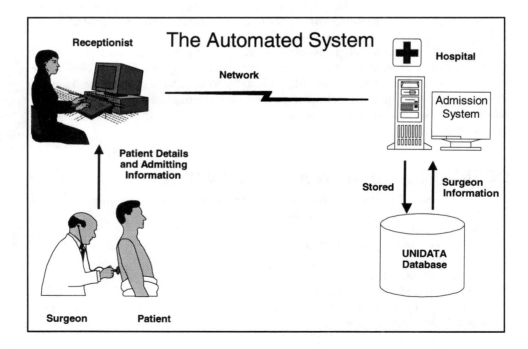

an Internet connection. Once the information is received by the hospital, it is stored in the admitting system.

Once a day, new information received by the Electronic Admitting System will be exported from the admitting database to the main database of the hospital (the UNIDATA database, linking accounts, forecasts, etc. together).

The main characteristics of the system would be:

- Graphical user interface for the admission form and any other interactive communication with the hospital; this should make it easy for users with low computer literacy;
- On-line query capabilities for surgeons to provide additional incentives to the use of the system;
- Data integrity between the admission system and the main UNIDATA database;
- Data verification in accordance with hospital rules and verification of the validity of codes used;
- Assistance in the 'Doctors' Audit', a procedure to obtain usage and other statistics; this includes query facilities and on-line reports in different sort sequences;
- Search engines to create and verify the codes required by the system, e.g. for the operative procedure codes (ICD9 code).

The new admission system would address the shortcomings of the manual system in five different ways.

1. *Efficiency and Accuracy:* Because data about a patient's admittance is only entered into the system once, and is done mainly by the surgeons themselves, it eliminates redundant procedures and reduces the probability of errors. Because the electronic form prompts for all the information/data needed logically for any given operations procedure, omissions of essential information would be largely eliminated.

2. *Increased Service to Surgeons:* On-line reports and queries are available to the users of the electronic admitting system. This would provide a means for reminding the surgeons when they have an operation to conduct at the hospital, and on which patient. Surgeons would be able to check this 24 hours a day.

3. *Security and Privacy:* Only hospital staff that need to know about specific patient details will have access to the information relevant to their needs.

4. *Compliance with Coding Requirements:* Usually, when admission forms are filled out, operation codes were not filled in because of the difficulty of memorising all possible ICD9 operation codes. As a result, there always was a probability that the hospital might prepare the operating theatre for the wrong operation, due to a misinterpretation of the admission form. A search engine that will select all the possible operation codes based on a keyword search provided for the user would address this issue.

5. *Labour Cost Savings for the Hospital:* With such a system, the hospital did not have to dedicate full time staff for patient admission. The routine of making sure that all required patient details are stated can very easily be carried out by an electronic admitting system. The staff hours previously spent on this administrative work could be better spent elsewhere. A consequence of using staff time for other purpose means cost savings for the hospital.

To minimise the cost and inconvenience for the surgeon, the system was developed to function as a client/server application. Using Internet browser software (such as *Netscape* or *MSExplorer)* would ensure that the client software could be implemented at the surgeons' practices on a common-standard, easily acquired platform. The receiving software at the hospital would consequently be implemented as server software, with a standard gateway to the admission database. In this fashion, any future extension of the system, using either the *Inter-* or an *intra*net would also be possible with minimal inconvenience for the surgeons.

DEVELOPING THE ARCHITECTURE

Following the new admission process, the basic information technology architecture of such an electronic admission system is simple and consists of the following building blocks:

- At the front end, where the surgeons interact with the system, all that was needed was a Web-capable machine, i.e. with an Intel 486 (or higher) processor and a minimum of 8 MB of memory.
- A browser client would be used to accept the Web pages. Any one of the established browsers would suffice, as long as it could understand and run JavaScripts.
- The back end firstly consisted of a Web server to manage the Web pages and the user interaction.
- Secondly, a relational database is required to store the admission details and all auxiliary data (e.g. the ICD9 codes).
- The interface between the Web server and the database is a further architecture element;
- A further interface between the admissions data and UNIDATA, the hospital's main data repository, is needed to integrate the admission system into the overall Hospital information technology architecture.

There are, however, a number of different ways to implement this basic architecture. The next step was therefore to develop and assess the options open to the hospital within the technical and economic constraints defined at the outset.

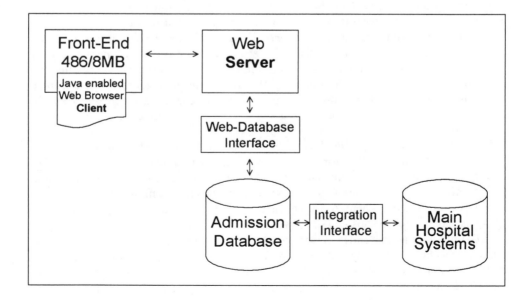

Architecture Options

Four options to realise the architecture and to deploy such a system were developed, each catering for different volumes of traffic and number of users. The four options are:

1. ISP "Hosting" – The Web site and the admission database are stored in an ISP's Web server located at the ISP's premises
2. ISP "Tele-Housing" – Tele-Housing foresees that the web-site and database stored on a hospital server. This server however, is located at the ISP's premises and is maintained by them.
3. Leased-line to ISP – The web-site and databases are stored on the server located at the hospital. A leased-line is used to connect the server from the Hospital to the Internet via an ISP.
4. Remote Access Dial-up – The web-site and the databases are both stored on the hospital's server, located at the hospital's premises. Users dial-up into the server to connect as remote clients.

The advantages and disadvantages of each option are described in the table below:

	Advantages	Disadvantages
ISP-Hosting	• No capital investment; the ISP will provide the necessary hardware and software to house the system. • Concurrent access by users; access is not limited by the number of telephone lines available. • 'Unlimited' storage capacity is provided by the ISP.	• No direct physical security control. The Web pages and the database are on the ISP's server. • Shared hard disk. Should the ISP's hard disk crash the hospital's database with all the vital and confidential patient information will be lost or breached.
ISP tele-housing	• Concurrent access by users because access is not limited by the number of telephone lines available. • Hospital owned server. The Web pages and database will be housed in the hospital's own server and are not shared with other ISP clients. • Maintenance and technical support is also not a concern for the hospital.	• No direct physical security control. This is because the Web pages, database & server are on the ISP's premises. • The storage capacity of the server is now a concern for the hospital. • Large initial capital investments. The hospital will be required to purchase the necessary hardware and software for the system.
Leased Line to ISP	• Full security control. Both the physical hardware and databases are located at the hospital's premises. • Concurrent access is available; the Web pages are essentially accessed through the World Wide Web.	• Large capital investments need to be made by the hospital to purchase the necessary hardware and software. • This solution is also the most expensive of the lot.
Remote Dial-up – no Internet	• Full security control is in the hands of the hospital, because the hardware & software are located at the hospital's premises. • No initial capital outlay because an existing computer can be used as a server machine initially, obviating the need for immediate capital outlay. • This solution is the cheapest among all the options. • No monthly expenditure as local calls are not charged.	• No concurrent access can be provided because dial-up as a point-to-point cannot support multiple users; • Capacity is limited because of hardware limitations and at the same time, this limitation might hinder the growth of the system.

SELECTION OF OPTIONS
AND TECHNOLOGY COMPONENTS

After a round of consultation and consensus within the hospital management and staff, the hospital decided in favour of the *'Remote Access Dial-up'* option. The decision was influenced by a number of considerations:

1. The hospital had never undertaken a project within this kind of information technology before and therefore assessed the development and implementation risks as significant;
2. In addition to the internal risk, the hospital could see a significant degree of uncertainty over the acceptance (i.e., the perceived utility and level of use) of such an electronic admission system by their customers, i.e., the surgeons using their operating facilities;
3. Given both those risks, selecting the option with the lowest cost seemed prudent – especially when the selected option also offers a number of advantages *eo ipso;*
4. Dial-up access offered the relatively highest level of access security, with the electronic admission system server computer fully and physically under the hospital's control;
5. The restriction of single-user access was felt as not significant initially, given the current volume of admission transactions (around 30 per day). Furthermore, extension of access from a single modem to a modem-bank is relatively trivial;
6. By using Internet technology in the development of the electronic admission system the dial-up access could be extended at a later stage at comparatively low cost; and if and when the acceptance of the system demanded it.

This decision on the architecture of the system was then defining the foundations for the actual systems design. The proposed systems architecture is shown diagrammatically in the figure below.

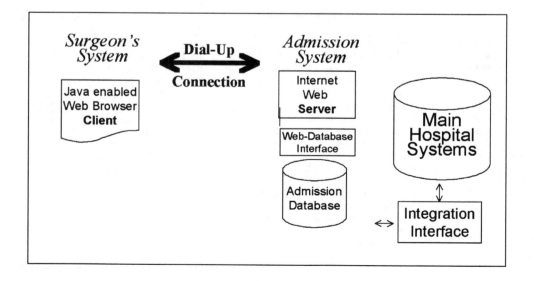

Software Selection

Having determined the technology configuration for the system, the next step was the selection of the actual software in which the system would be implemented.

The criteria for software selection needed to be set taking into account that this was initially a pilot project with the purposes of assessing how responsive surgeons would be to an electronic admission system introduced by the hospital. This system was also to be developed with a tight budget. Given these circumstances, suitable software would have to be:

- Inexpensive – This was the overriding criterion;
- Compliant with common, public and accepted standards—This was particularly important for the Web database interface elements of the software architecture; –
- Internet/World Wide Web capable; the interface at the surgeons' end was to be web based. Therefore, the software required to generate the data input displays must to be able to generate dynamic HTML[3] pages;
- Compatible with the existing UNIDATA system—Data captured by the electronic admitting system will eventually be exported to UNIDATA, which runs on a UNIX platform. Therefore, it was required that the admission system database must have the capability to generate data files for export to UNIDATA.

The two most important software elements for the selection process were the relational database management system (RDBMS) for the admission system on the one hand, and the 'middleware, i.e. the interface between the RDBMS and the data transmitted from the surgeons in the web-pages. Selecting the RDBMS of choice was not a difficult process as there are a number of options falling within the tight budget that the development team had to work on. However, selecting the middleware was not as straightforward. There are several products that would have satisfied the requirements, but all were outside the budget limits. For this reason, the offer of a software vendor to supply a new product at a considerable discount was taken up.

In retrospect, the choosing of these two pivotal software elements for the system should have depended more heavily on the functionality, maturity and maintainability of the software. Inadequate functionality such as lack of concurrent access to the RDBMS, cumbersome use and pedestrian performance of the middleware and the lack of ready integration between these two caused considerable problems during the development of the system. These considerations should have been paramount assessment criteria for the selection process.

In the following paragraphs, each software element is discussed in turn. A more detailed technical specification of the hardware and software used is attached in *Appendix B: Technical Notes*.

Databases

MSAccess was chosen as the RDBMS because it was cheap, easily obtainable and most of all, it was easy to use. Data from the Web pages had to be stored in the *MSAccess* database, necessitating a common interface between the browser, server and database software. A common standard for this interchange is the Open DataBase Connectivity (ODBC), with which *MSAccess* was compliant, thereby allowing any other ODBC-compliant software to manipulate data within a database. However, one drawback about *MSAccess* is that it does not handle concurrent users of a particular database well or securely, which restricts the number of users of the electronic admitting system to just one at a time.

Browsers

Because of the ubiquity of the Internet and its protocols, creating a Web-based solution was a favoured option for the design of the system. However, as mentioned above, the HTML language was originally designed for posting static information on the Internet. To use it interactively meant that additional programming would have to be carried out. The programming language *Java* has been developed to fit in with the Internet standards and protocols. Therefore, it was decided that Java and JavaScript were to be used to enhance HTML, thus allowing data entry type usage.

Initially, there were no preferences as to what browsers to use at the front end. However, *Netscape*'s *Navigator* software was selected because of their decision to support Java and JavaScript. The extensive software support for creating Java programs that comes as part of any *Netscape Navigator* product, V. 3.0 or above, was an additional argument in favour of *Netscape*.

Another consideration was that some of the surgeons were still using the Windows 3.xx operating systems platform. Therefore, it was rather important that the selected browser was a reasonably 'old' version.

Server Software

The Web server selected was a *Borland* product. The main reason for its selection was that the vendor had bundled it together with the middleware software chosen.

Middleware

Upon deciding on *MSAccess* for storing data and *Netscape Navigator* (Version 3.0) for the Web browser, there was the issue of getting data entered on the browser into the database. *MSAccess* is ODBC compliant. Therefore, it was necessary to choose a middleware that could interface with ODBC. Although there is a good selection of products on the market, the deep discount offered on the new *Borland* product *'IntraBuilder'* made this the preferred choice for the hospital. A key requirement of the middleware was that it provided a Fourth Generation Language (4GL) environment for rapid development. *Borland IntraBuilder* provided this environment and thus seemed to meet an important requirement. It was also ODBC compliant and was therefore suitable for channelling data from *Netscape* to *MSAccess*. It also generates the JavaScript pages requested by the remote user 'on the fly', i.e. it builds them as and when they are requested.

The diagram on the next page depicts the final software configuration and architecture for the admission system.

IMPLEMENTATION

The initial project brief stated that the project was to build a system to allow on-line registration of patients to the hospital. As the project went underway, the benefits of the electronic admission system quickly became apparent to the hospital's CEO. This very soon resulted in several requests for more functionality and often an extension of scope. The added functionality largely related to the provision of increased interactivity such as instant, up-to-date feedback to surgeons on their performance in the operating theatre as well as more extensive usage statistics for the hospital. Due to budget and time constraints, not all requests for added functionality were met.

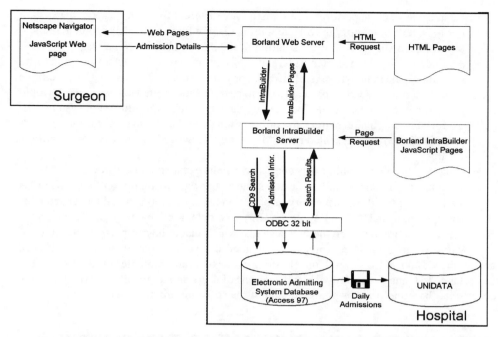

However, as development went on, the following features – outside the original specification – were added to the final version of Phase One:
- In put of Correct ICD9 codes
- User friendly search engine for ICD9 codes
- Keyword search on ICD9 codes
- Online report generation of surgeons operation statistics.
- Error checking for NHI and ICD9 codes
- Personalised Web pages for surgeons

The following examples illustrate how convoluted in technical terms some seemingly simple add-on requirements became during the development of the system.

Personalisation of Web Pages

One of the features that the hospital's CEO requested for was to have personalised Web pages. This means that upon login to the system, it should be able to identify the user and have the user's name printed on the Web pages. This seems like a very trivial task, but the ('free') *Borland* Web server used did not have the facility to maintain a user database. This meant that the Web server was not able to identify the different users and thus provide personalised Web pages. To get round this problem, meant that an additional field (check field) was added to the database record. This locked the database for the duration of the transaction, which in turn meant that the system no longer could allow concurrent users access to the database.

Online Surgeon Reports

Another technical difficulty faced by the development team was the request by the CEO to include on-line reporting of surgeon's performance statistics. This posed several issues.

- First, because these performance statistics are different for each surgeon, the system has to be able to identify the different users that are logged on. This problem seemed to have been solved with the resolution of the *personalised Web pages*.
- Second, data stored in *MSAccess* is relational and normalised to the third normal form, i.e. related data may span several different physical records. This meant that to retrieve data, a query is needed, and because it is to be done online, the *MSAccess* query would have to be generated 'on the fly', i.e., by the software in the admission system.
- To further complicate matters, the information generated by the Access query needs to be formatted and presented in HTML format. However, *MSAccess* does not allow for this;
- Finally, a number of online surgeons' performance statistic reports required data not captured by the electronic admitting system, but only available on the UNIDATA system. To provide the necessary information for online reporting, data needed to be transported from UNIDATA into the *MSAccess* database. There was, however, no on-line connection between the two systems, which made those reports impossible.

More powerful software would have obviated some of the complications experienced and described above. However, if only basic software tools are available, it is of even greater importance to manage carefully the expectations of users and to get all involved parties to agree on a 'baseline' for this phase/version of the software project in hand.

DIFFICULTIES AND CONSTRAINTS EXPERIENCED DURING THE DEVELOPMENT

The requirement to use only standard software and standard systems interfaces was initially seen as an advantage and a contributor to keeping the costs of the project at a minimum. However, the 'standard' interfaces were not always as standard as they would be expected to and the use of different software also caused unexpected problems. The main concerns and problems are set out below.

Database Constraints

The hospital's main database, 'UNIDATA', operates on a Digital Alpha computer under Unix. According to the database administrator at the Hospital, the database structure was mainly in 1st or 2nd normal form. There were also several primary fields required by UNIDATA, which were not necessarily being captured by the electronic admitting data-base. As shown in the diagram, both UNIDATA and the electronic admitting database are separate databases. They were both not connected electronically in any way. This was originally designed for security reasons. It also turned out to be like that for reasons of incompatibility. To minimise hardware and software costs, phase one of the electronic admitting system utilised a PC with Windows 95 operating system (OS), with a standard Microsoft® Office suite and several external applications. However, this did not readily communicate with UNIDATA under a Unix OS. Furthermore, data stored in *MSAccess* was relational, and data stored in UNIDATA was not. This meant manually generating a *MSAccess* export file and transferring data via diskette between the machines.

Another constraint was that a key field in UNIDATA for each record was not captured by the electronic admitting system, and UNIDATA would not allow a new entry to its database without this key field. To overcome this problem, during the export of the day's data, a dummy field was inserted to each record of the export file.

Security Concerns

As mentioned above, UNIDATA is the hospital's entire database system. It houses the most sensitive of information, from patient's records to the hospital's accounting information. Because phase one was considered a pilot project, purchasing a firewall was not considered. The CEO of the hospital felt that without a firewall, UNIDATA was susceptible to hacking and breach of security. This was the primary reason why both databases in concern were kept separate.

Web Interface and Relational Database Issues

The Internet and the World Wide Web have traditionally been used as a media for publishing static information to a large number of users. Although the HTML language allows for simple form filling, it is unable to "communicate" with a relational database without the assistance of some form of middleware. The backend database, on the other hand, needed to be a relational database because it had to facilitate and provide data for a wide variety of reports. In addition, the hospital's CEO required the web interface to be highly interactive, highlighting mistakes made by the surgeons during the form filling procedure. This interactivity was achieved by using *Borland IntraBuilder* (Version 1.0 and 1.5) as 'middleware' to create an ODBC link between the Web pages and *MSAccess*. This link was achieved after considerable programming by the development team.

The decision to use Borland proved to be somewhat of a mistake. The first version used was full of bugs and in many cases could not perform to its specified functionality. The Help and Support facilities were largely incomplete and seemed to rely on the problems reported by the development team to develop solutions. Although the next version did ameliorate some of the problems, it still did not restore critical, but dysfunctional features, such as an automated search engine. For example, a search engine for retrieving the ICD9 codes had to be built from scratch.

Search Engine for ICD9 codes

One of the major challenges of the system was to develop a search engine for it. The ICD9 code is an international coding system for diseases. It is very extensive and contains codes for every type of disease as well as any form of medical procedure. Although the electronic admitting system (because it was limited to surgical admissions at this phase) was only to use a small subset of the coding system, it still contained a large number of records. As indicated above, the Web interface does not provide a highly interactive user interface, neither does it provide for a dynamic keyword search through a relational database. Since Borland's *IntraBuilder* did not deliver on a search feature, the only other option would have been the purchase of commercial search engine software, but this would have exceeded the budget of the system excessively. There are Web sites that provide for this requirement, but because the system was not Internet capable at phase one, this was not an option.

CONCLUSION AND LESSONS

The final implementation of the system did meet the initial specifications, which were to allow surgeons to admit patients online via a Web interface. However, not all requests on the subsequent 'wish-list' could be provided. The main reason was that the development tools used as well as the budget constraints of the system did not allow for the very high level of interactivity wanted in the 'wish-list'.

The final system provided surgeons and the hospital with the following functionality:
- On-line admission of a patient from a remote location.
- Search engine for correct input of correct ICD9 codes on both keywords and the codes.
- Error checking for necessary fields in admission form.
- Personalised web pages for surgeons

From the beginning of the project to the final hand-over to hospital staff, the development team had clocked up some 1250 hours of work. Hospital staff estimated that they had spent a total of some 300 hours – including requirements work and supervision time, e.g. in steering group meetings.

The end users of the system, mainly the administrative staffs who were going to be in direct contact with the system were very pleased with the new system as it clearly met their daily work requirements. The CEO of the hospital was also pleased with the final implementation of the system although not all requests on the 'wish-list' were provided for. However, it was pointed out to him that further versions of the system could include those requests.

The lessons learned from this project are set out in the following paragraphs in the form of 'wisdoms' gleaned from the experience. They are set out as postulates and formulated in a sweeping fashion, as if they were generalised 'theory'. In this way, the result of the analysis of this case can be used as a vehicle to formulate hypotheses for future research.

The lessons are as follows:
- **Re-engineering needs leadership more than it needs technology:** The hospital implemented an automated procedure against its customers apathy and resistance – without having to resort to expensive, sophisticated and state-of-the-art technology. While this was mainly dictated by economic constraints, the lesson is that building something quick and with a small pilot group of users can be the best way to introduce a new information technology facility.
- **Standard, 'mass-market' development tools can be sufficient for a 'Phase One' system**: The case shows that the basic functionality required by an interactive, web-based information system could be implemented by a relatively inexperienced development team without any technical problems. . However, the difficulties that the development team encountered indicate that there are caveats to be heeded.
- **Cheap tools make simple systems**: The case has shown that it is possible to re-engineer an important business process using off-the-shelf, general-application type software and existing, mature hardware. However, it is essential to manage the user expectations and avoid 'function-creep', i.e. the problems encountered with users producing and ongoing, ever lengthening 'wish-list'. In the hospital's case – where the project's sponsor was the worst culprit! – the added requirements soon drove the system beyond the limits and capability of the available technology.
- **Simple systems are not always future-proof**: While it was possible to design a satisfactory system (i.e. one that fulfils immediate requirements) with cheap tools and a close-to-zero budget, there are negative consequences in terms of flexibility, i.e., the extent to which future extension of requirements can be accommodated. Examples in the case are the constraints in the interactivity and the limitations introduced by the single-user access to the system;

- **Free beta-release software is dangerous:** a hackneyed adage in information systems lore is that "garbage in" generates "garbage out". The hospital case showed that this not only works for data, but also holds true of the tools used to develop a system. Another saying that applies is that "a chain is only as strong as the weakest link". If the system is viewed as a chain, then it is only as good as the tools used to develop it. The tools used in this project were rather simple, but in the main robust, of predictable behaviour and with known constraints. Accepting untested and unsupported new software for free proved a serious stumbling block in the project. *IntraBuilder,* meant to be a developer's tool for providing connectivity between a browser and a back-end RDBMS, would only function as a cumbersome user interface for developing JavaScript Web pages. Another dysfunction of *Intrabuilder* virtually eliminated *MSAccess's* already weak concurrency features – which in turn severely limited the future utility of the system. Single-user access is not a serious constraint for the dial-up architecture. However, porting the system to an intranet or the Internet now means a redevelopment of the database (using a more robust database such as MS SQL Server) as well as a more powerful language for an interactive user interface (i.e., rewriting from *JavaScript* to *Java*). In this specific instance, where the system under construction was explicitly the first phase of a multi-stage development, the hospital should have remembered another saying, that sometimes "penny wise" turns out to be "pound foolish". Vendors provide free beta-release software to get developers "hooked" on their product. However, for developers, a thorough analysis into the suitability of the software platform to e used is imperative.
- Related to the previous lesson is the insight that **new, untested software (e.g. a 'beta-release') is unsuitable for a live project:** The cost in wasted effort, the lost time and the uncertain functionality are consequences that in the hospital case proved far more expensive than the software cost saved. However, it is important to analyse the different technologies that could be used to provide the functionality required by the users. Since Web technologies are improving rapidly, it is imperative that developers keep abreast of the capabilities offered by the different technologies. In the hospital's case, for instance, *Java* would have been better able (than *JavaScript* and *IntraBuilder*) to meet the user requirements (including those in the 'wish-list'). However, during the development of this system, *Java* was relatively new – and expensive.

The next phases of the system will be to develop it into an Internet-based communications medium to the surgeons. The lessons from this first phase will be a welcome set of guiding principles for this ongoing development.

Note: The chapter is based on a paper delivered at the Information Resources Management Association 1998 conference: "A Case for automating Patients Admission: Proactive Leadership in a Small Country", Hans Lehmann, Daniel Mar, Benson Soong, Terence Wee.

APPENDIX A: SURGEON'S SURVEY – DETAILED RESULTS

Surgeon's satisfaction with the current system	Response	%
No problems with current system	24	*73%*
Too much paperwork involved	2	*6%*
Response time from the Hospital is too long	4	*12%*
Other	3	*9%*

Admitting Method used by Surgeons	Response	%
Mail	10	*30%*
Fax	15	*45%*
Phone	23	*70%*
Surgeon's List (filled in at the Hospital)	8	*24%*

Surgeons' preparedness to use the system	Response	%
Would use it	6	*18%*
Would use if "forced"/required to	17	*52*
Would not use it	10	*30%*

APPENDIX B: TECHNICAL NOTES

Hardware

Server	Client
• Pentium 133 MHz Processor	• 486 66MHz Processor
• 128 Mb RAM	• 16 Mb RAM
• 2 Gb HDD	• 1 Mb Video Card RAM
• 1 Mb Video Card RAM	• 28.8 kbps Modem (or faster)
• 33.6 kbps Modem (or faster)	

Software

Server	Client
• Microsoft Windows 95/98/NT	• Microsoft Windows 3.1/95/98/NT
• Microsoft Dial-up Server	• Microsoft Dial-up Networking
• Borland IntraBuilder Server	• JavaScript capable Web Browser
• Borland Web Server	• Internet Explorer 2.0(or above)
• Microsoft Access 97	• Netscape Navigator 2.0 (or above)
• Microsoft ODBC	

ENDNOTES

1 In New Zealand, the *National Health Index* (NHI) provides a mechanism uniquely to identify healthcare users. Developed under the provisions of the Health Information Privacy Code of Practice (in the Privacy Act, 1993), it protects privacy in any linkage between healthcare information systems by replacing easily recognisable identifying details such as name and address with a 'string' of seven characters. The characters are randomly assigned and none have any codified meaning. Access to the NHI database (containing the link between NHI numbers and individual identities) is restricted to authorised users. (For more details see the New Zealand Health Information Service Web site at http://www.nzhis.govt.nz/publications).

2 The *International Classification of Disease, 9th* revision, (ICD 9) was originally published by the World Health Organisation (WHO). The version used in New Zealand is ICD-9 -Clinical Modification (ICD-9-CM). This was developed by the National Centre for Health Statistics for use in the United States (see http://www.cdc.gov/nchswww/about/otheract/icd9/icd9hp2.htm). A version ICD-10 (and ICD-10-CM) is in preparation.

3 HTML, the *Hyper Text Mark-up Language* is the common code mechanism for displaying data on the World Wide Web.

REFERENCES

Anonymous (1997). Two distinctly different paths to Web nirvana. *Infoworld*, 19(44), 19.

Benbasat, I., Goldstein, D. K. and Mead. (1987). The Case Research Strategy in Studies of Information systems, *MIS Quarterly*, September, 369-386

Eisenhardt, K.M. (1989). Building Theories from Case Study Research. *Academy of Management Review*, 14(4), 532-550

Evans, J. 919970. At KUMC, Inexpensive Web-based Diaqgnostic Imaging delivers Information and Images to any PC with a Browser. *Health Management Technology*. 18(5), 14-15.

Galliers, R.D. and Land, F.F. (1987). Choosing Appropriate Information Systems Research Methodologies. *Communications of the ACM*, 30(11), 900-902.

Hoyt, J. P.(1998). Putting Information Technology to Use. *Healthcare Executive*, 13(5), 52-53.

Jackson, W. M., Means, D. B., and Palvia, P. (1994). Determinants of Computing in Very Small Business, *Information and Management*, 27, 161-164.

Lee, A. (1989). A Scientific Methodology for MIS Case Studies, *MIS Quarterly*, 13(1), 32-50.

Lehmann, H.P. and Nin, D. (1995). 'Nr 8 IT - Creating An Information Intensive Business In NZ: A Single Case Study Approach'. *New Zealand Journal of Computing*, 6(1a), 163-170.

Myers, M. D.(1993). An Information System Disaster: An Interpretative Analysis of a New Zealand Case. *New Zealand Journal of Business*, 15, 19-33

Yin, R. K.(1989). *Case Study Research: Design and Methods*. Sage Publications, Newbury Park, Ca.

Zinatelli, N. And Cavaye, A.(1994). Case Study Research in Information Systems: Strategies for Success and Pitfalls to avoid. *New Zealand Journal of Computing*,5(1), 17-22.

Chapter VII

Transforming Legacy Systems into a Valuable Heritage: The Case of the FixIT Migration Tools in Finland

Mikko Korpela, Juha Mykkänen, Mika Räsänen,
Hellevi Ruonamaa and Marko Sormunen
University of Kuopio

A migration strategy can turn legacy systems into a valuable heritage. In Finland, most hospital information systems are based on the U.S. Department of Veterans Affairs FileMan/Kernel technology. By the mid-1990s, the user interface and system architecture had become obsolete. The University of Kuopio together with a consortium of vendors and hospitals developed a migration strategy and toolkit, Delphi-FixIT, to move the viable systems to the client/server architecture and graphic user interface. An alternative toolkit, Web-FixIT, was developed in 1998–99 to allow a further migration to the Web browser interface and Java applets. The next step in 2000–01 will be to encapsulate existing functionality into components. This will make it possible to replace even the FileMan database by an object database at some later time. The migration strategy will thus keep the systems always abreast with technological progress without major disruptions. The technological solution developed is argued to be scalable down to very small setups in Nigeria, and up to quite large setups in the USA.

INTRODUCTION

Large operational information systems, e.g., hospital information systems (HIS), tend to be surprisingly long-lived, far beyond the expectations of their original developers. If care is not taken, such systems become technologically and functionally outdated legacy systems. For instance in Finland, the most popular applications packages for patient information management in hospitals, the *Musti* family of packages, were developed some 15 years ago, and the *Finstar* package for health centers (primary healthcare) even before. Both of them are based on *dumb* terminal access to mainframe computers. Big university hospitals have calculated that it will take four to six more years to completely replace the terminal-based technology and move to client/server applications. In the USA, the hospital information systems of the Department of Veterans Affairs (VA) and the Department of Defense (DoD) are based on the same software technology as the *Musti* systems.

In this chapter we present a migration strategy and technology which was developed to move the viable *Musti* applications first to the Windows-based ("fat") client/server architecture and graphic user interfaces, and further to the Web browser-based ("thin") architecture and interface. The next steps and future challenges on the migration path are presented, and the wider applicability of the technology discussed. The objective is to describe the strategy and migration technology as well as their development processes in sufficient detail to allow systems developers and technology managers with other kinds of legacy technologies to adopt ideas for their own migration solutions.

BACKGROUND: LIFECYCLE MANAGEMENT OF HOSPITAL INFORMATION SYSTEMS

The overall lifecycle of large hospital information systems can be managed by basically two different long-term strategies. Firstly, one can try to freeze the HIS as much as possible until it has become obsolete, and then replace everything at one time. The second option is to design a migration strategy and apply stepwise renovation. With the latter option, the idea is to design, implement and update a plan for "modernizing" different parts and aspects of the overall HIS in a piecemeal manner and before any old part or aspect becomes a severe obstacle to further development.

More specifically, the following aspects of an HIS application package can be considered for renovation, with some degree of independence from each other:
- Functionality (the support provided to clinical and management purposes)
- User interface
- Internal software structure of the application
- Database
- Hardware platform
- Network infrastructure
- Application interfaces (the linkages between subsystems as well as interorganizational linkages)

It may be advisable to try to minimize the number of aspects that are thoroughly changed at the same time. For instance, if a given subsystem (application package) is not serving changing clinical purposes well any more, it may be better to freeze the user interface, software architecture and application interface technologies while redesigning the functionality and the database contents. Likewise, while the user interface technology is being thoroughly changed, it makes life easier for the users if the functionality and data contents are retained familiar. If most or all aspects of a system need to be changed at the same time, it is likely that it does not provide a sufficient basis for renovation, and it is cheaper and easier to replace it by a completely new one.

In the rest of this chapter, we illustrate the HIS renovation principles by presenting and discussing a case in which a migration strategy and technology were developed for a specific class of legacy systems in Finland. The user interface and software architecture were considered the most urgent aspects for renovation in this case, but the strategy and technology provide a path for gradually replacing all parts and aspects of the systems in a phased manner. Finally we discuss the wider applicability of the case in the USA and elsewhere.

THE PROBLEM CASE: FILEMAN-BASED DEPARTMENTAL SYSTEMS IN FINLAND

The majority of hospital information system installations in Finland make use of the *Musti* family of patient information systems. These systems originate from the mid-1980s and are based on the FileMan database management system (DBMS) and the Kernel utility software developed by the U.S. Department of Veterans Affairs. The Finnish core applications were developed in a joint project by three of the five university hospitals in the country, the Computing Centre of the University of Kuopio, and three vendors (Koskimies, 1985). Today half a dozen software firms offer applications packages and systems support within the *Musti* framework.

Three aspects have made the VA technology globally attractive in hospitals. Firstly, FileMan, Kernel and a number of VA applications packages are available in the *public domain*, i.e. free of charge (Hardhats organization, 1999). Secondly, they are based on the M technology which makes them highly *portable* from one hardware platform to the other, and *scalable* from stand-alone personal computers (PCs) to clustered mainframes. Thirdly, FileMan *outperforms* commercial relational databases in complex cases since it is a network DBMS, not relational by physical design, and makes use of the efficient physical storage of the M technology (Jeon, Kwak, Cho & Kim, 1998). In addition to the 170 hospitals of the VA itself, the same or similar technology is in use in the hospitals of the U.S. Department of Defense and in Finland, Germany, Egypt, Pakistan and Nigeria, among others (Bader & Fort, 1997; Daini, Korpela, Ojo & Soriyan, 1992; Dolezol, 1991; El Hattab & Dayhoff, 1995; Kolodner, 1997).

However, the VA technology is based on the hardware architecture of the early 1980s, i.e. on-line transaction processing with minicomputers and terminals. The architecture was becoming outdated in two respects. Firstly, the processing power of today's PC workstations could not be utilized. Secondly, modern graphic user interfaces (GUIs) could not be utilized.

By the turn of the 1990s, the biggest *Musti* hospitals felt that the technology was obsolete. Together with the other two university hospitals, they established a jointly owned software company to develop a completely new 'patient information system core' which would replace all the previous HISs in the country. The new system was to be based on the best client/server technology commercially available. In waiting for a complete replacement, the further development of the *Musti* applications in Finland stagnated.

However, it appeared to be more difficult than expected to start from scratch. A couple of years went by in selecting "the best" technologies and specifying the functional requirements which would satisfy all the hospitals. Half a decade after the beginning, no single subsystem was ready. Furthermore, hospitals realized that the introduction of the new system would be very expensive and laborious. Since the new system was the *core* which was needed by everyone in the hospital, it had to be interfaced with all other systems (which were not to be replaced) and deployed everywhere in the hospital at the same time. All the dumb terminals were to be replaced by PCs in advance, and typical Finnish hospitals still have two to three times more terminals than PCs. In the context of an economic recession, it was going to be a hard task to explain to political decision-makers why huge amounts of money should be spent in a change of technology without any major impact on patient care.

Even the selected technology, which was initially "the best", started to gradually be left behind the leading edge already before any subsystem was available. In this situation both vendors and mid-range hospitals, in separate developments, decided to search for alternatives, which attracted a couple of multinational HIS companies to enter the scene. By mid-1999, no hospital has yet purchased an entire new generation HIS, but it seems evident that the years of stagnated development and the waiting for a "complete replacement based on the best technology" severely threatened the Finnish software industry's initially strong position in the HIS core market.

However, the patient information system *core* is not the entire market. Besides the core, every hospital needs several specialized or departmental systems. Most of these are currently developed by local software companies who have thorough understanding of a narrow niche domain. Particularly in university hospitals some research-like or short-term systems should even best be developed in-house. A number of such departmental and specialized systems are currently based on the *Musti*, i.e. VA FileMan and Kernel, technology. Whether there is going to be domestic supply of systems in this market sector in the future depends now on these vendors' and hospitals' ability to migrate to a competitive, up-to-date technology.

THE SOLUTION: MIGRATION THROUGH CLIENT/ SERVER TO NETWORK COMPUTING

The leading vendor of laboratory information systems in Finland, Mylab Corporation, together with three university hospitals established a project in 1995 to develop a migration path from the *Musti* type of legacy technology to the 21st century (Korpela, 1998a). The implementation of the study was assigned to the Computing Centre of University of Kuopio. The objectives were as follows.

- First, the *architecture* for a new generation of applications was to be developed. After that, a set of systems development *tools and techniques* was to be selected or developed.
- The *client/server technology*, windowing, graphic user interfaces and high-productivity programming tools were to be applied.
- The investments made in the legacy systems were to be *conserved* as much as reasonable. The migration path was to be stepwise so that lengthy delays would be avoided.
- The main focus was to be on the modernization of *departmental* systems like the laboratory information system, while the HIS core market was left to other vendors.

First, existing and emerging technologies were surveyed which might be relevant in "modernizing" departmental *Musti* applications. The findings were analyzed and grouped into three alternative strategies, depending on how much of the existing technology and know-how would be conserved and how much completely new technology would be introduced (Karvinen, Korpela & Ruonamaa, 1996). The conclusion of the analysis was that the FileMan database technology was a strong foundation worth being retained—highly efficient, easy to manage, cheap, widely used and understood in Finnish hospitals, sufficiently open—while the user interface and the client software in general should be implemented in latest commercially available technologies.

The VA had meanwhile also studied the same issues and also arrived at a similar strategy. More precisely, the VA selected Borland's (currently Inprise) Delphi as the tool for the user interface layer, and decided to develop dedicated messaging software to link the client and the server in such a way that existing M software could be called from the client PC. The messaging software was tagged the Remote Procedure Call (RPC) Broker (U.S. Department of Veterans Affairs, 1996). The VA also announced that they would make available readily made FileMan/Delphi components (FMDC) to call FileMan database functions from the client software. The Finnish project fully approved of the VA's new architecture and decided to build on it.

The Client/Server Toolkit: Delphi-FixIT

While waiting for the Broker to be released, we developed a more detailed software architecture (Korpela, Kaatrasalo & Ruonamaa, 1997). The main principle of the architecture was to specify as high-level components as possible, from which applications can be composed. Figure 1 presents the various software layers and elements on the PC client and the M server (Korpela, 1998a). There are four layers, separated from each other by well-defined interfaces depicted by dashed lines in the diagram. The application programmer needs to develop the topmost level of code on the PC side and make use of existing application software on the M server side (depicted by bold-line boxes). All the rest is ready-made for him or her. The Finnish project's contribution is the upper half of the Pascal components layer (XFID components), the rest is developed by the VA.

We identified four major classes of functionality that almost every application will contain – firstly, system functions like log-in etc.; secondly, rudimentary functionality to browse, edit and enter file entries in the data base; thirdly, functionality to enter transactions; and fourthly, report-generating functions. We decided to develop high-level building blocks initially for the second class and next to the fourth class.

The first version of the toolkit made use of the VA's *FileMan/Delphi Components* (FMDC) directly. However, systems developers complained that too much "spaghetti programming"—as they called it—was needed on the application layer. Three major improvements were made to solve the problem (Figure 2; Korpela, 1998b).

Firstly, we completely replaced the FMDC visual components by equivalent ones which did not use the RPC Broker directly but through a hidden *data source* component, according to the standard model used with relational databases. Secondly, *form templates* were introduced which visually represented all the various master file/subfile structures which can appear in FileMan databases. Thirdly, specialized *Find*, *Zoom* and *Print* components were developed to visually implement the most innovative functions of FileMan—"learn-as-you-go" navigation, print templates, etc.–in a graphic form. The improved toolkit decreased the need for coding on the application level to a fraction (Figure 2), and thus provided a dramatic increase in programmer productivity in comparison with the VA's original way.

The toolkit described above was named *FixIT* and officially released as a 16-bit version in May 1997 and as a Windows 95/NT version in January 1998. Later improvements have included full English language support and a form wizard which further decreased the development time of straightforward forms into minutes. By mid-1999, the University of Kuopio itself has released seven small to medium size applications based on it, and vendors

Figure 1. The FixIT Software Architecture

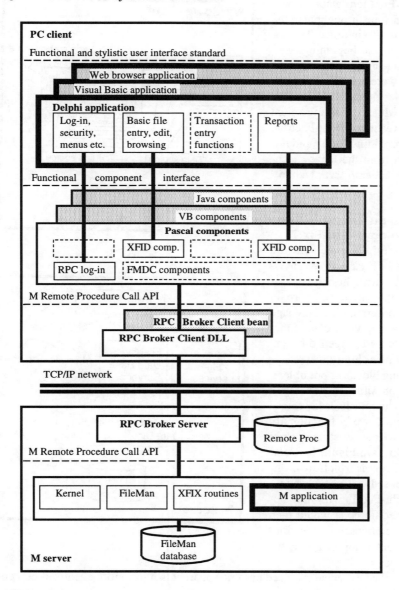

are developing a few larger ones. The results so far show that it is indeed very fast to develop visual interfaces to FileMan databases with it and the run-time throughput of the technology is also in order. The objectives set in the beginning were thus reached – an architecture and a set of tools were created which enable rapid development of modern GUI clients while conserving a great part of the investments in the FileMan databases, providing for a rapid migration path from the legacy technology to the client/server technology.

Further to the Browser/Java Technology: Web-FixIT

When designing the software architecture in Figure 1, we envisaged that need might arise to reimplement the client software in some other programming language after some time. With clear functional interfaces between different layers and with as high-level readymade building blocks as possible, it should be possible to develop a toolkit of Visual Basic or Java components which were functionally equivalent to the existing Delphi Pascal toolkit (see Figure 1). Data-driven applications which are originally composed of *XFID components* (Delphi-FixIT) with little application-specific code would then be easily re-composed of functionally equivalent components in the new language.

Figure 2. Ready-made Form Templates and Components vs. "Spaghetti Programming".

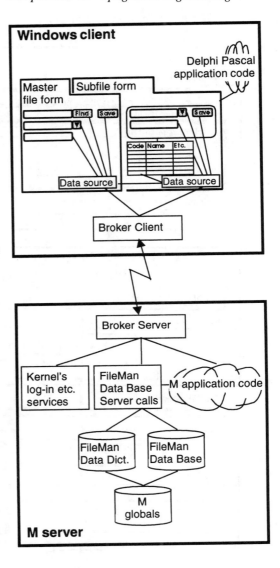

Sooner than expected it indeed became apparent that the entire client/server technology was being challenged by a new revolution (Korpela, 1998a; Pollard & Hammond, 1998). *Web browsers* have become a *de facto* universal user interface technology. Initially the Web technology was used for unidirectional information distribution, but today tools have appeared which make it possible to develop *operational transactions processing applications* as well, for instance hospital information systems, with this technology. In the browser technology, all that the client computer needs to have permanently installed is the browser, which will then load plug-in pieces of software (*applets*) from respective servers as need arises, in principle from anywhere around the world using the Internet.

The replacement of current "fat" clients by "thin" browser clients in operational information systems has two far-reaching implications. Firstly, the main disadvantage of the client/server technology, i.e. the high need for system administration, will at least be alleviated since the software will be stored in one place only. Secondly, when all applications needed in a given organization are available as "applets", cheap *Network Computers* (NCs) or *NetPCs* can be used instead of full-blown PCs.

The latter aspect could potentially be particularly important to hospitals. University hospitals in Finland currently still have 1,000 to 2,000 "dumb" terminals each, compared to 300 to 1,000 PC workstations each, respectively. The ratio of terminals over PCs is at least equally high in smaller hospitals. All terminals must be replaced by PCs before traditional client/server applications can be utilized throughout, which is a big financial burden with little apparent benefit to the patients. With browser-based applications, the terminals can in principle be replaced by NCs or NetPCs, which would cut the cost significantly. However, whether this can eventually be realized depends on whether cheap browser-based software and hardware will become widespread. So far the cheap hardware is still lacking.

In early 1998 the University of Kuopio, with public research funding and a consortium of university hospitals and vendors, established a new research and development project to transform the *FixIT* toolkit to the Web browser basis (FixIT Project, 1999). The project had the following main steps:

- *Survey of the requirements and potential technologies.* This step concluded in identifying a few typical use situations – citizens, mobile healthcare providers, extranet users, intranet users – and ways of realizing the client/server connection – CGI gateways, Java applets, distributed objects, etc. It was decided that the next *FixIT* generation shall focus on intranet and extranet users, and be based on the Java applet technology.
- *Development of a prototype of the Java-based toolkit.* This step was to produce a Java-component ("bean") version of the RPC Broker Client, as well as Java versions of the most important data source and visual components. By summer 1998, the prototype was ready and proved that the selected technological basis was feasible, although not without problems. A demonstration application was also developed using the prototype toolkit (Web-FixIT demonstration application, 1999).
- *Pilot projects.* The prototype toolkit was tried in practice and completed in a couple of small pilot projects in autumn 1998 to summer 1999.
- *Further research on user and application interfaces.* In parallel with the toolkit development, a research thread studied how the novel features of the network-oriented user interface (NUI) – e.g. hyperlinks – can best be utilized without compromising too much of backward compatibility with previous user interface styles. Another research thread focused on paving the way for the next phase on the migration path.
- *Dissemination.* The *Web-FixIT* toolkit was ready to be released to the consortium members in autumn 1999, and thereafter as a commercial product.

The prototype and pilot phases of *Web-FixIT* already showed that it indeed is easy enough to take a "fat" Windows application composed of high-level *Delphi-FixIT* components, and re-compose it into "thin" browser applets by making use of functionally equivalent Java components (cf. the parallel component layers in Figure 1). In one

Figure 3. Three User Interface Technologies Used in Parallel with the Same Server Application.

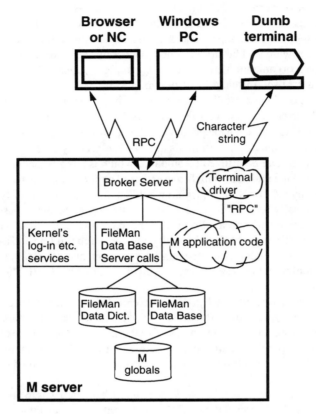

experiment, a system developer required five hours to rebuild a small Delphi-FixIT application he did not know before, consisting of five forms and a number of server-side reporting routines, into a browser-based version using Web-FixIT.

It is thus feasible to first develop a Windows user interface to existing terminal-based applications using the mature "fat" client technology, and then transform parts of the user interface further to the "thin" browser technology in a piecemeal way, where and when reasonable (Figure 3). The dumb-terminal, Windows and browser technologies can be used in parallel, without a need for changing everything at the same time.

Even the prototype phase also showed, however, that the browser/Java technology is not without its problems. Most importantly, the Java Development Kit standard and Java Virtual Machine implementations of various browser vendors are not yet mature enough for mission-critical applications in a large scale. The run-time throughput can be far from what the "fat" technology provides today. When database front-ends are disseminated to extranet or indeed ordinary Internet users, in contrast to current intranet users, various security issues become more critical – user authentication, data encryption, software certification, etc. All these new problems are solvable, but require some time before the browser-based technology will achieve the same level of maturity as the "fat" client technology. (Mykkänen,

Sormunen & Korpela, 1999)

Web-FixIT thus is a complement to the *Delphi-FixIT* phase on the migration path, not a replacement. More generally, it is currently reasonable to use the "fat" client technology in mission-critical intranet applications, and restrict the "thin" browser technology to where it provides an added value – to occasional users within the hospital and to extranet users (i.e. users who have a virtual intranet linkage through the hospital's firewall) outside of the hospital. Mobile healthcare providers, patients, citizens in general and other occasional Internet users are also a potential target group, but may be currently better served by traditional Web pages rather than a full-blown database front-end which *Web-FixIT* is.

The Next Phase: Opening Up Through Distributed Components and Transactions Management Middleware

Both the "fat" and "thin" technologies discussed so far are based on a two-tier architecture, consisting of a client and a server connected through a network. They are straightforward and efficient technologies for being used *within one application*. However, today's hospital information system increasingly consists of a great number of subsystems or applications which need to operate together. In the classical object thinking, each application can be seen as one big object which consists of data (database) and the methods (application software) required to manage that data (Figure 4). The application objects should communicate with each other only through strictly defined interfaces. It is thus not sufficient to renovate the *internal* structures only of a legacy application — the application must also be opened up to other applications by developing the interfaces. The migration strategy and technology discussed so far has not addressed this issue yet.

There are currently basically three ways of implementing the application interfaces.

- Firstly, the *SQL query language and ODBC standard* (Open Data Base Connectivity) provide the lowest level of interoperability. Such an SQL interface is available to the VA FileMan databases as well (Magee, 1999). However, with the SQL/ODBC technology, the external client application must know the internal structure of the server database exactly, which makes the interconnections burdensome to develop and hard to maintain. This interfacing technology is thus mainly applicable to *ad hoc* reporting needs within the organization and to transporting data routinely to a data

Figure 4. Applications as Objects

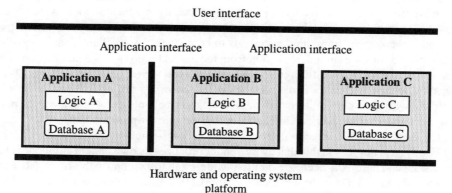

User interface

Application interface   Application interface

Hardware and operating system
platform

warehouse.

- Secondly, *standardized messages* can be used to transfer data between applications. EDI (Electronic Data Interconnection) and HL7 (Health Level 7) are the prime examples today. With this technology, interacting applications need not know about each others' internal logic any more since that is hidden behind the standard message syntax and semantics. However, composing and decomposing bulky messages makes this technology quite heavy and forces application interface developers to spend a lot of energy in the intricacies of data communication systems (Ohe, 1998). The HL7 and especially EDI technologies are thus mainly applicable to transferring bulk data in batches from one application or server to another.

- The third existing alternative is to use *distributed objects* or rather, distributed components (Leão, Madril, Mendonça, Lopes, Sigulem, Anção & Moura, 1998; Ohe, 1998). This means that the monolithic applications of Figure 4 are split up into autonomous components, which are made accessible to other applications. For instance, a laboratory application will usually need patient information from a core application. Instead of writing an SQL enquiry or sending an HL7 message to retrieve the patient information, in the distributed components world the laboratory system will simply *reuse* the core application's patient component. The latter can reside in the same server with the former, or even in another institution. Commercially available Object Request Broker (ORB) software is required as the infrastructure which will take care of all the intricacies of the linkage. There are three somewhat incompatible ORB technologies, namely CORBA (Common Object Request Broker Architecture), Microsoft's DCOM, and Enterprise Java Beans.

In the next phase of our migration strategy we will focus on opening up the FileMan-based, *Musti* type of departmental systems by developing a technology for component interfaces to them. This requires a move from the existing two-tier architecture to a three-tier architecture, in which an application server encapsulates relevant parts of the applications in a standard way into components (Figure 5).

There are three types of uses for the encapsulated components, within and between applications. Firstly, *"our own"* application's client side will now be composed of component representations. Secondly, "foreign" clients or server applications can also use "our" components. Thirdly, "our" application can make use of "foreign" components implemented in a completely different technology, as if they were "our own" components.

In Figure 5 we have depicted one possible alternative implementation, in which "our" components are making use of the existing Broker functionality. In this way four alternative front-end technologies, from dumb terminals to component-based clients, can coexist in parallel, providing for a smooth transition from the old technology to the newest one. The VA is also actively studying different encapsulation architectures (e.g., Yacobucci, 1999), which may not be based on the Broker. In the *Component-FixIT* project in 2000–01 we will experiment with two or three alternative implementation technologies within an implementation-independent framework architecture, and select one for production use.

The component-based technology has again very far-reaching implications:

- Firstly, it is not reasonable that every vendor produces its own patient component for instance. There is a need for industry-wide standardization of the main *business components* needed in the healthcare sector (CORBAmed, 1999), and also a need for localization or national standardization within the healthcare sector in each country, at least outside of the USA. The Brazilian national consortium for developing the core

Figure 5: Encapsulating Functionality into Components by Adding a Third Tier

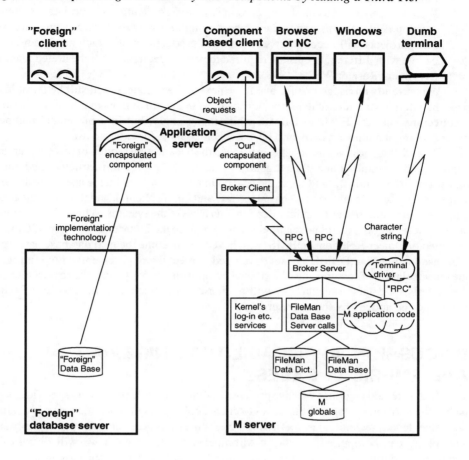

healthcare component interfaces is an excellent model (Leão et al., 1998).

- Secondly, it has been pointed out that ORB servers as such are not a sufficient infrastructure for distributed systems, but need to be complemented by *Transaction Processing monitors* (Cobb, 1998). The merger of component-based technologies and TP monitors is currently based on incompatible proprietary standards, and it may not yet be mature enough a technology for mission-critical applications.
- Thirdly, a logical further step is to store the component software and data in a unified way into an *Object-Oriented Database* (OODBMS), instead of managing and filing them in separate relational database systems (RDBMS). With this development, currently dominant relational databases are becoming a legacy technology as well. It seems probable, thus, that in the future the network model of the FileMan DBMS is not going to be replaced by the relational model, but by the object model. However, object databases are again a technology which is not yet mature enough for mission-critical applications.

- Finally, the distributed objects and component-based technologies together with the Web browser-based technology, represent a *paradigm change* in information systems development – a transition to the *network computing architecture*. System development projects will become more like movie productions, in which an ensemble of people with different talents are required to work together in an orchestrated manner (Lyytinen, Rose & Welke, 1998).

We currently envisage that for about the next half a decade, it will still be feasible to base the internal structure of departmental systems in the *Musti* lineage mostly to two-tier architectures and the FileMan DBMS, while increasingly, but in a piecemeal manner, encapsulating the relevant parts into business components for external usage.

Referring to the renovation aspects listed in the background section of this chapter, the vendors and hospitals should thus urgently work on the network infrastructure and client hardware (from terminals to PCs), in the next couple of years work on the user interface and software structure (from terminal-based to "fat" and "thin" clients), and then turn the main emphasis to the functionality and application interfaces of the systems. When all this is done, around the year 2005, it will be relatively easy to replace the FileMan DBMS by an Object-Oriented or Object-Relational DBMS, whichever will become the next database paradigm – in case the FileMan DBMS has not developed to meet the requirements of the future. If the encapsulation of features into distributed components is well done, the replacement of the underlying database technology will neither require much modification to the other layers, nor be noticed by the end users.

DISCUSSION: APPLICABILITY TO NIGERIAN AND AMERICAN CASES

In the previous sections we have presented a Finnish case dealing with a specific legacy technology. We have done that in detail to enable colleagues in other countries or dealing with other legacy technologies to assess whether some aspects of our migration strategy and technology can be applied to other environments. In this section we will discuss the applicability of our strategy and technology in a low-end and a high-end case in which the legacy technological base is the same.

Scaling Down: A Teaching Hospital's Information System in Nigeria

The University of Kuopio has collaborated for a decade with the Department of Computer Science and Engineering of the Obafemi Awolowo University (OAU), Ile-Ife, Nigeria, and the OAU Teaching Hospitals Complex (OAUTHC) of the same town in West Africa. A jointly developed hospital information system, based on the VA FileMan/Kernel technology, has been operational in the OAUTHC since 1991 (Daini et al., 1992). After some years, the need for major functional enhancements was identified, and in May 1998 a new joint project was established to develop an entire "Made-in-Nigeria Primary Healthcare and Hospital Information System" (Ife Project, 1999).

In terms of technology, the new system will be based on the existing base, but introduce modern user interface technologies. The VA's dumb terminal technology was initially highly appropriate to the constrained African environment since it scaled down well from VAX/VMS mainframes to a stand-alone MS-DOS PC running as a multi-user system (Soriyan, Akinde, Farewo, Adekunle, Orisatoberu & Korpela, 1996). Recently, however, it has become viable to move on to Local Area Networks (LANs) and the client/server architecture in Nigerian hospitals as well.

The *FixIT* toolkits automatically recognize the character set and language settings of the Kernel in the run-time environment, and all the programmer facilities use English. Only the System Developer's Guide needed to be translated and the VA FileMan/Kernel transported from MS-DOS to Windows NT to make the "fat" and "thin" client technologies accessible to Nigerian systems developers. The minimum configuration of the Made-In-Nigeria system will run the Windows/Delphi client and the M/FileMan database server on the same, stand-alone Windows NT computer. Scaling up from the minimum will require the addition of a LAN and one or more client workstations.

The "fat" *Delphi-FixIT* architecture has scaled down well from Finnish to Nigerian hospitals. With the absence of interorganizational Internet linkages, there is not that much need for the "thin" *Web-FixIT* technology as yet, not to speak about distributed components. However, the existence of a stepwise migration path provides Nigerian systems developers with a means to experiment with the technologies of the future, thus ensuring that the currently developed HIS is not a dead end but an open door.

Scaling Up: The VA, DoD and Indian Health Service in the USA

In the other extreme, slightly different versions of FileMan and Kernel provide the technological basis for the dozens of applications packages used in the hundreds of hospitals of the U.S. Department of Veterans Affairs and the Department of Defense, as well as the Indian Health Service. They established in early 1998 a joint *Government Computer-based Patient Record (G-CPR) Project* (1999), which was initially perceived by many VA developers as a total replacement initiative in the same way as the Finnish HIS core project of the early 1990s. However, the VA later clarified that their strategy is based on a stepwise migration ideology very similar to the one presented in this chapter.

The FileMan/Kernel technology will be used in these large U.S. institutions for at least the same half a decade as in Finland, if not more – it is simply not possible to move away from the existing technology faster than that. Indeed, the FileMan/Kernel technology can rather be seen as a valuable heritage which should be maximally benefited from, during a phased transition to the full Network Computing Architecture and to distributed business components with open standards interfaces.

During the transition, the migration technology being developed in Finland might attract the interest of vendors and hospitals in the USA and elsewhere around the world where the VA technology is being used. Technologically and functionally this would appear reasonable, since the *Delphi-FixIT* toolkit is based on a shared RPC Broker architecture, provides much higher programmer productivity than the VA's own FMDC components, and opens up an easy migration path to the browser/Java based "thin" technology. Moreover, both *FixIT* toolkits support different languages and are documented in English.

However, scaling up to several countries and organizational settings would require major managerial efforts, large-scale systems support, resources for adapting the technology to different settings, etc. It is impossible for a minor Finnish public-sector institution to provide the technological support for a global user base directly.

There are two excellent models of how useful software can spread around the globe even without a big transnational corporation selling it – the Internet and the Linux operating system, the latter even born in Finland. In both cases, the basic technology was cheap if not free and further developed by a user community, while commercial activities mushroomed around the technological support required by prospective users locally in each country.

The VA FileMan together with high-productivity systems development toolkits and an up-to-date migration strategy may have some potential for spreading in the Linux way, but the user community has a crucial role in realizing this potentiality. Such an organized user community exists in the form of the Hardhats Organization (1999). If the Finnish migration technologies should scale up to the USA, thus, the Hardhats should become the distribution center and clearinghouse, and systems support should be provided by American experts on a commercialized basis.

CONCLUSION

In this chapter we argued that a phased migration strategy building on the strengths of the legacy HIS technology is a better option than to let the HIS stagnate and become obsolete, and then replace everything at one time. We described in detail a phased migration strategy and technology for a specific case, namely the VA FileMan-based departmental systems in Finnish hospitals. In this case, it is possible to renovate the legacy systems in a piecemeal manner without abrupt crises – first the network infrastructure and client hardware, then the user interface and software architecture according to the "fat" model, gradually adding "thin" client portions, moving further to component-based technologies, and ultimately to object databases if need arises to replace FileMan around the year 2005.

We argued that the VA FileMan DBMS is a valuable heritage which provides a strong foundation for a migration strategy which can be scaled down to a stand-alone PC in a Nigerian teaching hospital, and scaled up to the hundreds of U.S. government institutions' hospitals. In order to make the migration strategy and technology globally viable and accessible, however, an international partnership among the user community is needed.

ACKNOWLEDGMENTS

The initial research and development work in 1995–96 was funded by the University Hospitals of Helsinki, Kuopio and Turku as well as by Mylab Corporation. The research and development in the *Web-FixIT* project in 1998–99 was funded by the same together with Compaq Finland, Medigroup Corporation and Novo Group Corporation as well as the National Technology Agency of Finland as the main financier. This chapter is modified and updated from a poster article published in HIMSS'99 (Korpela, 1999).

REFERENCES

Bader, E., & Fort, W. (1997). DHCP in Pakistan. *M Computing, 5*(1), 12–13.

Cobb, E. (1998). Issues when making object middleware scalable. *Middleware Spectra, 12*(Report 2), 36–41.

CORBAmed [Web pages]. (1999, September 1). http://www.omg.org/homepages/corbamed/

Daini, O. A., Korpela, M., Ojo, J. O., & Soriyan, H. A. (1992). The computer in a Nigerian teaching hospital: First-year experiences. In K. C. Lun, P. Degoulet, T. E. Piemme, & O. Rienhoff (Eds.), *MEDINFO 92* (pp. 230-235). Amsterdam: Elsevier.

Dolezol, W. (1991). System protection techniques within the hospital information system at the hospitals of the University of Würzburg. *MUG Quarterly, 21*(4), 27–32.

El Hattab, O., & Dayhoff, R. E. (1995). Automated medical records technology at the National Cancer Institute-Egypt: A case study in technology transfer. In R. A. Greenes, H. E. Peterson, & D. J. Protti (Eds.), *MEDINFO'95* (pp. 305–309). Edmonton: HC&CC.

FixIT project [Web pages]. (1999, September 1). http://www.uku.fi/atkk/fixit/

Government Computer-based Patient Record (G-CPR) project [Web pages]. (1999, September 1). http://www.ihs.gov/gcpr/

Hardhats organization [Web pages]. (1999, September 1). http://www.hardhats.org/

Ife project [Web pages]. (1999, September 1). http://www.uku.fi/atkk/ife/

Jeon, J. H., Kwak, Y. S., Cho, H., & Kim, H. S. (1998). The superiority of M-technology for the hospital information system: III. Comparison of system performance between relational database management system and M-technology [Abstract]. In B. Cesnik, A. T. McCray, & J.-R. Scherrer (Eds.), *MEDINFO'98* (p. 1346). Amsterdam: IOS Press.

Karvinen, K., Korpela, M., & Ruonamaa, H. (1996). Rejuvenation of legacy systems: The case of M/Kernel-based hospital information systems in Finland. *M Computing, 4*(1), 9–14.

Kolodner, R. M. (1997). *Computerizing Large Integrated Health Networks: The VA Experience.* New York: Springer-Verlag.

Korpela, M. (1998a, August). From legacy systems via client/server to Web browser technology in hospital informatics in Finland. In B. Cesnik, A. T. McCray, & J.-R. Scherrer (Eds.), *MEDINFO'98* (pp. 222–226). Amsterdam: IOS Press.

Korpela, M. (1998b, October 6). Why FixIT is a high-productivity toolkit [Web page]. http://www.uku.fi/atkk/fixit/why.html

Korpela, M. (1999, February). Moving a valuable heritage to the network computing architecture. In *Proceedings of the 1999 Annual HIMSS Conference, Vol. 3* (pp. 405–419). Chicago, IL: Healthcare Information and Management Systems Society.

Korpela, M., Kaatrasalo, M., & Ruonamaa, H. (1997). Application development with VA's FileMan: From terminals via client/server to Web. *M Computing, 5*(2), 13–21.

Koskimies, J. (1985). Use of U.S. Veterans Administration software in Finnish health care. In F. H. Roger, P. Grönroos, R. Tervo-Pellikka & R. O'Moore (Eds.), *Medical Informatics Europe 85* (pp. 246–250). Berlin: Springer-Verlag.

Leão, B. de F., Madril, P. J., Mendonça, E. A., Lopes, P. R., Sigulem, D., Anção, M. S., & Moura, L. (1998). The software challenge for the next decade: the global object scenario. In B. Cesnik, A. T. McCray, & J.-R. Scherrer (Eds.), *MEDINFO'98* (pp. 202–206). Amsterdam: IOS Press.

Lyytinen, K., Rose, G., & Welke, R. (1998). The brave new world of development in the internetwork computing architecture (InterNCA): or how distributed computing platforms will change systems development. *Information System Journal, 8*(3), 241–253.

Magee, K. (1999, September 1). Sure would like to view my VISTA data outside of VISTA [Web page]. http://www.hardhats.org/cs/vis_interdev/index.html

Mykkänen, J., Sormunen, M., & Korpela, M. (1999, March). Comparison between a Windows/Delphi and a browser/Java technology in hospital information systems. Paper presented in PEP'99, Sao Paulo, Brazil. http://www.uku.fi/atkk/fixit/xfi-pep.doc

Ohe, K. (1998). A hospital information system based on Common Object Request Broker Architecture (CORBA) for exchanging distributed medical objects – an approach to future environment of sharing healthcare information. In B. Cesnik, A. T. McCray, & J.-

R. Scherrer (Eds.), *MEDINFO'98* (pp. 962–964). Amsterdam: IOS Press.

Pollard, D. L., & Hammond, W. E. (1998). Object technology: Raising the standards for healthcare information systems. In B. Cesnik, A. T. McCray, & J.-R. Scherrer (Eds.), *MEDINFO'98* (pp. 217–221). Amsterdam: IOS Press.

Soriyan, H. A., Akinde, A. D., Farewo, F. O., Adekunle, M. A., Orisatoberu, A. O., & Korpela, M. (1996). M and Kernel as appropriate technology in health care in Africa. *M Computing, 4*(1), 15-19.

U.S. Department of Veterans Affairs. (1996). *RPC Broker User Manual* (Version 1.0). San Francisco, CA.

Web-FixIT demonstration application [Computer software]. (1999, September 1). http://www.uku.fi/atkk/fixit/Web/demo/

Yacobucci, B. (1999, September 1). Java/M 3 tier system solution [Web page]. http://www.hardhats.org/cs/java_corba/index.htm.

Chapter VIII

Disseminating Cost Information through a Corporate Intranet: A Case Study and Lessons Learned

Rajiv Kohli
University of Notre Dame and
Holy Cross Health System

David Ziege
Holy Cross Health System

INTRODUCTION

Changes in the healthcare business resulting from capitation and declining reimbursement have led to cost-cutting measures in all areas of healthcare delivery. In some cases, the failure of healthcare organizations to reduce costs can threaten their financial viability. The difficulty remains in identifying how and where to cut costs. In order to target cost-cutting measures, it is critical to get an accurate cost of chargeable items that take into account the activities and resources incurred in producing those chargeable items.

With the change in the market conditions resulting in managed care such as prospective payment system (PPS) and capitation contracts, the focus of managerial accounting has shifted from reporting, budgeting and planning to analysis of contracts and operations (Heshmat, 1997). Cost information is now an integral part of the decision making and is being used by department managers more than ever before (Eastaugh, 1987). However, this is not always the case because many cost information systems (CIS) were designed for reporting and they inadequately met the emerging demands for costs such as activity-based costing.

It has also been argued that one cost accounting system may not be sufficient for meeting the needs of an entire healthcare organization. Kaplan (1988) suggests that the purposes of the cost accounting systems are (i) inventory valuation, (ii) operation control of ongoing activities, and (iii) product costing information for decisions about the mix of products to be offered. Given that each of these purposes has different information requirements, Kaplan argues that one CIS may be insufficient (Kaplan, 1988). However, CIS discussed in the literature indicate that creating a well-planned CIS can accomplish the various cost information needs of a healthcare organization (Chan, 1993; Hiromoto, 1988).

Cost information is fundamental to assessing the profitability of the organization, its service lines, performance of the negotiated payer contracts, etc. (Kohli, Tan, Piontek, Ziege and Groot, 1999). As services are provided to patients, revenue is generated. The difference between the revenue and the costs associated with the revenue equate to the profitability of the organization, service line, procedure, etc. However, if accurate costs are not available, the profitability of the healthcare organization, a service line, or a procedure cannot be determined.

The enabler for the collection and processing of such data is the information system and the network that captures and processes financial and clinical data. For a health system that includes a number of healthcare organizations, the dissemination of such information can be a challenging task. Such are the challenges faced by Holy Cross Health System (HCHS). HCHS operates nine hospitals in five states, nine nursing homes and three residential facilities, each of whom are referred to as member organizations (MO).

In 1995, HCHS began a major initiative that resulted in the development of a cost management vision, an enhanced cost accounting methodology and the supporting information technology to support the new methodology. One of the primary objectives of this initiative was to develop accurate, timely, and relevant cost information that better addresses the health system's current business issues than the existing cost information system, which was developed and implemented in the mid-1980s.

This chapter presents a case study of the challenges faced by HCHS and how it responded to them. Throughout the chapter, we will present both cost accounting and information technology perspectives. We believe that readers will find the business and cost accounting overview valuable as it presents the project from the users' perspective. This also presents the backdrop against which the development for such an information system was warranted. Our experience suggests a compelling need for technologists to understand the 'business' of the users in order to develop an appropriate information system that the users will own and incorporate into their operations.

First, we present an overview of the cost management vision and the Web-enabled intranet infrastructure. The overview discusses the selection process, Web-enabled technology infrastructure, and the ensuing advantages resulting from the choice of the technology infrastructure. We then present the challenges, issues, and their resolution both in cost accounting and the technology areas. We conclude with the next steps in the HCHS project, future trends in managerial cost accounting, and conclusions from the case study.

OVERVIEW

This section will provide an overview of the business case driving the developments of the new cost accounting application, followed by an overview of the web-enabled intranet technology.

Business and Cost Accounting Overview

The costing process can be divided into four steps. Each step, listed below, is integral to producing accurate costs and affects the accuracy of the succeeding step(s).

    a) Valuation: capturing accurate labor, supplies and other costs from the general ledger,

    b) Allocation: allocating expenses for overhead departments to the revenue producing departments,

c) Cost Calculation: computing procedure-level and per unit costs, and

d) Application: applying the procedure-level per unit costs to each patient encounter.

The case study reported in this chapter focuses on an application developed for the cost allocation (CA) process (step b).

HCHS responded to the challenges of a competitive marketplace by initiating a cost information system (CIS) project with the development of a cost management vision. Approved by the senior management in 1995, the cost management vision strives to produce accurate cost information through information systems built to support it. The project was geared toward meeting the managed care needs of its MOs.

Following approval of the vision by senior management, a cost management team (CMT) was created. The CMT consisted of individuals from both the corporate office and the individual hospitals. The team composition included finance as well as information resources personnel. Creating a team that incorporated a mix of individuals from these two functional areas allowed the team to address both the functional and technical components of implementing a new costing methodology and also agree upon supporting applications that are needed to accomplish the vision.

The CMT developed detailed features of the new costing methodology and evaluated vendor-supported software. With no off-the-shelf systems available in the market that met the needs of the health system, a decision was made to design and develop the costing applications internally. Some key elements of the new costing methodology were:

i) Relative Value Units (RVU) methodology, instead of microcosting (Finkler, 1987),

ii) Expanded categories of fixed and variable costs,

iii) Ability to reclassify expenses from one department to another,

iv) Unit cost information for patient support departments; i.e., admitting, medical records. This feature is referred to as non-revenue costing. Under the old methodology, these departments were considered overhead,

v) Unit cost information based on quarterly averages rather than year-to-date average. This feature is referred to as "periodicity costing". Under the old costing methodology, procedure level unit cost results would be recalculated each month to represent average year-to-date activity.

The implementation process of the cost information system (CIS) began with two pilot MOs in 1996 while other MOs began implementation in 1997. Several months into the implementation process, one pilot MO had to change its status to a non-pilot location due to significant challenges it faced, primarily involving internal accounting and technology related issues. More information on this issue will follow under the *Challenges, Issues and Solutions* section of the chapter. The one pilot MO completed the implementation in late 1997 while the remaining organizations completed their process by mid-1998.

Since the implementation, each MO continues to review and update information in order to improve the overall integrity of the information. Further, each MO is beginning to shift its focus to analyzing the cost results and documenting these findings. Some examples of the utilizing cost information are:

a) Service-line analysis,

b) Payor profitability analysis,

c) Case management analysis: identify potential cost savings if patients were discharged in accordance with the Health Care Financing Administration's geometric mean

average length of stay, and
d) Process redesign initiatives.

Information Technology Overview

Each MO populates this application with General Ledger expense information along with allocation rules. The corporate information systems receive patient and procedure level volume information from the admissions, discharges and transfers (ADT) and billing systems via interfaces. This information is housed in the decision support system (DSS), which stores unit cost information, patient encounter data, payor contract modeling data, physician information and other key operational, clinical and financial managerial information. DSS is built on an IBM mainframe environment, while CA resides within the OnLine Analytical Processing (OLAP) environment located in the corporate office. More information on OLAP is provided below.

The CA system is accessed via the HCHS Intranet through which the cost personnel remotely trigger cost allocation models and also access the resulting allocated costs. The allocated costs calculated within CA are exported to the DSS for unit of service level cost calculation. Figure 1 shows a DSS screen showing the unit costs. Once the procedural level unit cost results have been produced and reviewed by cost accountants for reasonableness, these results are then applied to the patient encounter data stored within DSS and made available for the decision makers in various clinical, financial, and administrative departments.

Figure 1: A sample screen showing the total and variable costs available in the Cost Calculator. The numbers have been changed for confidentiality purposes.

```
 PMQ02260            ***** DECISION SUPPORT SERVICES *****
 < 6 more         - Costs by Period by Department/SIM (QC6) -          1 more >

                              Total          Total         Total          Total
 Dept # Item Num  Volume    Indirect       Variable        Fixed          Cost
 ------ --------- ------ ------------- -------------- ------------- -------------
 15300  14292163             13.30          20.70         93.62         124.33
 15300  14292164             27.62          18.51         45.81          64.33
 15300  14292167            129.62          22.59         41.46          74.05
 15301  14292168             35.78          34.11         70.36         104.47
 15300  14292170            198.18         307.65        102.22         609.88
 15300  14292171             28.71          20.86         48.73          69.60
 15301  14092172             26.11          16.07         40.67          56.75
 15300  14292173             11.03          13.01         11.25          24.27
 15300  14292174             29.09          22.05         49.30          71.36
 15300  14292175              0.00           0.00         10.00          10.00
 15300  14292178             13.50          41.66         20.10          61.76
 15300  14292179             28.65          72.59         29.65         102.24
 15300  14292180             10.80          12.24         11.01          23.26
 15300  14292181             30.23          23.34         53.88          77.22
 Entr: 01 *Faci: 01 *Dept: 15300_ *SIM: _____  *Per: 3_ Omit inactive SIMs: _
 Enter-PF1---PF2---PF3---PF4---PF5---PF6---PF7---PF8---PF9---PF10--PF11--PF12---
        Help  RAPS  Retrn Quit  Print      Bkwrd Frwrd Dnld  Left  Right Main
```

SELECTION PROCESS OF THE COST ALLOCATION (CA) ARCHITECTURE

To implement the CA application, the CMT had to make recommendations in two areas: (i) selection of application software and hardware, (ii) physical layout or architecture through which access to the application will be provided to geographically diverse users.

For the selection of application software and hardware, the CMT considered On Line Analytical Processing systems, in addition to traditional database applications. Software applications based upon OLAP enable users to selectively extract and view data from different points of view. For example, a manager can request that data be analyzed to display a spreadsheet showing all of a hospital's cost within the radiology department for the second quarter. Then, the manager can compare these results to the third quarter. This analysis can be conducted within the OLAP environment for any department by changing the department dimension and then retrieving the new data from the database.

To facilitate this kind of analysis, OLAP data is stored in a "multidimensional" database. Whereas a relational database can be thought of as two-dimensional, a multidimensional database considers each data attribute (such as cost, department, and time period) as a separate "dimension." OLAP software can locate the intersection of dimensions and display them. Attributes such as time periods can be broken down into sub-attributes such as months (Whatis.com, 1999).

The CMT selected the OLAP-based software for the CA application because of its ability to pre-calculate cost allocations and to present multiple dimensions such as time periods and departments. This is most suitable for the healthcare business environment where datasets can be large, and therefore processing intensive, with multiple dimensions of time, payers, departments and physicians. The CMT also considered other OLAP application software. The factors evaluated in the selection of the OLAP software were user interface, cost, hardware platform and HCHS' existing technical environment. An option to locate OLAP servers at each Member Organization (MO) linked by the corporate Wide Area Network (WAN) was also considered. However, this option was rejected because it would require technical personnel at each site for maintenance and trouble shooting.

WEB-ENABLED COST ALLOCATION ARCHITECTURE AND PROCESS

The CA system at HCHS operates in a client-server environment and is also used for other financial applications such as payroll and general ledger. The access to the CA system is web-enabled and users in MO's across the country access the CA application through the desktop Web browsers. The telecommunications network access is provided through server based computing software (SBCS). SBCS are third party add-on software that extend the Windows terminal servers with additional client and server functionality — including support for heterogeneous computing environments, enterprise-scale management and desktop integration. The SBCS at HCHS uses a thin-client approach between the users (client) and the CA server. It also provides additional features such as access through the World Wide Web (WWW), client printing, and load balancing among servers.

Figure 2 presents an overview of the architecture of CA application. Following the figure from bottom up — the user at a MO's Local Area Network (LAN) selects the Web

Figure 2: A diagram representing the Information Technology architecture of the Cost Accounting System

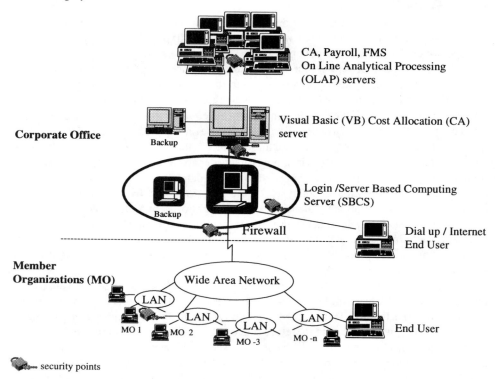

address of the HCHS intranet. Processed via the WAN, the request presents the intranet-based Web page from the log-in server at the corporate office. The intranet-based Web page provides links to various applications available at the corporate office. The log-in server is the first point of entry into the corporate computing environment and is protected by an electronic 'firewall'. A firewall is a set of related programs located at a network gateway server that protects the resources of a private network from users from other networks (whatis.com, 1999). One of the choices on the intranet Web page is the link to the CA application. Alternatively, the users also have the capability to access the applications through dial-up to the corporate office.

Plans are underway to extend access to CA and other intranet applications through the Internet. An authorized user will then be able to access the CA application through any provider of Internet service without having to dial-in directly to the HCHS Intranet. Data security concerns have delayed implementation until a secure environment can be created.

Through the log-in server, the request is passed to the CA application server, which is designed using Visual Basic. The CA server creates a batch of user requests and forwards the batch to the OLAP database server for further processing. The output is then passed back to the CA application server and ultimately to the user.

Advantages of the IT Environment

The OLAP environment uses a commonly used electronic spreadsheet application as the user interface. All CA users are well versed in using this electronic spreadsheet thus minimizing training requirements. The OLAP environment also allows users to navigate through the data and quickly identify high cost areas. The increased mobility within the data set allows managers to better utilize their time and creativity in finding solutions.

The client-server architecture, particularly with SBCS, provides several advantages:

i) Changes or upgrades can be made centrally without having to send computer technicians to MO sites,

ii) Balancing the processing load when a large number of simultaneous users log on,

iii) Adding processing power when the user base grows, especially with WWW access,

iv) Troubleshooting from a central location,

v) Built-in system redundancy for backup, and

vi) Effective security enforcement through firewall, log-in server, and field-level security (as described above).

For the service and support personnel, the SBCS utility providing user 'shadowing', through which the users' computer screen can be replicated, is very appealing. When a user has difficulty in executing a processing task, the support personnel can remotely view the contents of a user's screen and even take control of the process, thus providing better troubleshooting and support.

CHALLENGES, ISSUES AND RESOLUTIONS

The success of an information system depends upon the successful resolution of the challenges and issues resulting from the application as well as the supporting technological architecture. As is usually the case, the issues in our case study arose from the cost application as well as the Web-enabled technology infrastructure. In this section we discuss the cost accounting, project management and information technology issues and resolutions.

Cost Accounting Issues and Resolutions

Cost information systems should have the ability to provide detailed cost data including fixed and variable, direct and indirect departmental and overhead costs for the item (Carr, 1993). However, it is challenging to accurately produce the various categories of cost information because of the following issues:

Patient Severity: Two patients receive the same services; however, the resources required for providing these services will probably be different as a result of the patient's acuity.

General Accounting Policies and Procedures (GAPP): For GAPP and financial reporting purposes, accounting policies and procedures are primarily focused on ensuring that financial statement integrity exists. As a result, many account-level transaction issues go unresolved because they have no impact on the overall integrity of the financial statements. However, these issues can adversely impact cost and managerial information, given that the general ledger is the source of expense information used for the cost process.

Management's Knowledge of Cost Information: The management team, as a whole, typically has minimal understanding of cost information and its practical applications towards assisting them with managing operations. In order to reach the long-term objective of incorporating cost information into operations, it is vital that management personnel understand how cost information can assist with managing operations.

Project Management Issues and Resolutions

Project management challenges and issues encountered during CA development and implementation include:

Sponsorship: Now that enhanced cost information is being generated, the organizations are struggling with putting the information to proper use due to a lack of sponsorship from senior management. This issue frustrates the CMT because they know that the cost information can add value to managing operations. To overcome this issue, the corporate office team members are persuading corporate senior management to champion the cause of using cost information across all MOs.

Insufficient Project Management Resources: During the cost management initiative, we struggled with accountability and setting and managing expectations due to insufficient resources devoted to the project management. These issues did not involve lack of commitment on the part of the individuals fulfilling the role of project leadership and management. On the contrary, they were very committed to the cost management vision and the implementation of the new costing methodology. The problem involved availability, or lack of it.

Our resolution of this problem was twofold. First of all, a decision was made to staff the project management role with a resource devoted to this project full time. And secondly, this project was eventually moved up in priority, resulting in adequate project leadership. Once these issues had been resolved, realistic expectations were developed and effectively communicated to the project's constituents. Team members were held accountable for fulfilling their responsibilities.

Internal Application Development: As indicated earlier, we decided to develop the application software using internal and consulting resources. The CA system was outsourced to a consulting company, while internal programming staff assumed responsibility for developing the unit cost application, referred to as the cost calculator application within the DSS. Unfortunately, we struggled with the development of the cost allocator. HCHS staff allowed the consulting company to select the individuals assigned to the project and manage the development process within their organization with insufficient HCHS oversight. The consulting development staff was not assigned full time to the CA project and had other responsibilities. It was not until two weeks before user training that we realized that the development project was behind schedule. As a result, the allocation development process was extended by several months causing the project to miss deliverable dates. Ultimately, HCHS decided to replace the CA developed by the consulting company with one redesigned by HCHS. Since cost allocation is an early step in the costing process, the technical issues encountered also delayed the cost calculator development process within DSS. In order to meet the pilot organization's timeline, we moved the CA system into production without sufficient testing. In essence, we were testing the CA system using live data. In hindsight, this was inappropriate and caused user dissatisfaction with the CA system.

Would we be willing to consider developing software internally in the future? Yes, as long as the development process is managed effectively and the developers held accountable to the milestone dates. The key to effective management of software applications development is to manage the deadlines associated with each detailed task. We believe managing overall milestone dates without looking at the individual task dates first will probably result in similar issues as HCHS encountered with this initiative.

Cost Production and Ongoing Maintenance of the Information: Since the conclusion of the implementation process in 1998, we have struggled with shifting the workload from processing and maintenance to analysis. The reasons for this struggle include:

1. Cost information is currently being under-utilized within some of the organizations resulting in minimal expectations as to when the quarterly cost maintenance and processing should be completed. This also delays ongoing review and revisions of the data assumptions.

2. Other responsibilities assigned to the cost management resources have received higher priority than cost processing and maintenance. These other responsibilities extend overall processing cycle time, reduce the available time for cost maintenance, and ultimately will impact the integrity of cost information.

To stress the importance of completing the cost process in a timely manner, HCHS corporate staff is developing a 30-calendar-days processing standard with the expectation that everyone will be held accountable to it. As for cost maintenance, all assumptions will be reviewed annually to ensure they are still relevant to ongoing operations.

Information Technology Issues and Resolutions

A critical issue involves keeping the data and systems secure from unauthorized access. Other issues involve maintaining the infrastructure and anticipating growth in the number of the users.

Security: Given that the data contains patient-related and cost-based competitive information, confidentiality of data is of paramount importance. Security checks and validations begin from the site of the user. As indicated in Figure 2, first-level security is enforced when a user accesses the password-protected LAN. In some cases the users have to use a workstation at a predefined location, in addition to the password, to access the LAN. Next, the user workstation has to be authorized to communicate through the WAN.

The second-level security is enforced at the corporate office through a firewall. Only authorized users are allowed to go through the firewall. Once the user request to access an application is passed through the firewall, the login server verifies the username and password. Following this verification, the user's authorization for applications is checked to verify whether the user is a valid OLAP user, and if so, the authorized module(s). Once within the OLAP application, the security extends to the database such as read only, read and write, calculate; and to the field level such as the department and accounts. For instance, the manager of the Pathology Laboratory should be able to look at the costs of the Pathology Laboratory department and salaries of those individuals who directly report to him or her. Each database and network access is recorded in a log file that is periodically reviewed by network management personnel. Any questionable access is reported to the department manager for follow-up action.

Maintaining Availability During Growth: The access to the CA and other applications through the WWW is expected to lead to an unusual growth in the number of users. This places a strain on the network and processors and increases the demand for stronger security measures. In the past, the WAN access architecture had not posed any major security issues.

Increasing Database Complexity: As the users' data needs rise, their expectations of data set and number of dimensions also rise. This will inevitably increase the size of the OLAP database. Larger databases can lead to greater complexity, increased processing times, and increased effort required in navigating the data. There are plans for enlarging these databases to include dimensions such as payers and health plans.

Managerial Buy-In: Managerial buy-in is fundamental for the CIS to have an organization-wide impact. When additional applications are implemented, user education and training in managerial reporting are also increased.

Although the above challenges will require additional resources, the cost team does not believe that they are insurmountable. Technical and finance personnel have continued to keep abreast of the Web-based network and add-on tools that can facilitate and better manage the growth. Meanwhile, senior management is being constantly updated on the increasing user demands and anticipated resources requirement to meet such demands.

NEXT STEPS

Cost Accounting

Although the CMT has accomplished much from the successful implementation of the new costing methodology and its supporting applications, we still have more to accomplish. Some of the tasks to be addressed in the future include:

- Develop cost information for business segments that fall outside of the acute care arena (the initial implementation process focused on the acute care business only). Examples of the non-acute businesses that we still need to create detailed cost information for include: home health, physician offices, long-term care, and free-standing ambulatory services.
- Integrate cost information into the budgeting process, and
- Develop education programs to assist managers in better understanding the benefits and uses of cost information towards managing operations at the departmental level.

Information Technology Environment

To understand the future direction of the IT architecture, we surveyed end users, business analysts and network engineering personnel. We summarize the comments from the three constituencies below.

End Users: With the ongoing reduction in healthcare reimbursement, there has never been a greater emphasis among providers to cut costs. Healthcare financial and clinical end-users expect applications that would help identify areas of cost savings. Furthermore, cost savings will be seen in the light of improved quality and patient satisfaction outcomes. For instance, the information system should be able to indicate that the cardiology department has negative income. Once the department is identified, the systems should be able to identify specific diagnostic related groups (DRG) of high-cost treatments and the associated physicians. Currently, decision-makers spend considerable amount of time attempting to locate areas of improvement.

Business Analysts: Business analysts find it challenging to identify the data analysis needs of the user community. Once the analytical needs are identified, an appropriate database can be created. However, often the end users and department managers are hesitant to ask for help for fear of not understanding the technology. Business analysts believe that "a day in the life of the user" can be a rewarding approach in identifying potential application areas for Web-enabled OLAP applications. Future applications are expected to be clinical in nature as opposed to the financial applications that currently dominate the OLAP environment.

Technical Analysts: From a technical perspective, the implementation of Web-access and associated tools will require continuous upgrading. As the user base increases, the dependence on the Web as an ubiquitous interface will also increase. The development of predefined customized templates available through the Web browser will allow the decision-makers to monitor departmental costs at the level of detail that they require. In this regard, the CA and other applications will have an executive information systems (EIS) interface for access of timely and relevant data in a user-defined format. Currently, the flow of information is one-way, i.e., data is provided through the Web browser to the users. In the near future, applications will allow the users to upload data through the Web into applications. A potential application is the corporate budgeting process in which each department manager submits a budget to be incorporated in the organization's budget. Techniques are being studied to logically partition the database in a number of smaller databases. Advantages of such partitioning are enhanced speed of processing, effective troubleshooting, and ease of maintenance and backup of data.

From the business and technical perspective, the corporate network personnel believe that the architecture is built on a sound foundation with a potential for growth. They expect that the current architecture to support new applications that facilitate collaboration and decision-making, thereby providing the organization an opportunity to respond to the market demand.

FUTURE TRENDS

The future of managerial cost accounting will be determined in part by the market conditions and the needs of the information business decision-makers. Just as the prospective payment system led to changes in the objectives of costing, market dynamics will continue to shape how cost information will be generated (Butters and Eom (1992); Forgionne and Kohli, 1996). It is, however, clear from the pace changes in healthcare that the cost information will be needed faster and in greater detail of sub-specialty, payer, contract, and other operational information. These changes imply that information technology will have to be implemented more effectively in the calculation and dissemination of cost information. For instance, during the negotiations with a payer, if the contract manager needs the costs of a heart bypass procedure, the cost system should be able to identify costs associated with recent patients who have undergone that procedure, and make them available through the Internet.

Another model for the future of cost accounting can be viewed in the Japanese context. Instead of the cost systems determining the price of the product or service, the Japanese model first determines the price that the market can bear and then applies the cost accounting system to develop processes, products and services to achieve the required costs to meet the price (Hiromoto, 1988). In recommending activity-based costing, Drucker suggests that although cost accounting is the sum of all costs in individual operations, the cost that matters is the cost of the entire process. Drucker further argues that price-led costing can only be successful if organizations know and manage the entire cost of the economic chain (Drucker, 1995).

CONCLUSIONS

There were several lessons learned from this experience of implementing a corporate-wide Web-enabled cost allocation system. We found that, contrary to common belief, technical issues were not as critical as the business and organizational issues.

As information technology becomes increasingly central to financial systems, we recommend that organizations bring together members of information systems departments and user departments from the planning phase onward. Our experience also suggests the need for strong and visible corporate sponsorship. Further, project management is also critical to keep the users interested in the project.

To meet the demands of the competitive environment, accounting and other business functions will be required to be proactive in producing information that can be used to effectively manage operations as well as seek new business. However, HCHS experience indicates that although a significant effort went into the development of the methodology and the supporting information systems, the use of such information at the grassroots level has been limited. Furthermore, with the cost-cutting measures prevalent at healthcare organizations, human resources for creating and maintaining the cost systems are being threatened. While progressive organizations recognize the value of cost information, there is need for educating potential users so that cost information finds its way into the decision-making scenarios of the managers.

As managed care and capitated contracts become the norm, healthcare organizations will be held responsible for the costs incurred in the entire continuum of care including care dispensed at physician offices, home health, etc. Therefore, we expect the scope of the cost information systems to grow in the future. With it we see an increased opportunity and responsibility for the information technology to integrate systems across a number of organizations.

REFERENCES

Butters, S. and Eom, S. (1992). Decision support systems in the healthcare industry. *Journal of Systems Management, 43*(6), 28-31.

Carr, L.(1993). Unbundling the cost of hospitalization. *Management Accounting*, November, 75(5), 43-48.

Chan, Y. (1993). Improving hospital cost accounting with activity-based costing, *Health Care Management Review, 18*(1), 71-77.

Drucker, P. (1995). The information executives truly need. *Harvard Business Review, 73*(1), 54-62.

Eastaugh, S. R. (1987). Has PPS affected the sophistication of cost accounting, *Health Care Financial Management*, November, 50-52

Finkler, S., (1987). A microcosting approach, *Hospital Cost Accounting Advisor, 2*(12), 1-4.

Forgionne, G. A. and Kohli, R. (1996). HMSS: A management support system for concurrent hospital decision making, *Decision Support Systems, 16*(3):209-229.

Hemeon, Frank E.,III. (1989). Productivity, cost accounting, and information systems, *Topics In Health Care Financing. 15*(3). 55

Heshmat S. (1997). Managed care and the relevant costs for pricing. *Health Care Management Review, 22*(1), 82-85.

Hiromoto, T. (1988). Another hidden edge - Japanese Management Accounting, *Harvard Business Review, 66*(4), 22-28.

Kaplan, R. S. (1988). One cost accounting system isn't enough, *Harvard Business Review, 88*(1), 61-66.

Kohli, R., Tan, J.K., Piontek, F.A., Ziege, D. E., and Groot, H. (1999). Integrating cost information with healthcare management support systems (HMSS): an enhanced methodology to assess healthcare quality drivers, *Topics in Health Information Management, 20*(1), 80-95.

http://www.whatis.com

ACKNOWLEDGMENT

The authors wish to thank Bill Quig, Hank Groot and Charlie Shelley for helping to create the cost management vision; Gail Borlik, Mandy Whitcomb, Anne Doyle, Jim Carrier and Peter Kubiaczyk and cost accounting personnel at HCHS hospitals for their support in building the cost management system.

Section III: Web-Based Clinical Applications

In the last decade a major emphasis in healthcare computing has been on the digitalization and integration of clinical data to support clinical decision making. The evolution of the computer-based patient record (CPR) is central to many of the applications that have been developed. Clinical or medical applications may include patient management systems, patient monitoring, clinical decision support systems, nursing information systems, and laboratory information systems, among others. With the emergence of Web technologies, many of these applications and much of their data can be further integrated to improve healthcare delivery quality and accessibility. The four chapters in this section describe Web-enabled clinical applications that are in use or are under development today.

Grütter, Stanoevska-Slabeva, and Fierz discuss the complexities of knowledge management in a healthcare environment where both legacy and external knowledge sources in a variety of formats must be integrated. After a comprehensive overview on knowledge media, they illustrate a multi-center clinical trial scenario, the Swiss HIV Cohort Study (SHCS), and design a Web-based solution for effective data integration. The SHCS collects and analyzes clinical, laboratory, and socio-economic data with the intention of improving healthcare services to HIV-infected patients in Switzerland. The authors describe in detail the various users and processes involved in knowledge generation and dissemination. They present the technical architecture for the Web-enabled knowledge management system, and address several managerial issues including security and privacy. The authors assess the current state of their project and extend their discussion to include future plans and directions.

Forgionne, Gangopadhyay, and Adya develop a conceptual architecture for a Web-based decision technology system that can aid in the detection and treatment of breast cancer. Using a client-server infrastructure, the Breast Cancer Analytic System (BCAS) integrates geographic, demographic, environmental, clinical, and outcome data from multiple information sources. The system links several different platforms over a secured network including a geographic information system (GIS), executive information system (EIS), and expert system (ES) with a large data warehouse. The entire application uses a Web-based interface for researchers and clinical decision makers in disparate locations to access and analyze data. The goals of the proposed system include improving health outcomes through widely accessible and highly integrated decision support tools that can enhance breast cancer detection and intervention. The authors discuss the major challenges to implementing the system, such as process re-design issues and user resistance. They conclude with future directions and suggest several opportunities for further research.

Warren and Noone demonstrate how the Web-enabled integration of clinical practice guidelines with real patient data can improve clinical decision-making and health outcomes. They describe the objectives and design of a Web-based application called the Care Plan On Line (CPOL) with respect to the SA Healthplus Coordinated Care Trial, a program enrolling 4500 chronically ill South Australians. The authors begin with a review of the literature on clinical practice guidelines and decision support systems. They present the mission and goals of the SA Healthplus Coordinated Care model and describe the integration of CPOL into the model's infrastructure to support clinical decision making. In an initial study of

CPOL usage among general practitioners, preliminary findings suggest that benefits to the system include cost savings and improved patient outcomes for some patient groups. The authors conclude with an assessment of the system including its applicability to other healthcare environments, and provide an outlook for the future.

One of the most important issues concerning clinical practice guidelines is how to motivate physicians to adopt and use them in clinical decision making. Poor incentives, complex regulations, quality of information, and a lack available resources are just a few of the barriers cited by Anderson, Casebeer, Kristofco, Carillo, and Smith in the final chapter of this section. The authors assess a variety of clinical practice guideline dissemination strategies that are currently in use. They develop a prototype for an interactive, Web-enabled system designed to improve the adoption of clinical practice guidelines. The authors report their preliminary findings on the effectiveness of this strategy in influencing clinical decision making and reducing medical treatment variation. They conclude with the expansion plans for this project and recommend areas for further research.

Chapter IX

Enhancing Knowledge Management in a Multi-Center Clinical Trial by a Web-Based Knowledge Medium

Rolf Grütter and Katarina Stanoevska-Slabeva
University of St. Gallen

Walter Fierz
Institute for Clinical Microbiology and Immunology

The healthcare industry is essentially knowledge based. The quality and efficiency of work performed in healthcare institutions depends on their ability to both manage internally created knowledge about patients, e.g., healing practices, and available expertise as well as to enrich and integrate it with relevant external knowledge created worldwide by related institutions (pharmacy research teams, international health organizations, etc.). Efficient management of knowledge in healthcare requires, therefore, concepts and solutions for management, cooperation, and sharing of knowledge within and between institutions (Greiner & Rose, 1997).

Despite this fact, until now, knowledge management and processing techniques are mainly used in the form of isolated (e.g., expert) systems for very specific domains. The basic processes of knowledge generation and exchange across domains and locations are not supported by integrated information systems. Under the growing pressure on quality assurance and cost reduction, innovative concepts and technologies to support the management of knowledge are increasingly gaining attention from hospital workers, physicians, pharmacists, health insurance companies, and patients.

Knowledge management is a systematic approach to improve the way organizations, groups, and individuals handle their knowledge in all forms, in order to improve their effectiveness, innovation and quality. This implies effective creation, capturing, sharing, and managing of knowledge. Several approaches and guidelines for organizing knowledge management (Probst, Steffen and Kai, 1997; Davenport 1998) and technologies, such as organizational memory (Stein and Zwass, 1994; Conklin, 1996) or document-management systems, have been developed in order to guide knowledge management projects and enable knowledge management. The basic feature of these approaches is the focus on specific aspects of knowledge management. They do not provide a holistic approach dealing with all critical aspects of knowledge management (Schmid & Stanoevska, 1998) starting from developing a vision and finishing with a concept for an appropriate technical platform.

The complexity of the knowledge management problem in healthcare requires a holistic approach, which integrates conceptual and technical aspects of knowledge management, supports modular and evolutionary development, and considers existing (legacy) internal and external knowledge sources. In this chapter we will introduce the concept of the knowledge medium as defined by Schmid (1999), which goes beyond existing solutions for knowledge management, and will demonstrate its applicability to the healthcare domain through the example of a multi-center clinical trial. The project is a joint effort by the Swiss HIV Cohort Study, the Patient-Oriented Medical Information System Initiative of Walter Fierz, MD, and the Institute for Media and Communications Management, University of St Gallen, Switzerland.

In the next section, the Swiss HIV Cohort Study and its requirements regarding data processing and knowledge management will be described. Then, the concept of the knowledge medium as a framework for the design of knowledge media in multi-center clinical trials is introduced. We relate the concept to the application context and describe the implementation of a knowledge medium in the Swiss HIV Cohort Study. Finally, the achieved results are discussed and conclusions with an outlook of further plans are given.

THE SWISS HIV COHORT STUDY

The Swiss HIV Cohort Study (SHCS) was initiated in 1987
1) to collect clinical, laboratory, and socio-economic data with the intention of analyzing the prevalence and progression of the HIV-infection in Switzerland,
2) to promote and facilitate clinical research, and
3) to improve the healthcare services provided to HIV-infected patients (Ledergerber, Von Overbeck, Egger & Luthy, 1994).

SHCS involves outpatient clinics of center hospitals (referred to as "Cohort Centers") located in the cities of Basel, Berne, Geneva, Lausanne, Lugano, St Gallen, and Zurich as well as the Coordination and Data Center in Lausanne. In recent years, increasing numbers of private practitioners joined the study to complement the Cohort Centers. Currently, the technical infrastructure supporting the SHCS includes various legacy laboratory systems at the Cohort Centers and a relational database system at the Coordination and Data Center.

Throughout the study, data from HIV-infected patients are collected at the Cohort Centers and selected sets thereof are anonymously stored in a central database system at the Coordination and Data Center. The whole process of filling in the pre-formatted study form, sending the form to the Coordination and Data Center, and entering the data into the database system is paper-based and handled manually.

The collected data provides a central common repository of the involved Cohort Centers and provides the basis for statistical analysis and planning of clinical studies. The knowledge created from the study is distributed through publication in scientific journals, at the occasion of conferences, and through informal, bilateral contacts. Primarily because of the considerable time delay, the database system has so far not been fully exploited for the daily clinical care of the patients. With advances of antiretroviral[1] therapy, information on past treatment and laboratory data is becoming increasingly important.

The current redesign project aims at (1) improving the availability of data for timely research planning and (2) providing the clinicians with explicit knowledge for daily patient care. With respect to knowledge management this entails the following goals:

- to provide support for the representation of internally generated knowledge and for the integration of internal and external knowledge sources;
- to provide more sophisticated dissemination techniques for newly generated knowledge (e.g., push strategies and personalization);
- to foster knowledge sharing and collaboration at the project level by introducing a virtual discussion space.

To achieve the above goals, a new concept for knowledge management, i.e., the knowledge medium (Schmid, 1999), is applied as a conceptual framework in order to structure the design process. It will be described in more detail in the next section.

THE CONCEPT OF THE KNOWLEDGE MEDIUM

To increase the understandability of the concept of the knowledge medium, first the basic terms related to it will be explained. We define the term *knowledge* as the internal state of an agent resulting from the input and the processing of information. This definition implies that knowledge, in a narrow sense, must be associated with an agent (Schmid, 1999). Before knowledge can be shared, it has to be externalized on an external carrier (Nonaka, 1991). Therefore, we avoid using the crude term for knowledge when it is related to a (stateless) carrier. Instead, we use "explicit knowledge," or simply "information," in such cases. Information is distinguished from data by its high-level semantics, referring to real-world objects, as opposed to the low-level semantics of data, i.e., elementary data types, indicate only whether a given bitstream should be interpreted, e. g., as a character, an integer, etc.

Knowledge management refers to all management activities necessary for effective creation, capturing, sharing, and managing of knowledge. Knowledge management is substantially enhanced by information and communication technology.

Origin of the Knowledge Medium Concept

The term knowledge medium was introduced by Stefik (1986) as an information network with semi-automated services for the generation, distribution, and consumption of knowledge. According to Stefik, the goal of building a knowledge medium is to tie expert systems and communication media together into a greater whole. He furthermore pointed to the following research questions that had to be answered as a necessary prerequisite for building knowledge media (Stefik, 1988):

- development of common vocabularies, i.e., terminologies for important domains, and translators, which, based on common vocabularies, are capable of translating concepts from one expert system in another and for combining knowledge from different sources;
- development of transmission languages in addition to representation languages, which enable sharing, transportation, and integration of knowledge from different sources;

- development of knowledge markets with market coordination mechanisms for distribution and renting of knowledge.

First attempts to realize the above concepts have been conducted at Stanford University by joint research of four labs: the Center for Information Technology (CIT), the Logic Group, the Knowledge Systems Laboratory, and the Database Group. The result of the joint effort is the Knowledge Query and Manipulation Language (KQML) (Labrou and Finin, 1997; Finin, Labrou and Mayfield, 1997) and the concept of ontologies (Gruber, 1993). *KQML* is a general purpose communication language, i.e., a transmission language, enabling interoperability and the communication of software agents. *Ontologies* are defined as controlled vocabularies providing the basic terminology necessary for representation of a domain of discourse (Gruber, 1999). Ontologies are considered the basic elements of knowledge media. A knowledge medium is defined as *"a computational environment in which explicitly represented knowledge serves as a communication medium among people and their program"* (Gruber, Tenenbaum and Weber, 1992). In summary, the Stanford approach for knowledge media has concentrated on the realization of the first two points mentioned by Stefik and on the development of a very specific coordination mechanism for distribution and exchange of knowledge between artificial agents.

The concept of the knowledge medium proposed by Schmid (1999) extends the Stefik and Stanford approach for building knowledge media in three directions: First, it not only considers expert systems, but generalizes knowledge sharing for all kinds of knowledge sources. Second, it explicitly includes the agents who create and use the knowledge medium by introducing the concept of community. Third, it explicitly considers not only agent communication processes but any kind of organizational structure and coordination processes required and applied by the community creating and exchanging knowledge. Because of its more general approach, the concept of the knowledge medium of Schmid (1999) was chosen for structuring our redesign project.

Definition and Components of a Knowledge Medium

Schmid (1999) defines a knowledge medium as a sphere for the management and exchange of knowledge within a confined community of human and artificial agents. It is composed of the following components (for a detailed and formalized derivation see Lechner and Schmid, 1999; Lechner, Schmid, Schubert, Klose and Miler, 1999; Schmid, 1997; Schmid, 1999; Schmid and Stanoevska, 1998):

- a *logical space*, which defines the common syntax and semantics of the knowledge represented in and managed by the medium.
- a *system of channels*, i.e., carriers containing explicit knowledge capable of transporting knowledge over space and time barriers.
- an *organizational structure* consisting of roles describing the behavior of the agents in the medium and of protocols describing the interaction between the agents and the medium.

In the following section, the components of a knowledge medium will be explained in more detail in accordance with Lechner et al. (1999).

Logical Space

Language is the necessary prerequisite for the externalization and exchange of knowledge and a binding element in a community. The logical space of the knowledge medium provides the language, which is used in order to capture and code knowledge. It comprises the syntax and the semantics. The *syntax* defines the rules according to which correct sentences must be constructed and, in a broader sense, also the set of valid symbols and constructs. The *semantics* determines the meaning of the used language constructs, e.g., by reference to real-world objects or by operational semantics. The logical space provides a formal representation of a possible world. The optional character of the world reflects the fact that the representation may be incomplete and that various worlds can be represented by the same description. For instance, in the context of SHCS, taken alone, a given viral load is not predictive for a unique progression of the HIV-infection, i. e., for a single reality or world. In computer-mediated spaces the language has to be interpretable by machines. This machine-interpretable representation provides the basis, e.g., for the automated classification, retrieval, and combination of explicit knowledge thereby allowing machines for mimicking human intelligence (Schmid & Stanoevska, 1998).

System of Channels

Channels are the carriers containing explicit knowledge, which is exchanged between the communicating agents. Carriers can provide some interactivity.

A *carrier* includes a physical medium (sound waves in the case of human speech) and applies a language (syntax and semantics) for the logical representation of the contents. In the context of the knowledge medium, we allocate syntax and semantics to the logical space.

Interactivity means that the carrier can respond to some extent to inputs and inquiries. This feature distinguishes it from traditional channels like paper documents. In the context of the knowledge medium, we particularly refer to those carriers resulting from the convergence of information and communication technology and traditional media.

Interconnected channels provide a communication space, which can be used by agents to exchange knowledge. Filled with content, channels turn to interactive, ubiquitous, and multi-medial information objects. These objects can further include meta-information such as the author and address of the receiver or sender which are necessary for control of the communication.

Organizational Structure of the Medium

Communities of agents have an organizational structure which is defined by roles and protocols (Lechner et al., 1999). *Roles* define the required capabilities, rights, and obligations of agents participating in the community. *Protocols* are a set of rules that govern the interaction of agents. Protocols are defined for roles and not for agents. The organizational structure (as well as the system of channels) can be represented in the logical space of the knowledge medium allowing for automated reasoning over roles and processes.

Relationship Between the Components of the Knowledge Medium

The above described components of the knowledge medium are related to each other and form a single entity of human and artificial agents exchanging explicit knowledge within a common semantic space. Taken together, they furthermore represent a complete mapping, i.e., a metaphor, of the real-world environment and the community onto an artificial world based on information and communication technology and capable of mimicking human knowledge generation and exchange. Agents of the community can enter the medium by taking over one of the predefined roles defined in the organizational structure (Lechner et al., 1999).

The knowledge medium created, using the chosen language, is a representation of the world as observed by the community. Different communities can model any given world using different languages. If a semantic connection between the resulting knowledge media can be established, the exchange of explicit knowledge between them can be facilitated by automated translation from one language into another. In this case, the different knowledge media form a knowledge media *net*. An example of a knowledge media net for the scientific community is described by Handschuh et al. (1998).

RELATING THE CONCEPT OF THE KNOWLEDGE MEDIUM TO THE SWISS HIV COHORT STUDY

In this section, we will apply the concept of the knowledge medium as a framework in order to structure SHCS and to identify the requirements for the re-design project.

The necessary design steps can be summarized as follows:

- identification of the communities;
- analysis of the communities with respect to organizational structure, i.e., processes;
- identification of the objects being exchanged through the system of channels.

Identification of the Communities

As shown earlier, SHCS represents a dynamic and complex real-world setting including various communities and processes with intense communication of different objects, i.e., data, descriptive information, explicit knowledge, and combinations thereof. In accordance with the objectives (1) through (3) specified, SHCS can be structured in the following way:

- *Study nurses* and data managers collect, process, and validate the study data (e. g., laboratory results);
- *epidemiologists* perform analyses of the prevalence and progression of the HIV-infection in Switzerland, based on descriptive information on patients, classifying the data collected throughout the study (e. g. patients with a similar socio-anamnesis such as Intravenous Drug Users (IDUs));
- clinicians (and laboratory physicians) in the temporary role as *project managers* use descriptive information on patients or patient groups for clinical research planning;
- clinicians (and laboratory physicians) in the temporary role as *analysts* (or epidemiologists by order of the clinicians) perform clinical studies based on the collected data;
- *clinicians and private practitioners* apply explicit knowledge created from clinical studies and acquired from sources external to SHCS, while providing healthcare services to HIV-infected patients.

Identification of Processes, Objects, and Requirements Specification

The communities of SHCS are involved in the following processes: data processing, analysis of the prevalence and progression of the HIV-infection in Switzerland, clinical research planning, performance of clinical studies, and healthcare provision to HIV-infected patients.

Data processing includes the collection, selection, transcription, transmission, entry into database, and validation of data. This process is in part performed at the Cohort Centers, in another part at the Coordination and Data Center. As a requirement, the user-interface of the system to develop should provide significant support for the study nurses and data mangers to efficiently and accurately fulfill their tasks.

Analysis of the prevalence and progression of the HIV-infection in Switzerland implies an area-wide collection of descriptive information from a representative sample on a repetitive basis for a sufficient length of time. Currently, this is done in accordance with a predefined study protocol by the various Cohort Centers. The collected descriptive information, together with the data, are transmitted to the Coordination and Data Center where they are stored in a central database. At this point, the requirement is specified that alternate study protocols should be supported by the knowledge medium.

Clinical research planning is initiated on an ad hoc basis. It requires updated descriptive information on patients meeting the specified inclusion criteria. As this information is also available from the central database at the Coordination and Data Center, a periodically actualized data pool and – as a precondition – a seamless flow of information between the Cohort Centers and the Coordination and Data Center is required. This same requirement also applies to the *performance of clinical studies*, particularly including the accuracy of the collected data.

Despite the recent advances of antiretroviral therapy, *healthcare provision to HIV-infected patients* is still far from the establishment of a good clinical practice (GCP). As a consequence, clinicians and private practitioners must be committed to continuing education regarding the activity and tolerance of new drugs or combinations thereof, administration procedures, dosages, and adverse events. This knowledge is created from clinical studies. It is complemented by explicit knowledge available from external sources such as publications in scientific journals, conferences, Web sources, and informal bilateral contacts. This dynamic aspect is complemented by the complexity inherent in providing healthcare to HIV-infected patients such as the management of follow-ups and patients' adherence to drug administration prescription. As a consequence, not only is it a requirement that the newly created knowledge be fast and easily communicated, but also that this knowledge be explicitly represented in the system.

Summary of the Requirements for a Knowledge Medium

Table 1 summarizes the communities, processes, and objects which are part of SHCS, as well as the derived requirements for the implementation of the knowledge medium:

With regards to knowledge management, the different requirements are further

Table 1. SHCS and the Requirements for the Knowledge Medium

Community	Process	Object	Requirement
study nurses	data processing	data (and descriptive information)	user-friendly interface
epidemiologists	epidemiological analysis	descriptive information	flexible protocol
project managers	clinical research planning	descriptive information	availability of information
analysts	clinical study	data	accuracy of data
clinicians, private practitioners	healthcare provision	explicit knowledge	knowledge representation

related: improving the availability of descriptive information and data reduces the duration of clinical studies, thereby speeding up the creation of new knowledge. Based on a redesigned technical infrastructure, this new knowledge can, in turn, be represented in the system and made available faster to the points of care.

The identified requirements are part of the specification for the implementation of our knowledge medium. Therefore, following the description of its implementation, we will evaluate whether the requirements are being met.

IMPLEMENTING A KNOWLEDGE MEDIUM IN THE SWISS HIV COHORT STUDY

Technical Issues

Based on the integrated and theoretically motivated concept of the knowledge medium and on a Web-based systems architecture (Figure 1), which was designed during a preliminary feasibility study, we developed the Electronic Study Form (ESF) application as

Figure 1: Systems Architecture

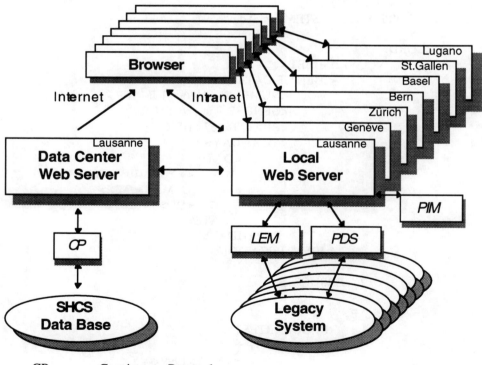

CP	Consistency Protocol
LEM	Local Enterprise Manager
PDS	Patient Dossier Server
PIM	Patient Identification Manager

common middleware and made a first step towards encompassing computerization (Fierz & Grütter, 1998; Grütter, Stanoevska-Slabeva and Fierz, 1999). The ESF is a client/server application for the automated input of laboratory data, which are already electronically available, and for the manual entry of additional data. For its development eXtensible Markup Language (XML), Dynamic Hypertext Markup Language (DHTML), and JavaScript were used.

XML is a simplified subset of Standard Generalized Markup Language (SGML, ISO 8879), created particularly to support distributed computing on the World Wide Web (WWW) (Bradley, 1998; Connolly, 1997; Light, 1997). It was accepted under the recommendation of the WWW consortium (W3C) in February 1998. This document-based approach has been chosen in order to deal with the long lifecycle of information created throughout the study (XML documents are both man- and machine-interpretable (see Figure 2) and to ensure independence from proprietary software systems in a distributed and heterogeneous environment. Furthermore, as a Web-based technology (cheap, short development cycles, ubiquitous access), it allows for easy integration of private practitioners with the knowledge medium.

Figure 2. XML Document (excerpt)

```
<?xml version="1.0"?>
<!DOCTYPE SHCS SYSTEM „esfel.dtd">
<SHCS>
<RECORD>
        <COVERSHEET>
                <IDENTIFICATION>
                        <NUMBER>47436</NUMBER>
                        <GENDER>male</GENDER>
                        <HEIGHT>167</HEIGHT>
                        <BIRTHDAY>
                                <DATE>
                                        <YYYY>1947</YYYY>
                                        <MM>10</MM>
                                        <DD>09</DD>
                                </DATE>
                        </BIRTHDAY>
                </IDENTIFICATION>
                ...
        </COVERSHEET>
        ...
        <LAB>
                <REGULARTESTS>
                        <DATE>
                                <YYYY>1999</YYYY>
                                <MM>09</MM>
                                <DD>16</DD>
                        </DATE>
```

```
                    <HEMATOLOGY>
                            <LEUKOCYT>5700</LEUKOCYT>
                            <HEMOGLOB>15</HEMOGLOB>
                            <PLATELET>217</PLATELET>
                    </HEMATOLOGY>
                    <SUBPOPULATIONS>
                            <DATE>
                                    <YYYY></YYYY>
                                    <MM></MM>
                                    <DD></DD>
                            </DATE>
                            <LY-ABS>1360</LY-ABS>
                            <CD3-ABS>1030</CD3-ABS>
                            <CD4-ABS>420</CD4-ABS>
                            <CD8-ABS>590</CD8-ABS>
                            <LY-REL>24</LY-REL>
                            <CD3-REL>75</CD3-REL>
                            <CD4-REL>30</CD4-REL>
                            <CD8-REL>43</CD8-REL>
                    </SUBPOPULATIONS>
                    <VIRALLOAD>
                            <RNA>50000</RNA>
                            <LIMIT></LIMIT>
                            <METHOD>ultrasensitive</METHOD>
                    </VIRALLOAD>
                    <SEROLOGY>
                            <P24>100</P24>
                            <ICDP24>2</ICDP24>
                    </SEROLOGY>
                    <BODYWEIGHT>65</BODYWEIGHT>
            </REGULARTESTS>
                ...
        </LAB>
            ...
    </RECORD>
</SHCS>
```

The XML template was programmed in accordance with the preexisting paper-based study form using an SGML authoring tool requiring some manual adaptations. Until recently no Web-browsers were available, which fully supported XML, so a Web client had to be developed. In its current version, i.e., in September 1999, an off-the-shelf XML parser is used to parse the exchanged documents. This parser is implemented as a Java applet. The document components are presented according to an object model (which is an Application Programming Interface, API) and are accessed by JavaScript. The scripts together with the Java applet are embedded in DHTML, the latter being presented by a commercial browser. In order to support the user in the processing of data, various checks for invalid and missing data are performed. In a like manner, a help file supporting a low level of context-sensitivity has been integrated with the user-interface.

To integrate data from legacy laboratory systems, comma-separated text files are generated and embedded in DHTML using Microsoft's ActiveX-based data-binding technology.

The communication between client and server within the local intranet employs the Hypertext Transfer Protocol (HTTP). The communication between applications across intranets is managed using the File Transfer Protocol (FTP).

Managerial Issues

Being a multi-center clinical trial, the structure, processes, and responsibilities of SHCS are very different from traditional hierarchical settings, found in monolithic enterprises, as the participating Cohort Centers are autonomous and committed to the study on a temporary and free basis. In this respect, SHCS mirrors the rather recent concept of the virtual organization, as it has the appearance of organizations in knowledge-intensive industries or functions such as R & D. Typically, a variety of experts work together on an interdisciplinary and temporal basis in order to solve complex problems with uncertain outcome.

When applied to our redesign project this implies two things. First, the implementation of our knowledge medium has to carefully consider the existing structures, processes, and responsibilities at the Cohort Centers and to map them onto the medium in an adequate and appropriate manner. Second, we have to deal with a pronounced demand regarding the communication with all participants in order to establish a common basis of agreement. This approach is not an integral part of our Western European culture, where decisions are often enforced on a hub and spoke basis. As a consequence, it presents both a great challenge but also an opportunity to learn more about cooperation.

When starting with the project, a discussion forum including representatives from all centers was established to support the communication among the participants. Although being helpful for the distribution of project deliverables, the discussion forum has so far not provided a sufficient degree of communication to contribute substantially to the establishment of a common basis of agreement. Additional face-to-face meetings were necessary to achieve this. This may in part be due to the rather low level of experience most participants have with this kind of electronic communication. In addition, and more important, it may reflect the fact that the physical presence of people participating in a discussion cannot be easily substituted, at least not in such cases where sensitive issues are on the agenda.

State of the Project

The current state of the project includes a Web discussion forum supporting the communication among the project partners and a distributed prototype consisting of the following components:

- the ESF application at one of the Cohort Centers (St. Gallen);
- an interface to the relational database system at the Coordination and Data Center in Lausanne—this interface comprises a lean version of the ESF application and uses proprietary "stored procedures" of the Oracle 7.x database system, which are accessed by JavaScript;
- an Internet connection between the Cohort Center and the Coordination and Data

Figure 3. User-Interface of the Electronic Study Form Application

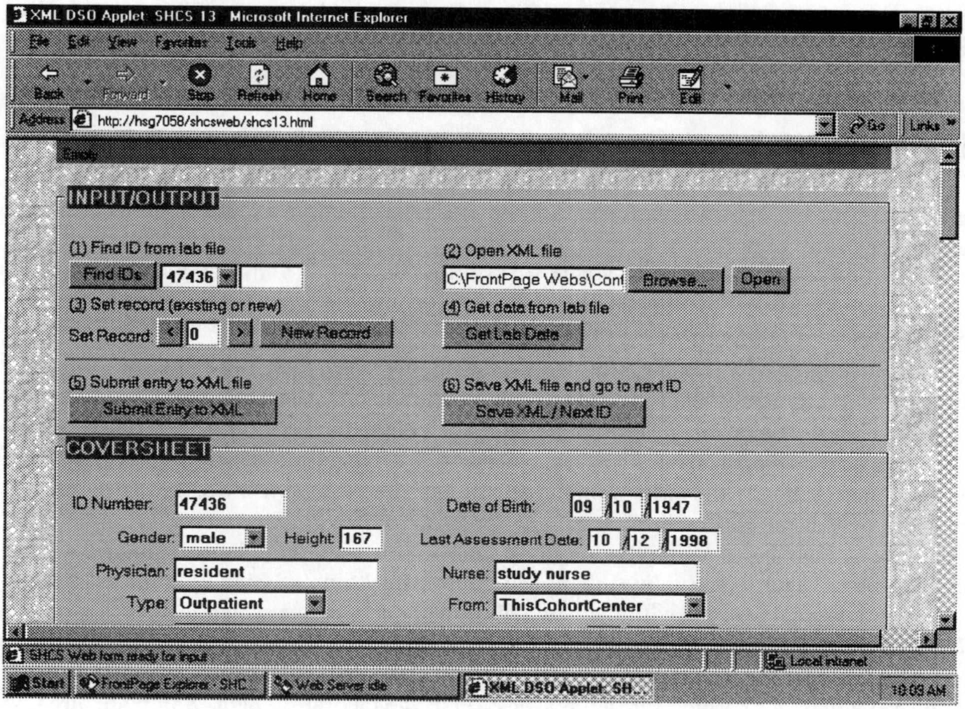

Center.

Currently, different XML database systems for the storage of individual patient information and data at the Cohort Centers are being evaluated (see Patient Dossier Server in Figure 1).

Likewise, a Web site at the Coordination and Data Center for the provision of cumulated study data and statistical figures is under construction (see Data Center Web Server in Figure 1).

The study nurse working with the ESF application processes all data from the Web browser (Figure 3). First, she looks for the patients with new laboratory data ("Find ID from lab file"). Currently, new laboratory data are placed on the Intranet Web server in a batch every two weeks. Since only anonymous data are processed, patients are represented by their unique Cohort IDs. Then she loads the corresponding XML file ("Open XML file"). For convenience, the files are named by the Cohort IDs (e.g., 47436.xml). As we have adopted a one-file-per-patient paradigm, the loaded file usually contains one or more records with data from previous visits. She then appends a new record to the XML file ("Set record (existing or new)"). Alternatively, she may browse through the existing records in order to read or edit data from previous visits. While appending a new record, the (descriptive) patient information is automatically copied from the last record and pasted into the new one. The input of the new laboratory data is also automated ("Get data from lab file"). If additional data are required, she manually completes the form. While submitting the entered data to the XML file various data checks are performed ("Submit entry to XML file"), the most important of which is the check for identity of the Cohort ID from the laboratory file with that of the XML file. Finally, the study nurse saves the data to file ("Save XML and go to next ID"). By doing so, the pointer in the laboratory file automatically switches to the next ID allowing the study nurse to proceed with the next XML file.

DISCUSSION

In this section, we will evaluate to what extent the requirements specified earlier are met by the current implementation of our knowledge medium. In addition, some considerations regarding security issues will be made.

The user-interface has been developed in close cooperation with a study nurse, thereby assuring a basic level regarding quality of design and functionality. However, an evaluation after a period of productive usage has to follow.

The support of a flexible protocol means among other things that the frequency of Cohort visits can easily be adapted to changing requirements (the current protocol foresees regular Cohort visits on a six-months-interval basis). In addition, the integration of intermediate, primarily laboratory results into the database should be supported. This requirement is met by the current implementation if the average workload per patient and visit can be reduced both at the Cohort Centers and at the Coordination and Data Center. The resulting savings in terms of work capacity can then be used to implement changes to the study protocol such as the above mentioned. Preliminary figures comparing the old paper-based and manual process with the new redesigned one were expected to be available in October 1999.

With respect to the availability and up-to-date of information (and data), substantial improvements are expected for two reasons. First, the laboratory data, which are already electronically available at the Cohort Centers, are processed without intermediate manual transcription to paper. Second, the data, which are not yet electronically available, are entered into the system only once. However, the entire workflow of data collection, transmission, and entry into the database still follows a batch procedure, the data are not accessed "online" in the strict sense. This results from maintaining the established study design of leaving the process ownership at the Cohort Centers, i.e., the processing of data is triggered from the periphery. The arguments are detailed.

The requirement of accurate data (and descriptive information), of course, also applied to the preexisting study design and was met by the implementation of the four-eyes-principle for data control (i.e., two-step validation). New to the current knowledge medium is the mentioned reduction of manual transcription, which is expected to significantly reduce the occurrence of errors.

With respect to knowledge representation and easy access to explicit knowledge, the current implementation will be complemented by additional components. These will be outlined in the next section.

An important issue of the project relates to upholding appropriate security measures in order to guarantee the privacy of the patient data. A key element for this purpose is the continuation of the existing Cohort design, in which the names of the patients are kept solely at the Cohort Centers, and separated from the database at the Coordination and Data Center. They are only connected to the data "on the fly" at the time of data usage. A second issue is the restriction of access to the FTP server at the Coordination and Data Center, which is used for data exchange. Thus, access to a password-protected domain is restricted to a number of registered clients. Although these measures provide a sufficient level of security for the prototype, the application of data encryption (Secure Sockets Layer, SSL) is being considered as soon as the ESF application will be deployed to other Cohort Centers. With respect to SSL there is a special situation outside the United States in that the common Web browsers are subject to an U.S. export law limiting the key length supported by the browsers. In order to use longer, and therefore more reliable, keys, the browsers must be upgraded with software patches.

OUTLOOK

Regarding the knowledge representation requirement of our knowledge medium, the Coordination and Data Center has recently initiated a Web site project. The idea is to exploit the Web integration features of Oracle 7.x in order to provide the Cohort Centers with a set of query options on their password-protected domains of the central database. Likewise, some general statistical figures should be made available. In addition, the Web site hiv.ch (http://www.hiv.ch/), which is edited by Markus Flepp, M.D., head of the Zurich Cohort Center, will be integrated into the knowledge medium. This Web site serves as a portal to a rich variety of explicit knowledge on HIV and AIDS. In order to provide the maximum of acceptance and support, the integration of these Web sites into the user-interface must be as seamless as possible. Since the use of Web technology by the current knowledge medium provides the advantage of the user working with a single application, i.e., with a browser, the integration is merely a question of user-friendly design. This interface can in a further step be personalized according to the individual preferences of the user. For instance, software agents can be applied to remind the user via an e-mail message as soon as contents are added according to his or her interests. This will allow for the selective browsing of updates according to predefined profiles.

In the first step of applying the concept of the knowledge medium to SHCS, we have adopted a bottom-up approach. Based on existing isolated information sources, an exchangeable object including descriptive information and data has been designed and implemented.

A next step will be the installation of local database systems at the Cohort Centers to store and manage the XML documents. By the use of object-oriented or hierarchical database systems implementing the structure of the documents as a database structure, it will be possible to navigate through the database and process (structural) semantic queries (besides, e.g., full-text retrieval). Medical (and administrative) personnel will access the contents using different filters reflecting their role within the community and/or the state of the process of healthcare delivery. Capable of drawing inferences from their contents, these database systems will act themselves as agents and, thus, participate in knowledge management. In addition, the user-interfaces can be enriched with additional (comfort) features to ensure not only context sensitivity but also interactive learning from individual user habits.

Once the clinical and laboratory data are available at the local Cohort Centers, the knowledge medium can be extended to also include on-line libraries of expert knowledge, such as the above mentioned portal site, and expert systems. As mentioned in the Introduction, such systems already exist but are usually isolated applications and not well integrated in the process of healthcare delivery. The leverage of the knowledge medium will support the healthcare providers in their daily work with HIV-infected patients and ensure that the patients take advantage from up-to-date and accurate diagnostic and therapeutic procedures.

Apart from these rather content-oriented aspects of knowledge medium development, the process aspect might become more important in the future. Thus, it will not suffice to exchange single contents (referred to as propositional knowledge) but also to add *procedural* knowledge on how the contents must be processed when received by an agent (see also the notion of the process template in XML/EDI (Webber, 1998)). Again, these procedures have to be automated as far as possible.

At the Coordination and Data Center tools with flexible Online Analytical Processing (OLAP) capabilities can be integrated with the central database system besides traditional tools for statistical analysis. These will allow for a dynamic planning of clinical trials thereby reducing coordination time and cost. A possible technology to develop such tools has been described (Geyer, Höhener, & Stanoevska-Slabeva, 1993a; Geyer, Höhener, & Stanoevska-Slabeva, 1993b and in the context of clinical trials Geyer & Grütter, 1996; Grütter, Geyer, & Schmid, 1998).

ACKNOWLEDGMENTS

It is particularly due to the detailed work on the presented concept of Professor Dr. Beat F. Schmid, chair of the Institute for Media and Communications Management that we were inspired to adopt this framework for our development attempts. Likewise, the careful reading of the manuscript by Martin Rickenbach, MD, and Pascal Janin from the Coordination and Data Center, SHCS, Lausanne, is gratefully acknowledged. Furthermore, we would like to thank Ms. Brigette Buchet, editor of *"The International Journal of Electronic Commerce and Business Media"*, for her help in maintaining a high quality of English throughout. The project presented in this chapter is generously granted by the Swiss HIV Cohort Study (SHCS).

REFERENCES

Bradley, N. (1998). *The XML companion.* Harlow, Essex, UK: Addison-Wesley.

Conklin, J.E. (1996). Designing Organizational Memory: Preserving Intellectual Assets in a Knowledge Economy, retrieved September, 1999 from the World Wide Web: http://www.gdss.com/DOM.htm.

Connolly, D. (1997). *XML: Principles, Tools, and Techniques.* World Wide Web Journal 2(4). Sebastopol, CA: O'Reilly.

Davenport, Th. (1996). Some Principles of Knowledge Management, posted April, 1996, retrieved September 1999 from the World Wide Web: http://www.bus.utexas.edu/%7Edavenpot/kmprin.htm.

Fierz, W. & Grütter, R. (1998). The use of a structured XML document to integrate distributed heterogeneous computer systems in a multi-centered clinical study. In E. Greiser & M. Wischnewsky (Eds.), *Methoden der Medizinischen Informatik, Biometrie und Epidemiologie in der modernen Informationsgesellschaft* (pp. 324-326). 43. Jahrestagung der GMDS, Bremen. München: MMV Medien & Medizin Verlag.

Finin, T., Labrou, Y. & Mayfield J. (1997). KQML as an agent communication language.

In Jeff Bradshaw (ed.), *Software Agents*. Cambridge: MIT Press.

Geyer, G. & Grütter, R. (1996). First step towards a quantitative knowledge medium for knowledge management in clinical studies. In *Proceedings of the first international conference on practical aspects of knowledge management*. Basel: PAKM.

Geyer, G., Höhener, T. & Stanoevska-Slabeva, K. (1993a). Acquisiton and processing of quantitative information within a distributed heterogeneous environment. In Hamza M. H. (Ed.), *Proceedings of the eleventh IASTED international conference: applied informatics* (pp. 143-146). Annecy: IASTED.

Geyer, G., Höhener, T. & Stanoevska-Slabeva, K. (1993b). Representation, normalization and processing of quantitative information. In *Proceedings of the 5th UNB AI Symposium, Fredericton,* (pp. 207-217). Canada: UNB AI Symposium.

Greiner, C. & Rose, T. (1997, September). Knowledge Management in Global Health Research Planning. In *Proceedings of the Workshop Knowledge-Based Systems for Knowledge Management in Enterprises, 21st Annual German Conference on AI ,97,* Freiburg, Germany, retrieved September, 1999 from the World Wide Web: http://www.dfki.uni-kl.de/~aabecker/Freiburg/Final/Greiner/greiner.html.

Gruber, T. (1993). *Toward Principles for the Design of Ontologies Used for Knowledge Sharing, Technical Report KSL 93-04*. Stanford University: Knowledge Systems Laboratory, retrieved September, 1999 from the World Wide Web: http://ksl-web.stanford.edu/KSL_Abstracts/KSL-93-04.html.

Gruber, T. (1999) *What is an Ontology?* Retrieved April 22, 1999 from the World Wide Web: http://www-ksl.stanford.edu/kst/what-is-an-ontology.html.

Gruber, T., Tenenbaum, J.M. & Weber, J.C. (1992). Towards a Knowledge Medium for Collaborative Knowledge Development. In J.S. Gero (ed.), *Proceedings of the Second International Conference on Artificial Intelligence in Design, Pittsburg, USA, June 22-25, 1992.* pp. 413-431. Boston: Kluwer Academic Publishers.

Grütter, R., Geyer, G. & Schmid, B.F. (1998). Konzeption einer ELIAS-Applikationsarchitektur für das klinische Studiendatenbanksystem der L.A.B. Neu-Ulm. *Zeitschrift Wirtschaftsinformatik, 4,* S. 291-300.

Grütter, R., Stanoevska-Slabeva, K. & Fierz, W. (1999). Implementing a Knowledge Medium in a Multi-centered Clinical Trial. In Sprague, R.H. (Ed.), *Proceedings of the 32nd Hawaii International Conference on System Sciences (HICSS-32)*. Los Alamitos, California: IEEE Computer Society.

Handschuh, S., Lechner, U., Lincke, D.-M., Schmid, B. F., Schubert, P., Selz, D. & Stanoevska, K. (1998). The NetAcademy - A New Concept for Online Publishing and Knowledge Management. In Margaria, T., Steffen, B., Rückert, R. & Posegga, J. (Eds.) *Services and Visualization – Towards a User-Friendly Design*, (pp. 29-43). Berlin/Heidelberg: Springer Verlag.

Labrou, Y. & Finin, T. (1997). *A Proposal for a new KQML Specification*. Baltimore: TR CS-97-03 of the Computer Science and Electrical Engineering Department, University of Maryland, Baltimore. Retrieved September, 1999 from the World Wide Web: http://www.cs.umbc.edu/kqml/papers/.

Lechner, U. & Schmid, B.F. (1999). Logic for Media – The Computational Media Metaphor. In Sprague, R.H. (Ed.), *Proceedings of the 32nd Hawaii International Conference on System Sciences (HICSS-32)*. Los Alamitos, California: IEEE Computer Society.

Lechner, U., Schmid, B.F., Schubert, P., Klose, M. & Miler, O. (1999). Ein Referenzmodell für Gemeinschaften und Medien – Case Study Amazon.com. Accepted for publication in the proceedings of the Workshop „Gemeinschaften in neuen Medien" GeNeMe'99.

Ledergerber, B., Von Overbeck, J., Egger, M. & Luthy, R (1994). The Swiss HIV Cohort Study: rationale, organization and selected baseline characteristics. *Soz Praventivmed, 39*(6), S. 387-394.

Light, R. (1997). *Presenting XML.* Indianapolis, IN: Sams.net Publishing.

Nonaka, I. (1991, November-December). The Knowledge Creating Company, *Harward Business Review,* pp. 96-104.

Probst, G., Raub, S. & Rohmhard, K. (1997). *Wissensmanagement – Wie Unternehmen ihre wertvollste Ressource optimal nutzen.* Wiesbaden: Gabler Verlag.

Schmid, B. F. (1997) The Concept of Media. In *Electronic Markets Workshop.* Maastricht, The Netherlands.

Schmid, B. F. (Hrsg.) (1999). *Wissensmedien.* Wiesbaden: Gabler Verlag.

Schmid, B.F. & Stanoevska, K. (1998, June). Knowledge Media: An Innovative Concept and Technology for Knowledge Management in the Information Age. In *Proceedings of the 12th Biennal International Telecommunications Society Conference - Beyond Convergence.* Stockholm, Sweden: IST'98.

Stefik, M. J. (1986, Spring). The Next Knowledge Medium. *AIP Magazine, 7.*

Stefik, M.J. (1988). The Next Knowledge Medium. In: Huberman, B. A. (Ed.), *The Ecology of Computation* (pp. 315-342). Amsterdam: Elsevier Science Publishers B.V.

Stein, E.W. & Zwass, V. (1995). Actualising Organisational Memory with Information Systems. *Information Systems Research,* 6 (2), 85-117.

Webber, D.R.R. (1998). Introducing XML/EDI frameworks. *EM - Electronic Markets: the International Journal of Electronic Commerce and Business Media,* 8(1), 38-41.

ENDNOTE

1. Antiretroviral: directed against retroviruses (the HIV-virus is a retrovirus).

Chapter X

A Decision Technology System to Advance the Diagnosis and Treatment of Breast Cancer

Guisseppi A. Forgionne, Aryya Gangopadhyay and Monica Adya
University of Maryland Baltimore County

INTRODUCTION

Geographical variations in cancer rates have been observed for decades. Described spatial patterns and trends have provided clues for generating hypotheses about the etiology of cancer. For breast cancer, investigators have demonstrated that some variation can be explained by differences in the population distribution of known breast cancer risk factors such as menstrual and reproductive variables (Laden, Spiegelman, and Neas, 1997; Robbins, Bescianini, and Kelsey, 1997; Sturgeon, Schairer, and Gail, 1995). However, regional patterns also may reflect the effects of Workshop on Hormones, Hormone Metabolism, Environment, and Breast Cancer (1995): (a) environmental hazards (such as air and water pollution), (b) demographics and the lifestyle of a mobile population, (c) subgroup susceptibility, (d) changes and advances in medical practice and healthcare management, and (e) other factors. To accurately measure breast cancer risk in individuals and population groups, it is necessary to singly and jointly assess the association between such risk and the hypothesized factors.

Various statistical models will be needed to determine the potential relationships between breast cancer development and estimated exposures to environmental contamination. To apply the models, data must be assembled from a variety of sources, converted into the statistical models' parameters, and delivered effectively to researchers and policy makers. A Web-enabled decision technology system can be developed to provide the needed functionality.

This chapter will present a conceptual architecture for such a decision technology system. First, there will be a brief overview of a typical geographical analysis. Next, the chapter will present the conceptual Web-based decision technology system and illustrate how the system can assist users in diagnosing and treating breast cancer. The chapter will conclude with an examination of the potential benefits from system use and the implications for breast cancer research and practice.

BACKGROUND

Environmental contaminants tend to be clustered geographically (Chen, 1996; Grimson and Oden, 1996; Oden, Jacquez, and Grimson, 1996). Studies that link breast cancer with environmental factors, then, have focused on geographical analysis.

In a typical geographic analysis, the researcher will utilize clustering techniques and other statistical methodologies to identify abnormal concentrations of breast cancer. Abnormality usually is defined as a concentration that deviates significantly from expected patterns. Sometimes regression and other multivariate statistical analyses will be used to isolate the independent and joint effects of environmental and other variables on breast cancer incidence and mortality. Customarily, the statistical analyses will be based largely on metric data and be single-equation in form. Other times, qualitative evaluations will be used to test the hypothesized relationships. Ordinarily, these evaluations will rely to some extent on the judgment and experience of the researcher and/or other experts.

Researchers and policy makers recognized that information technology could be used to facilitate the desired geographic analysis. Such recognition and subsequent lobbying efforts resulted in legislation that mandated the development of this technology. The National Institutes of Health's National Cancer Institute (NCI) recently sought a geographic information system (GIS) to support breast cancer studies mandated by public law (Geographic Information System for the Long Island Breast Cancer Study Project, 1998).

Geographic Information System (GIS)

In the GIS sought by the NCI, researchers and other interested parties would utilize computer technology to process available inputs into desired outputs. Inputs would include a database that captures and stores spatial and attribute data for the geographic areas defined by the breast cancer studies. Spatial data, which includes longitude and latitude coordinates that are used to draw on study area maps, can be obtained from state and local government base map files, U.S. Postal Service ZIP Code files, U. S. Geological Survey hydrology data files, and U.S. Bureau of the Census TIGER (Topologically Integrated Geographic Encoding and Referencing) files (Fischer and Nijkamp, 1993). Attribute data, which, among other things, consists of pollution measures, population characteristics, and healthcare provider and patient statistics, can be obtained the U.S. Bureau of the Census, the U. S. Healthcare Financing Administration, the National Health and Nutrition Examination Surveys, state-specific public health data files, and state and federal survey data files on pollution-source emissions.

There is also a model base that contains statistical procedures and location formulas. Some statistical procedures are used to categorize attribute data within the study areas and to calculate summary statistics for the demographic, environmental, healthcare, and other pertinent variables within the areas. Other procedures analyze the data for spatial and temporal patterns and for space-time interactions. A third set of statistical procedures are used to perform selected health-related analyses, including cluster detection of breast cancer incident and mortality, assessment of disease risk from nearby environmental hazards, and genetic activity profiling. Location formulas are used to convert various geographic coordinate systems into alternative forms and to make corresponding map projections.

The decision maker (a scientist or public health official) uses available computer technology to organize the collected spatial and attribute data, structure the study area maps, locate breast cancer incidents on the maps, and simulate spatial, temporal, and spatial-temporal patterns. Spatial and attribute data created during GIS processing can be captured and stored as inputs for future processing.

Processing automatically generates visual displays of the outputs desired by the scientists or public health officials. Outputs include study area maps and associated breast cancer incident and mortality reports. The maps define the boundaries of the study area, give the road and street patterns, identify important landmarks, locate the patterns within the study area, and color the concentrations on the study area roads and streets. Reports list the breast cancer incident and mortality statistics by user-selected pattern categories. The reports also summarize key patterns for the study area, including high-incidence and high-mortality clusters, temporal trends, and spatial-temporal relationships, including key incidence and mortality indicators.

The user can utilize the outputs to guide further GIS processing before exiting the system. Typically, the feedback will involve sensitivity analyses in which the user extends or modifies the study area boundaries and observes the effects on breast cancer concentrations and on key spatial and temporal indicators.

MAIN THRUST OF THE CHAPTER

There are several issues, controversies, and problems associated with the NCI GIS concept. An analysis of these issues recommends a Web-based technology solution.

Issues, Controversies, and Problems

Much of the relevant spatial and attribute data needed for the geographic studies are captured and stored on a variety of distributed data sets. In addition, these data are not organized into the variables needed to perform the breast cancer studies. Moreover, required data are collected, captured, and recorded in various formats, and often in an incomplete manner. There is little (if any) sharing of information between the collection sources and the NCI-supported geographic breast cancer study process. To be useful for this process, then, captured data must be located, accessed, and converted into the appropriate format for the analyses and evaluations.

After the relevant data formats have been created, researchers and other analysts will use data mining methods to manually identify spatial and temporal data patterns (Abraham and Roddick, 1998; Davidson, Henrickson, Johnson, Myers, and Wylie, 1999). These methods, however, will not explain the specific environmental and other potential causes of the detected breast cancer patterns. A statistical model will be needed to determine the pattern determinants and their relationship to mortality and morbidity (Borok, 1997; Burn-Thornton and Edenbrandt, 1998). Researchers and analysts must use their insights, analytical and creative abilities, knowledge and experience to formulate the model, test hypotheses, and derive explanations. As new data become available, the models should be updated in terms of parameters and variables. A high level of expertise will be required to perform the model updating and derive the pattern explanations (Hornung, Deddens, and Roscoe, 1998; Makino, Suda, Ono, and Ibaraki, 1999).

All potential users of the prototype GIS are unlikely to possess the necessary analytical and information technology expertise. Even then, the proposed GIS will not have the functionality to perform the required data management, modeling, and presentation tasks. To achieve the desired functionality, additional information systems will have to be developed and linked to the prototype GIS. Modeling assistance, for example, will require a decision support system (Tan and Sheps, 1998). Another important requirement of such a system is the ease of accessibility of data to users, which would require a wide area intranet or Web-based Internet environment.

Solutions and Recommendations

The NCI can have several stand-alone systems to provide the decision analyses and evaluations (Tan, 1995; Tan and Sheps, 1998). Integrating the stand-alone functions, however, can enhance the quality and efficiency of the segmented support, create synergistic effects, and augment decision-making performance and value (Forgionne and Kohli, 1996). A Web-based information system, called the *Breast Cancer Analysis System (BCAS)*, can deliver such integrated and complete decision support. The BCAS will consist of the GIS, an executive information system (EIS), and a decision support system (DSS), with the architecture shown in Figure 1.

Inputs

The BCAS has a database that captures and stores geographic, demographic, environmental, health outcome, and healthcare data. There is also a modelbase, or organized repository of models and algorithms, captures and stores a multiple-equation statistical model along with the GIS, health, and other statistical models required and desired in the National Cancer Institute Specified GIS-H Functions table. As a package, these models compute and estimate breast-cancer-relevant variables, describe and explain the spatial, temporal, and space-time relationships between the variables and breast cancer development, and use the relationships to simulate breast cancer incidence and mortality.

In addition, there is a knowledgebase that captures and stores spatial and temporal profiles linked to breast cancer incidence, development, and mortality patterns. Profile data will be available from the sources identified in the NCI Specified Initial Datasets.

Processing

Interested investigators and officials use the BCAS computer technology interactively to perform analyses and evaluations that include: (a) organizing data into parameters needed for the spatial, temporal, and space-time beast cancer analyses, (b) structuring models that represent and simulate breast cancer development patterns in an integrated and complete manner, and (c) simulating breast cancer incidence and mortality under specified healthcare, health outcome, demographic, and environmental profiles.

Pertinent hardware includes a standard personal computer, Internet (or network) connectivity devices, storage equipment sufficient to accommodate the large volume of spatial and attribute data likely to be processed by the system, and compatible display devices sufficient to show cartographic, interactive visual, map, tabular, plotted, text, and multimedia processing results in hard and soft copy form. Software includes a windowed operating system, a Web-browser, and an integrated application software suite that will accommodate data warehousing, spatial and temporal data analysis, and decision support.

The embedded GIS serves as a front-end to the processing of the profile data. This system extracts the pertinent data from an Internet (or intranet) based data warehouse, links the data to spatial dimensions, and transfers the linked data to the embedded executive information system (EIS).

An implanted executive information system is used to (a) filter the profile data, (b)

Figure 1: BCAS Architecture

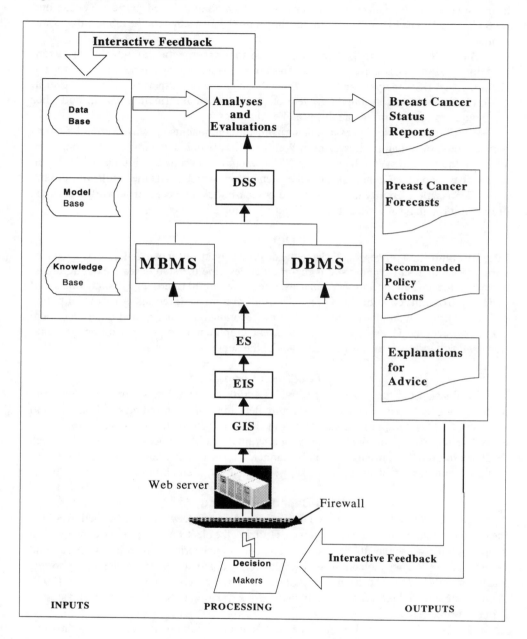

form BCAS's database, (c) focus the filtered information, and (d) communicate deviations from expected breast cancer development patterns among affected parties (Keegan and Baldwin, 1992). The EIS also will provide the focused data needed for the DSS analyses and evaluations.

The DSS and Expert Systems (ES) guide the investigator through the intelligent modeling and the modelbase, database, and knowledgebase management needed for the GIS, EIS, and DSS analyses and evaluations. Such embedded expertise assists the user in a virtual manner in performing the epidemiology, statistical, information system, and other tasks required to perform the analyses and evaluations.

BCAS supports Web access to clients using the components shown in Figure 1. Clients request static or dynamic files using a Web browser, which are transmitted through the World Wide Web to a Web listener (an HTTP daemon that runs continuously). The Web listener passes on the client request to the Web server, which sends the results back to the client. Transaction security is supported using secure socket layers and network security is provided through a firewall, shown in Figure 1, using a proxy server.

Outputs

By controlling processing tasks in the desired way, the user can generate: (a) visually attractive tabular and graphic status reports that describe the study area's existing breast cancer incidence and mortality summaries, track meaningful trends, and display important patterns, (b) claims condition and other electronic commerce forecasts, (c) provider policy and payer program simulation results, and (d) recommended claims and other electronic commerce actions. The system also depicts, in a graphic manner, the reasoning (explanations and supporting knowledge) that leads to the suggested actions.

Feedback Loops

Feedback from the processing provides additional data, knowledge, and enhanced decision models that may be useful for future decision activities and tasks (Kalakota, and Whinston, 1997). Output feedback (often in the form of sensitivity analyses) is used to extend or modify the original analyses and evaluations. All processing (including each feedback loop) is done in a user-friendly manner, with artificial intelligence (mainly expert system) technology, that meets the decision styles and requirements of participating parties.

Web-Based Technology

The BCAS will be a Web-based technology. A Web site will be established to collect the pertinent data from the various sources. Utilizing the electronic commerce concept, data suppliers will access the BCAS Web site and select appropriate screen icons (Gerull and Wientzen, 1997). These selections will automatically obtain the data from the supply source and transfer the elements to a data warehouse (Tsvetovatyy, Gini, and Wiecckowski, 1997). A component called *integrator* is responsible for extracting data from the GIS and storing it in the warehouse.

The BCAS's EIS will extract the pertinent data, capture the extractions in user-oriented data marts, and make the marked data available for ad hoc queries by: (a) principal investigators and other scientists; (b) public health officials; (c) private health practitioners; (d) individual investigators; (e) public interest groups, and (f) the public at large. Ad hoc queries can be made at the users' sites in an easy-to-use, convenient, and interactive manner, utilizing the Web-based BCAS. Results will be displayed in formats (tabular, graphic, and maps) anticipated by the requesting parties.

The system will provide an open and scalable on-line analytical processing (OLAP) solution using the thin-client architecture. The clients generate and view reports and graphs of data stored in the multidimensional database server (MDDB), which derives the raw data from the data warehouse located at the database (DB) server. Users can run queries and generate reports using with any HTML-based browser without having an application session being run on the client. The multidimensional database (MDDB) server is used to enable IT personnel to build, maintain, and optimize multidimensional data. This architecture would reduce the cost of client-server management by centralizing the data and applications on the server, and make it simple to distribute and upgrade applications and add new OLAP users.

FUTURE TRENDS

Web-based environments that provide universal access, via the Internet or an intranet, to integrated health information from a variety of sources is an emerging trend that can benefit the healthcare community and the nation in a variety of ways. Such access enables the healthcare organization to be proactive rather than reactive. For example, through this access, healthcare organizations can process expected outcomes and compare them against actual patient outcomes. Such comparisons can help predict: (a) patient problems; (b) required healthcare interventions; (c) time required for implementation of healthcare services; (d) accessibility of healthcare services; (e) quality of healthcare services, and (f) cost of healthcare services.

The BCAS concept provides a vehicle to utilize the emerging Web-based access for proactive breast cancer diagnosis and treatment. Without the BCAS, breast cancer detection involves a very complex process that requires extensive training for researchers and policy analysts. By decreasing the volume of documentation, by simplifying the educational process, and by simplifying and automating much of the process, the BCAS can be expected to save the medical community millions of dollars per year in breast cancer diagnosis and treatment costs. Based on the experience in a previous, and similar, project, it is anticipated that the BCAS can be developed and implemented for a small fraction of the potential cost savings (Forgionne, 1997).

From a diagnosis perspective, the manual search for breast cancer patterns, morbidities, and mortalities is a tedious process that often results in inaccurate, incomplete, and redundant data. Such data problems can leave cancer victims inadequately diagnosed and treated. With the BCAS, the researcher or analyst identifies all data relevant to the breast cancer analysis process, and the system provides a mechanism that facilitates data entry while reducing errors and eliminating redundant inputs. Reports from the BCAS also offer focused guidance that can be used to help researchers and policy analysts in performing breast cancer searches, diagnoses, and treatments.

Challenges

Realizing the strategic potential will present significant challenges to the traditional healthcare organization. Tasks, events, and processes must be redesigned and reengineered to accommodate the Web-based universal access. Clinicians and administrators must be convinced that the access will be personally as well as organizationally beneficial, and they must agree to participate in the effort. Finally, the organizational changes will compel substantial informational technology support.

When implemented fully, the innovation will alter the work design for, and supervision of, breast cancer diagnosis and treatment. Requisite operations and computations will be simplified, automated, and made error-free. Training requirements will be reduced to a minimum. Processing efficiency will be dramatically increased. User-inspired creative study-area and public health policy experimentation will be facilitated and nurtured. Management learning will be promoted. Knowledge capture will be expedited.

In short, BCAS's usage would substantially reshape the organizational culture. Faced with significant time pressures and limited staff, healthcare leadership may be reluctant to take on this burden at the present time. In addition, public health officials have developed and cultivated strong and enduring relationships with practitioners and vendors. These practitioners and vendors also have important contacts and allies within the government agencies that oversee healthcare programs. For these reasons, it may be politically wise for public health officials to preserve these practitioner and vendor relationships.

Future Research Opportunities

There are a number of future research opportunities presented by the BCAS. To ensure that the information system accurately replicates the inputs, the final version of the BCAS should be tested against Web-collected data from existing institutions study areas. In the testing, warehoused data should be compared against actual values. Statistical tests should be conducted on the estimated models. There should be evaluations of user satisfaction with: (a) the speed, relevance, and quality of ad hoc query results, (b) the system interface, (c) model appropriateness, and (d) the quality of the system explanation. Simulations should be statistically tested for accuracy, and confidence intervals should be established for the results. Tests should also be conducted on the system's ability to improve the decision making maturity of the user.

The BCAS concept can also be adapted for a variety of adjunct healthcare applications. Similar systems can be applied to the diagnosis and treatment of other forms of cancer, mental disorders, infectious diseases, and additional illnesses. Effectiveness studies can be done to measure the economic, management, and health impacts of the additional applications.

Another potential area for future research is the use of artificial intelligence techniques for model calibration and optimization. In a domain such as breast cancer diagnosis and treatment, there will often be a need to optimize models, especially as newer models emerge through BCAS processing. These emerging models should undergo a rigorous process of optimization and calibration. Empirical evidence suggests that genetic algorithms are superior to traditional search and optimization methods (such as hill climbing), and even neural networks, for such tasks (Kao et al., 1995; Kim, 1998).

CONCLUSIONS

The BCAS architecture is based on a combination of database, modeling, data mining, and mapping techniques. Its deployment can enable the NIH to realize significant economic and political benefits. Future enhancements promise to increase the power of the BCAS to further improve the nation's ability to manage its cancer resources.

The BCAS delivers the information and knowledge needed to support breast cancer detection in a comprehensive, integrated, and continuous fashion. In theory, the comprehensive, integrated, and continuous support from the BCAS should yield more decision value than the non-synthesized and partial support offered by any single autonomous system. Improvements should be observed in both the outcomes from, and the process of, strategic claims and other electronic commerce decision making (Lederer, Merchandani, and Sims, 1997). Outcome improvements can include advancements in the level of the users' decision-making maturity and gains in organization performance (Whinston, Stahl, and Choi, 1997). Process improvements can involve enhancements in the users' ability to perform the phases and steps of decision making.

Regardless of BCAS's legacy, the application offers useful lessons for Web-based healthcare decision technology systems development and management. The system is effectively delivering to the user, in a virtual manner, embedded statistical, medical, and information systems expertise specifically focused on the healthcare problem.

The virtual team characteristics and the organizational culture impacts also suggest that a hybrid project-technology organization may work well for Web-based decision technology system design, development, and implementation in a healthcare environment. The organization would be virtual rather than physical. A project team would be established and administered by the practicing healthcare professional. Team technology specialists would be drawn from within and outside the organization to match the expertise needed for the specific project. Telecommuting and distributed collaborative work would be allowed and possibly encouraged.

REFERENCES

Abraham, T., & Roddick, J. F. (1998). Opportunities for knowledge discovery in spatio-temporal information systems. *Australian Journal of Information Systems*. 5(2), 3-12.

Borok, L. S. (1997). Data mining: Sophisticated forms of managed care modeling through artificial intelligence. *Journal of Healthcare Finance*. 23(3), 20.

Burn-Thornton, K. E., & Edenbrandt, L. (1998). Myrocardial infarction-pinpointing the key indicators in the 12-lead ECG using data mining. *Computers and Biomedical Research*, 31(4), 293-303.

Chen, R. (1996). Exploratory analysis as a sequel to suspected increased rate of cancer in a small residential or workplace community. *Statistics in Medicine* 15, 807-816.

Davidson, G. S., Hendickson, B., Johnson, D. K., Meyers, C. E., & Wylie, B. N. (1999). Knowledge mining with VxInsight: Discovery through interaction. *Journal of Intelligent Information Systems: Integrating Artificial Intelligence and Database Technologies*. 11(3), 259-285.

Fischer, M. M. and P. Nijkamp (Eds.) (1993). *Geographic Information Systems, Spatial Modeling, and Policy Evaluation*. New York: Springer-Verlag.

Forgionne, G. A. (1997). HADTS: A decision technology system to support army housing management. *European Journal of Operational Research*, 97, 1120-1135.

Forgionne, G. A. and Kohli, R. (1996). HMSS: A management support system for concurrent hospital decision making. *Decision Support Systems*. 16, 209-223.

Grimson, R. C. and N. Oden (1996). Disease clusters in structured environments. *Statistics in Medicine* 15, 851-871.

Geographic Information System for the Long Island Breast Cancer Study Project (LIBCSP) (1998). National Cancer Institute's Electronic RFP Number NO2-PC-85074-39. Bethesda: National Cancer Institute.

Gerull, D. B. and Wientzen, R. (1997). Electronic commerce: The future of image delivery. *International Journal of Geographical Information Systems*, 7(7) 38-51.

Hornung, R. W., Deddens, J. A., & Roscoe, R. J. (1998). Modifiers of lung cancer risk in uranium miners from the Colorado Plateau. *Health Physics*, 74(1), 12-21.

Huxhold, W. E. (1991). *An Introduction to Urban Geographic Information Systems*. Oxford: Oxford University Press.

Kao, C., Chen, L.-H., Wang, T.-Y., Kuo, S., & Horng, S.-D. (1995). Productivity improvement: efficiency approach vs effectiveness approach. *Omega, International Journal of Managment Science,* 23(2), 197-204.

Kalakota, R. and Whinston, A. B. (1997). *Electronic Commerce: A Manager's Guide*, Reading, Massachusetts: Addison-Wesley.

Keegan, A. J. and Baldwin, B. (1992). EIS: A better way to view hospital trends. *Healthcare Financial Management,* 46(11), 58-64.

Kim, W. (1998). Data mining: Promises, reality, and future. *Journal of Object-Oriented Programming*, 11(4), 61-62+.

Laden, F., Spiegelman, D., and Neas, L. M. (1997). Geographic variation in breast cancer incidence rates in a cohort of U. S. women. *Journal of the National Cancer Institute* 89, 1373-1378.

Lederer, A. L., Merchandani, D. F., and Sims, K. (1997). The link between information strategy and electronic commerce. *Journal of Organizational Computing and Electronic Commerce*, 7(1), 17-25.

Makino, K., Suda, T., Ono, H., & Ibaraki, T. (1999). Data analysis by positive decision trees. *IEICE Transactions on Information and Systems*, E82-D(1), 76-88.

Oden, N., Jacquez, G., and Grimson, R. (1996). Realistic power simulations compare point- and area-based disease cluster tests. *Statistics in Medicine* 15, 783-806.

Regional Variation in Breast Cancer Rates in the U. S. – NIH. National Cancer Institute's Electronic RFA Number CA-98-017. Bethesda: National Cancer Institute, 1998.

Robbins, A. S., Brescianini, S., and Kelsey, J. L. (1997). Regional differences in known risk factors and the higher incidence of breast cancer in San Francisco. *Journal of the National Cancer Institute* 89, 960-965.

Sturgeon, S. R., Schairer, C., and Gail, M. (1995). Geographic variation in mortality rates from breast cancer among white women in the United States. *Journal of the National Cancer Institute* 87, 1846-1853.

Tan, J. K. H. (1995). *Health Management Information Systems*. Gaithersburg, Maryland: Aspen.

Tan, J. K.H., and Sheps, S., Editors (1998). *Health Decision Support Systems*. Gaithersburg, Maryland: Aspen.

Tsvetovatyy, N., Gini, M., and Wieckowski, Z. (1997). Magma: An agent-based virtual market for electronic commerce. *Applied Artificial Intelligence.* 11(6), 501-509.

Whinston, A. B., Stahl, D. O., and Choi, S. (1997). *The Economics of Electronic Commerce*. Indianapolis, Indiana: Macmillan Technical Publishing.

Workshop on Hormones, Hormone Metabolism, Environment, and Breast Cancer, New Orleans, Louisiana, September 28-29, 1995. *Monographs in Environmental Health Perspectives* supplement 1997, 105(3), 557-688.

Chapter XI

Web-Enabled Integration of Patient Data and Clinical Guidelines for Coordinated Care

James R. Warren and Joseph T. Noone
University of South Australia

INTRODUCTION

A variety of forces are encouraging change in the healthcare systems of developed countries. Chief among these is perception of high (and rising) cost. The arsenal of tests, medications and procedures at the hands of Western medicine is ever-increasing. This, in concert with an aging population, has brought the health expenditures in the U.S., EU, Japan and Australia edging to just under 10% of GNP. Furthermore, there is concern about waste of resources, principally through lack of coordination between healthcare facilities resulting in redundant investigations. A more subtle force comes from the rise of evidence-based medicine (EBM), as illustrated, for instance, by the extensive consolidated clinical reviews of the Cochrane Collaboration. EBM highlights that typical medical practice is not necessarily efficient or effective in all cases as compared to well-established findings of randomized controlled trials (e.g., Sydney GPs have been observed to over-prescribe antibiotics, which is both a waste and a community health hazard [Bolton et al., 1996]).

Happily, as motivations for change rise, we see the emergence of technologies with great promise for implementing solutions. The most obvious of these is of course Web technology. Cimino et al. (1995) illustrated (at a time that can now be considered early in the brief history of the Web) that intranet-based Web technology could provide a break-through in ease of integration of legacy information systems within a hospital environment, and thus be the basis for innovative clinical workstations within the hospital walls. More recently Cimino et al. (1998) have illustrated technical solutions to control the security and confidentiality risks associated with external access to the hospital intranet data. Moreover, as one uses an intranet for integration of patient data, they can simultaneously access internal (intranet) and/or external (Internet) decision support resources (such as access to Medline illustrated by Cimino et al., 1995).

Given that we have the technical means to make patient data and clinical decision support knowledge available, we are now left with a design problem: how to devise clinical workstation environments that leverage the available information resources and engender a superior process of patient care. Of course, many subsidiary questions follow from this framing of the design problem. Just what patient data do we collect and share? What decision support guidance is most important? What exactly might be a superior process of care? And who, if anyone, controls this process?

In this chapter, we describe the Care Plan On Line (CPOL) system, which provides clinical guidance to general practitioners (GPs) tailored by the electronic patient record. CPOL supports the SA HealthPlus Coordinated Care trial, enrolling 4,500 chronically ill South Australians across a range of disease-specific projects. The architecture leverages a central database that integrates diverse data sources to form a disease-specific, purpose-built chronic care record. CPOL provides an intranet gateway to this record and integrates it with clinical guidelines compiled for SA HealthPlus by focus groups to give contextualised decision support. CPOL helps the GP to consider the latest evidence-based thinking to devise a holistic and proactive plan of services. Furthermore, the guidelines have a transparent and layered structure that encourages the GP to 'opt in' on the HealthPlus care rationale. The architecture allows profound central modification of guideline and patient record elements without modification to the client installations.

The objectives of this chapter are:

• To illustrate the features and principles of clinical user interface design wherein patient data and practice guidelines are integrated with one another and with the model of care;

• To describe the technical architecture of the CPOL system that realises such integration;

• To describe the SA HealthPlus model of Coordinated Care as a concept of interest in its own right for its GP-controlled, patient-centred approach to proactive care of the chronically ill; and

• To emphasise the power of Web/intranet-based systems to focus data, decision knowledge and control on particular health professionals (in this case chiefly the GP) to suit the requirements of a given theory of patient care.

CLINICAL GUIDELINES AND DECISION SUPPORT

David Eddy of Kaiser Permanente has said (1990) "All [evidence] confirms what would be expected from common sense: The complexity of modern medicine exceeds the inherent limitations of the unaided human mind." Ergo, there is an opportunity to improve medical practice by appropriate provision of practice guidance to support clinical decision making.

Lam (1994) defines *practice guidelines* as statements that recommend appropriate practice of patient care for specific clinical circumstances. Leape (1990) puts forth the more specific definition that practice guidelines are standardized specifications for care developed by a formal process that incorporates the best scientific evidence of effectiveness with opinions of experts in the fields. Wide variations in clinical practice exist, for example:

• In Vermont, rate of removal of tonsils during childhood varied from 8% to 60% between communities (Eisenberg, 1986);

• In Maine, regional differences in prostatectomy rate for men under 85 can vary from 15% to 65% (Wall, 1993);

- In Iowa, hysterectomy by age 70 can vary from less than 20% to over 70% (Eisenberg, 1986);

While many factors influence these rates, there can be little doubt that not all practices would be classified as "best practice" to any specific guideline standard. In general, guidelines have been developed in an effort to reduce escalating healthcare costs (which in part can be due to the large variations in clinical practice) without sacrificing quality (Lobach, 1995). When successfully implemented in practice they have been shown to improve healthcare outcomes (Grimshaw & Russel, 1993).

The acceptance and utilisation of the guidelines by clinicians depends on several factors. Awareness of the existence of guidelines and their acceptance does not guarantee effective use. To be effective, guidelines need to be integrated into the physician's decision-making process in daily practice (Lam, 1994). Even assuming they have time to read the current reams of paper-based guidelines, physicians reading the guidelines is not sufficient. Physicians need to understand what they are reading, then decide it has some merit and is justified and agree with the guidance. Furthermore, once they have decided that a piece of guidance is relevant and useful to both themselves and their patients' care, they must implement the guideline into their process of care. An example of a shortfall in implementation is the guidelines introduced in the NIH consensus development program, where Kosecoff et al. (1987) found the guidelines reached their target (i.e., they were read) but did not influence practice.

Lomas, Pierre and colleagues (Lomas et al., 1989; Lomas et al. 1991; Pierre, 1991) investigated the effect of guidelines on care. The initial study by Lomas et al. found obstetricians who were given new guidelines on cesarean-section indications felt their practice had changed as a result of the guidelines. The cesarean rates, however, for the same obstetricians did not change. Lomas et al. (1989) and Pierre et al. suggest that while the guidelines may prompt the physician to consider changing their practice behaviors, compliance may need to be re-enforced by further incentives or efforts. The subsequent study by Lomas et al. found compliance by the obstetricians was greatly enhanced when an influential leader within the group/department of obstetricians promoted the guidelines.

The methods used to develop guidelines influence their success. Guidelines need to be developed by thorough reviews of literature and the development of supporting guidelines by consensus of opinion by the all types of healthcare workers that will use the guidelines. The guidelines then need to be evaluated, validated and updated through physician input. There needs to be a plan for successfully implementing the guidelines, which should include customisation of the guidelines and the opportunity for feedback and modification.

For guidelines to be successfully integrated into decision-making processes, those physicians who decisions are supposedly being influenced need to be part of the development process. Without the user input there will be little chance of their acceptance and subsequent use. Specialists have developed most of the available practice guidelines with little input from primary care practitioners. They are perceived to be inflexible when applied to the complexity of individual patient situations. These and other barriers to accepting the guidelines in daily practice need to be resolved prior to implementation (Lobach & Hammond, 1994). Moreover, most current guidelines are implemented in printed form, or as direct translations of the printed text-based narrative (Liem et al., 1995), which may not be the most amenable form for integrating the guidelines with daily practice.

There have been a number of recent attempts to provide effective electronic representations of clinical guidelines (Barnes & Barnett, 1995; Bouhaddou et al., 1994; Jenders et al., 1995; Lam, 1994; Liem et al., 1995; Lobach, 1995; Quaglini, 1997). It has been recognized that the guideline statements should be linked to the actual patient data, and that their utility can be enhanced by using interactive data entry to direct the user on the basis of entered information. Thus, integration of guidelines with the electronic medical record systems and their use at the point of care is of special importance. The highest probability of an effective guideline implementation occurs when patient-specific advice is provided at the time and place of a consultation (Grimshaw & Russel, 1993; Shiffman, 1997), and in particular "when the guideline is made accessible through computer-based, patient-specific reminders that are integrated into the clinician's workflow" (Zielstorff, 1998).

The term *Decision Support System* (DSS) usually refers to a computer program that supports a manager in making decisions when facing ill-structured problems (Klein & Methlie, 1995). A computer-based medical DSS is a computer program designed to help health professionals make clinical decisions (Shortliffe, 1987). This broad definition allows one to classify as medical, DSSs programs that range in functionality from merely displaying relevant medical data to the most advanced expert systems. A *passive* DSS aims to provide the system user with the right information at the right time, like an up-to-date clinical record, results of laboratory tests, information on latest methods of treatment, standard clinical protocols and guidelines, etc. Even a simple database management program can be used as a passive DSS. In contrast, active DSSs apply medical knowledge to a specific patient's data and recommend a specific conclusion or course of action (Barnett et al., 1987). Development of such systems represents a considerable challenge. Existing active DSSs include expert systems, computer reminders and alerts (Jenders et al., 1995; Silverman, 1997), dosage calculators, ECG analysis systems, and clinical guideline and protocol navigation systems (Liem et al., 1995).

Reviews on the effect of DSSs have shown improvement of physician performance, including appropriateness of drug dose, diagnosis accuracy, and overall quality of care, as well as demonstrating the utility of preventative care reminders (Sullivan and Mitchell 1995, Johnson et al., 1994). Lindberg and Humphreys (1998) find that the combination of computers, networks, on-line medical information and patient data can improve healthcare decisions, prevent dangerous oversights and reduce unnecessary cost. Computerised alert and order entry systems, in particular, have shown (Bates et al., 1998; Raschke et al., 1998) significant reduction in the number of adverse drug events and number of errors that lead to adverse drug events. In a recent review, Hunt et al. (1998) find an increasing number of studies in support of the hypothesis that clinical DSS can enhance clinician performance regarding drug dosage and preventative care, but the results were less convincing with respect to diagnosis. Additionally, they found there were insufficient numbers of studies on the impact of DSSs on patient outcomes.

While the evidence mounts in support of the utility of clinical guidelines (notably electronic guidelines that integrate with physician workflow), we need to carefully consider the exact role of the computer in the clinical decision making process. Traditional medical expert systems (rule-based reasoning programs) have existed, and been known to be effective for narrow clinical domains since the 1970s. Their utility suffers, however, due to a 'Greek Oracle' mentality (Miller & Maserie, 1990) – expert systems are substitute experts and with that carry a sense of authority. This is difficult to accept, since actual responsibility rests with the human practitioner. Situations where the user blindly follows the computer's suggestions or works in fear of being blamed for a "wrong" (counter to system advice) decision are highly undesirable (Pew, 1988). Administrative support of the formalized model can readily lead to real disincentives for physicians to use their own reasoning if it runs counter to the system (e.g., if the insurer only pays for the recommended treatment). Rather, the physician should be guided in making his/her own decision by being shown the relevant patient data, chain of reasoning and supporting evidence. In this way, we leave room for the broader quality of human decision making (as well as legitimate professional disagreement and discretion). This approach to decision support also serves to educate the physician such that ultimately they make more of the right, evidence-based decisions for themselves without the need for alerts or consultation to the DSS, leading to greater efficiency and professional satisfaction.

THE SA HEALTHPLUS COORDINATED CARE MODEL

Relatively new to Australia is the concept of *Coordinated Care*, which is being introduced by the Commonwealth Government as a range of trials. "The primary aim of the Coordinated Care trials is to examine whether coordinating care for people with complex needs through individual care plans and the pooling of funds from existing Federal, State and joint programmes will result in improved client care and well-being within current resource levels" (Wooleridge, 1996). The largest trial is within South Australia, under the control of the SA HealthPlus unit of the SA Department of Human Services (formerly the South Australian Health Commission), with 4500 patients enrolled. The trial focuses on patients with chronic and complex health problems that currently require high service use. Within the Healthplus trial there are individual projects based on region and health problem. Specific project foci include diabetes, cardiac, aged care, lung disease, somatization, back pain and complex illness. The trial began enrolling patients in July 1997 and runs through to the end of 1999.

Although the name may vary from country to country (as 'Managed,' 'Community,' 'Shared,' 'Integrated' or 'Coordinated' Care), the concept is of course nothing new to the developed world. Care Net Illawarra, an Australian Coordinated Care trial encompassing a region south of Sydney, sets out motivating issues for coordinated care that include (Foulston, 1997):

- GPs referring to higher levels of care because of patient expectations and absence of incentives for GPs to manage
- Poor communications between service providers
- Service providers powerless to solve inter-provider isolation

Perhaps the most fundamental objective is facilitating the proactive planning of interventions instead of a crisis reaction approach.

At the heart of such coordination is interchange of information, and thus it is natural to expect electronic patient records and related data networks to play a major role. A 'Shared Care' electronic patient record system in western Devon, UK, aims to address coordination issues by modeling more than just the historical medical record (Rigby & Robins, 1996). The system also models a proactive component, indicating the *care plan* and future treatment objectives. Moreover there is an emphasis on the aims of treatment, looking holistically at the patient, transcending the constraints of diagnoses and treatments per se. In the context of U.S. 'Managed Care,' The Personal Care Adviser programs (by the Patient InfoSystems company in conjunction with the Meridian Managed Care Corporation [Patient InfoSYSTEMS, 1997]) support management of asthma and diabetes. These programs provide ongoing personalized support for patients with chronic conditions through care services, compliance support and healthcare information. Focus on chronic diseases (which lead to high annual healthcare costs) is evidently a common theme for systems integrating computer-based patient records and decision support. In South Australia, Medical Communications Associates has developed diabetes and asthma management systems in collaboration with area hospitals, featuring decision support for patient assessment, and patient-specific color printouts of medication explanations to form part of the patient's care plan (Addams et al., 1997; Braund et al., 1997).

In the SA HealthPlus model of coordinated care each patient is designated a general practitioner (GP) as their Care Coordinator. This Care Coordinator formulates an individualised Care Plan designed to keep the patient as healthy as possible. Each HealthPlus patient is also assigned a Service Coordinator, generally a nurse with disease-specific training, that assists the GP in assessing and monitoring the patient. SA HealthPlus stresses proactive, evidence-based care and a holistic approach to the patient where the GP is encouraged to treat the patient's entire set of "problems," not just the principal diagnosis. Toward this end, Problem and Goal (P&G) statements in the patient's own words, are collected by the Service Coordinator, and progress on these patient-defined issues is monitored throughout the trial. A Base Care Plan of services – including domiciliary care, physiotherapy, and pathology – is set in accordance with condition severity, as determined by a program-specific Initial Medical Assessment. The Care Coordinator works with the patient to modify this base plan to suit the patient's individual needs. Medication management is also a major focus. Figure 1 illustrates the basic HealthPlus process, wherein cost containment is put aside initially, in order to deliver well-being that provides savings in the long run.

To fulfill the Care Coordinator role, the GP is provided with a broad profile of information on the patient (for which the patient has given informed consent). In particular, the HealthPlus Information System (HIS) draws together Commonwealth Health Insurance Commission data to track all reimbursable health expenditures made on the patient (in the Australian healthcare system this includes most drugs, pathology, hospital/emergency and health consultation services). This data is complemented with hospital database extracts and various other local sources (such as domiciliary care records), as well as the HealthPlus specific documents as per Figure 1. Periodic monitoring by the Service Coordinator also adds to the HIS record.

Figure 1: The SA HealthPlus Care Planning Process.

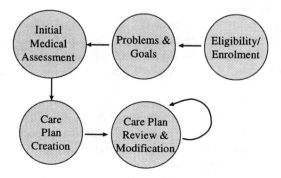

Each HealthPlus disease-specific program has a team of Care Mentors, including specialists, GPs, nurses and other health professionals. These care mentor groups have invested considerable effort to devise program-specific resources including guideline manuals, as well as the Base Care Plans and Initial Medical Assessment forms. The guidelines represent a consolidation of advice based on broad literature survey as well as the wisdom of the care mentor group. For instance, the guidelines for the Southern Chronic Lung Disease project (one of the 10 HealthPlus programs) cite European, British, American and Canadian, as well as Australian, sources. The odds of achieving implementable and accepted guidelines are maximized by using local opinion-leading health professionals who represent the spectrum of Coordinated Care service providers (not just specialists) and who understand local conditions.

The Base Care Plan (BCP) is a series of Level A services, dictated by the patient's severity level. Unless the GP has a specific reason to withdraw the service, all patients in a given project with a particular severity level receive the same Level A service. These services may include regular GP visits, diagnostic investigations (lung functions, blood sugar) and vaccinations. Based on a patient's specific problems, both clinical and personal (as expressed in the P&G statement), the GP may assign further B-level services. As an example: a moderate Respiratory patient will be assigned (as A-level services) two specialist visits and four GP visits per year, with education and physical assessment at each of these sessions. The GP may recommend that the client, due to mobility problems, requires physiotherapy sessions (a B-level service); and they may have eating difficulties, so a dietician visit will be built into the care plan (another B-level service). Additionally, the GP visits may be scheduled with a higher proportion of the visits falling in the winter or spring months, depending on whether cold weather or pollen most exacerbates this patient's problems. The result of tailoring the BCP is the Individual Care Plan.

CPOL ANALYSIS AND DESIGN

The systems analysis for CPOL revealed several key features of the system environment that the design must address:

1. **Patients are the central concern.** This is an obvious axiom of anything billed as Coordinated Care, but must not be lost in the details.

2. **The GPs face a number of forces which must be managed if they are to accept the system.** Despite involvement of GPs and nurses in Care Mentor groups, the HealthPlus model is pressing "best practice" guidance on the GP coordinators, which can be viewed as an affront to the GP's own knowledge, abilities and personal style. Despite all good intentions, cost is a huge concern, and from the Health Commission side there is a very apparent interest in showing that Coordinate Care satisfies its financial goals. Australian GPs are not especially technophillic – in a recent survey, only 14% were using computerized patient records (Bomba, 1997). In designing an innovative technical solution, we must not create a further obstacle for the GP. Cox and Walker (1993) assert that a "good tool" should be *transparent* to the user – they should be focused on the task, not the tool. With respect to each of the pressures of Care Mentors, Health Commission and Technology, we must create a solution that does not hinder the GP's ability to focus on the patient and to pursue a care solution that suits his/her individual style. The design of CPOL presents an opportunity to balance the external

pressures and possibly provide a degree of insulation from them.

3. **Information integration is a key benefit.** The SA HealthPlus framework provides a wide range of information sources, including those that are patient-specific (Initial Medical Assessments, Problem & Goal statements, hospital in-patient records, etc.) and those that are project-specific (care guidelines). As collections of paper forms and documents, they constitute an untidy jumble (or at least a very thick folder). Results from the HealthPlus core Information System (HIS) can (at least potentially) be accessed via specific computer applications using modem and/or CD ROM distribution; however, the resulting on-line information is not integrated with the care planning process. All relevant information sources must be brought onto the doctor's desktop in a coherent format.

4. **GP education is an objective.** Both the Care Mentors and the Health Commission express a desire to "educate" the GP on best practice, patient-centered care. There is a perceived need to transform GP behavior to be less focused on short-term clinical outcomes – to treat the whole patient – and to enhance GP awareness of the latest techniques. This effort must not be perceived as patronizing (or as a threat) and GP rejection of specific tenets from the Care Mentors must not result in rejection of the whole system. Education may be explicit or subtle, and both approaches are needed to suit the range of GP attitudes. Moreover, the GP may take an interest in self-education at any time – it may be a planned activity at the end of the day, but it may just be a sudden curiosity taken at the spur of the moment. The system must be supportive of an immediate divergence by the GP to pursue guidance information.

5. **Cost control is an objective.** The trial is not a success unless it can be defended as being at least cost neutral. The GPs must be cost aware as they plan care.

6. **The system must not be disease specific.** SA HealthPlus incorporates a range of chronic illnesses. Moreover, patients may present with more than one major illness (e.g., cardiac disease and respiratory disease are not at all uncommon to occur in the same patient). GPs can potentially work in more than one HealthPlus project. For all these reasons, we want one single coherent system that addresses all the HealthPlus projects. Even beyond this, however, HealthPlus is a trial: the overall scope of the HealthPlus solution (including its support software) should not be limited to the current range of disease foci.

7. **Decision support knowledge must be separable from the interface "engine."** This distinction came to the fore as a way to resolve the intellectual property rights of the various participants. However, it also is a sensible principal to achieve the needed flexibility and system maintainability.

In addition, several observations dictate the principles for our decision support strategy in CPOL. Our foremost design principal for CPOL is User Control (which is "good tool" principal number one by Cox and Walker [1993]). This arises for a number of reasons:

1. **The GP is responsible.** They are the Care Coordinator. It is their job to come up with the best possible Care Plan, and they have the right to remain in control of the task.

2. **A high degree of control is the only thing the GP will accept.** The GPs know they are responsible and they (not wrongly) have ego about their knowledge and firsthand experience. They do not want to be replaced by machines. They want control.

3. **The GPs are accustomed to control of their information resources.** While the GPs are not accustomed to access to as much information as they have in HealthPlus, a

Figure 2: CPOL System Architecture

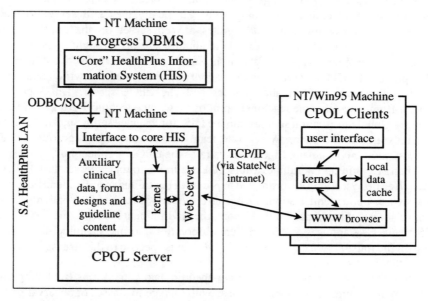

paper-based patient record or collection of forms does not tell the GP in which order they must read or work. GPs are used to organizing their work to their own personal style.

4. **GPs vary in the way they order the information.** When interviewed, GPs gave differing responses as to what information they would view first in formulating a care plan. Some would first look to medications, other to diagnosis, others to recent health events (e.g., hospital admissions). Since the patients are already diagnosed at the time of care planning, the task is less structured than a conventional consultation which might proceed in SOAP (Subjective, Objective, Analysis, Plan) order (Weed, 1969).

CPOL ARCHITECTURE

As mentioned briefly in the discussion of the SA HealthPlus coordinated care model, a HealthPlus Information System (HIS) was created to serve the basic needs of the HealthPlus trial. This HIS is not the CPOL system, but does serve as part of its infrastructure. The HIS was established using a conventional Windows NT-based relational database package (Progress DBMS). The principal purpose of the HIS is to collect information for the eventual evaluation of the HealthPlus trial. Since the trial has hypotheses concerning resource consumption, it is important that actual resource use is collected. This is done by matching of HealthPlus patient details to reimbursement records from the Commonwealth Health Insurance Commission and to area hospital databases. In fact, the HIS receives data updates from an ambitious statewide hospital data integration service based on the OACIS data integration tool. Care plan and patient Problem & Goal data are also recorded in the HIS to track other HealthPlus evaluation criteria: the extent to which actual services match planned ones, and the extent to which patients achieve their individual goals.

The CPOL system leverages the program evaluation data of the HIS to provide a clinical decision support tool and general on-line interface to SA HealthPlus. The CPOL system consists of server and client components. Physically, the CPOL server is a machine at the SA Health Commission that operates a Web server on the South Australian government's intranet (which is accessible to authorized staff throughout the state). This machine, running Windows NT, exists on the same Local Area Network as the HIS. Via ODBC queries, the CPOL server extracts patient data from, and can write updates to, the HIS. Clinical guideline information resides with the CPOL server. This separation is beneficial from a systems management point of view. One technical group can focus on integrating global information sources into the HIS (for instance setting up HL7 messaging to hospitals around the state). A separate team concentrates on supporting the CPOL decision support environment. Figure 2 illustrates the CPOL architecture.

When a HealthPlus coordinator (nurse, GP or administrator) accesses the CPOL server via their Web browser, they are prompted to provide HealthPlus specific identification code and password. Upon identification, the user is provided with a list of the patients for which they have access. When a patient is selected, the environment launches the CPOL client – an MS Visual C++ application – and patient observations, forms and guideline updates are sent down the line to invoke a session of CPOL that is specific to the disease-program and status of the given patient.

The CPOL server represents program-specific data entry forms (including clinical guidelines) in a common relational database with linkage to classes of observations made on patients (see Figure 3). When a patient is requested by a CPOL client, the server combines the latest relevant forms given the patient's status (for instance, whether they yet have a finalized Care Plan). The forms are populated with the known observations for the patient of the classes required by the forms. Many observations are in fact computed (derived) from other observations, including alert triggers, using prefix notation expressions stored in the same relational database.

Figure 3: Semantic Network Overview of CPOL Data Structures for Forms and Observations

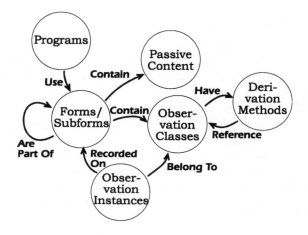

With this architecture, forms (such as for medical assessment) can be centrally updated without modification of the CPOL client. In fact, whole new data sources can be added to the HIS (such as the recent addition of domiciliary care data) and the CPOL server can be modified to query this new source and create a populated form which will appear as an information tab on the client. Fine adjustments can also be made centrally, such as deciding that two rather than three repeat measures of a diastolic blood pressure greater than or equal to 90 merits consideration of drug therapy. In addition, the "passive content" from Figure 3 can include URLs of HTML content held either locally on the CPOL server or at external sites. This is especially useful for the narrative "evidence" component of the clinical guidelines.

DECISION SUPPORT IN CPOL

Some authors suggest that guidelines are not intended to be taken literally but that rather they specify a "mixture of procedural and criterion-based knowledge, which the clinicians are tacitly expected to adjust and adapt according to the specifics of a case" (Gordon et al., 1997). As we had stated earlier, situations where the user blindly follows the computer's suggestions are highly undesirable, and medical practitioners hold the ultimate responsibility for their treatment decisions, and should quite rightly reject systems that try to force decisions they themselves are not comfortable in accepting. Certainly the present culture of Australian general practice does not permit dictating rigid care protocols. For this situation, CPOL provides decision support based on two principal methods:

- Contextual "flags" or warning markers that are persistently visible as the GP does care

Figure 4: CPOL Main Screen with Service Selection Tab

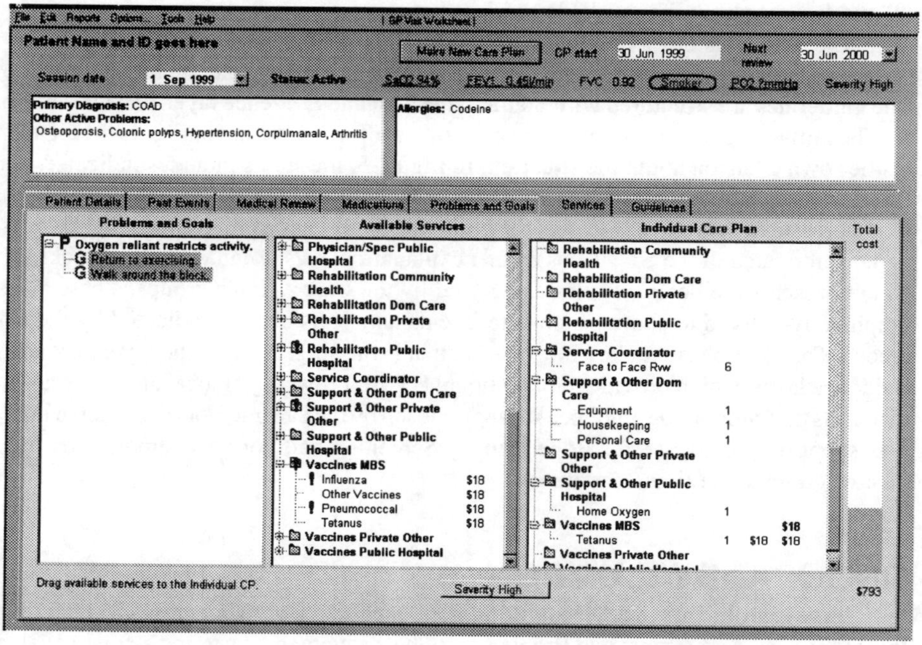

Figure 5: Status Section of Guideline in CPOL

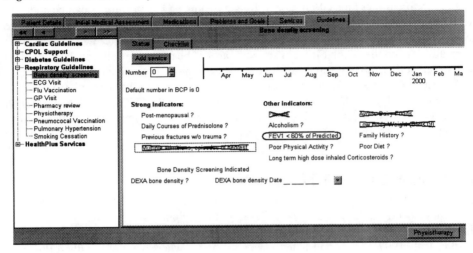

planning and encourage him/her to investigate relevant guidelines; and

• Random access to any part of the patient record or to any guideline at any time.

The central activity of SA HealthPlus care planning is establishing (and maintaining) the individualised schedule of service. The CPOL screen for this activity is shown in Figure 4. The top section provides key information that is to be always visible (such as allergies), including a set of program-specific indicator measures. These measures, plus the list of available services, are prime spots for guideline alert flags. Several appear on Figure 4 (the "!" mark symbols on the available services list).

The GP consults a guideline by right-clicking an alert flag, a service, or any observation that is linked to a specific guideline, or simply by selecting the Guideline tab. The guidelines are structured with Status, Checklist and Evidence layers (see Figures 5 and 6). The initial display is of problem-specific status information, encouraging the GP to make his/her own decision about the situation. In Figure 5, the status includes indicators for the Bone Density Screening service; the status display often includes a trend graph (e.g., for blood pressure or weight). Note that the guideline doubles as a problem-oriented worksheet or data entry area. If the GP wishes further explanation, he/she can view the Checklist layer which presents the decision rules as devised by the Care Mentor groups. These rules are graphically marked to show which antecedents and decisions are indicated by the patient record. The "?" flags mark key information that is missing. Finally, the GP can consult the Evidence layer, which provides conventional HTML browsing of local and external source materials that support the guidance strategy chosen by the care mentors (not shown in Figure 5 as supporting evidence for Bone Density Screening had not been supplied by the care mentor group at the time of writing).

ONGOING EVALUATION

Initial enrolments to SA HealthPlus were undertaken with paper forms, including the Initial Medical Assessment and Problems & Goals statement. As a first stage in evaluation

Figure 6: Checklist Tab — Cholesterol Guideline

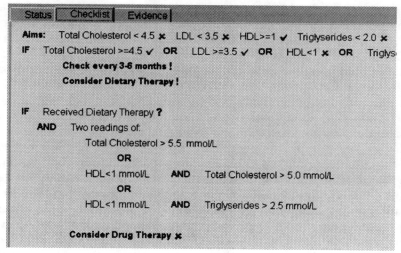

of CPOL, we have randomly selected 21 patients who have been manually care planned from the two respiratory disease programs is SA HealthPlus. For these patients, the initial medical assessment and P&G forms have been entered into CPOL and we have examined what services are flagged by the system. The forms were also given to three respiratory specialist Care Mentors.

We examined the B-level services flagged by CPOL in comparison to the recommendations of the Mentors and the assignments made by the actual Care Coordinators. In particular, nine B-Level services were examined: Dietician, Physiotherapy, Smoking Cessation, Flu Vaccination, Pneumococcal Vaccination, Pharmacy Medication Management (PMM), Bone Density Screening, Pulmonary Hypertension, and Blood Pressure. While some of these "services" represent direct specialist referrals or pathology tests, most also include monitoring, counselling and drug therapy activities. For each of the nine services, the system may provide an alert flag ("?" indicating that the service is possibly indicated and recommending that the GP consider the service guideline in more detail, or "!" indicating the service is clearly recommended according to the guidelines developed by the Care Mentors). The Mentors could decide to recommend the service, not recommend it, or that there was insufficient information to make a decision. The actual care plans developed previously by the Care Coordinators would either have the services included in the care plan or left out.

Totalling the three Mentors' decisions, there are 294 decisions where CPOL and the Mentor are in agreement (CPOL triggers a flag where the Mentor says Yes to the service, or CPOL makes no response where the Mentor says No) and 72 decisions where there is disagreement. There are 144 decisions where the Mentors judge there is insufficient information, and 91 cases where the CPOL had insufficient data input to cause a trigger. More specifically, there was 100% agreement between the Mentors and CPOL on the indication for Smoking Cessation, and 87% and 89% agreement on Influenza Vaccine and PMM service, respectively.

When comparing the decisions of the CPOL to those made by the Care Coordinators on paper, it was found there were 81 (out of a total of 147) decisions where the CPOL and CC were in agreement and 35 where there was disagreement, with the highest levels of agreement between the CC and CPOL on the Influenza Vaccination, Pneumococcal Vaccination and Smoking-Cessation services. In 29 cases, CPOL flags a service that the Care Coordinator did not put in the care plan, the majority involving Pneumococcal Vaccination, Bone Density Studies and the Dietician service. The Mentors' judgements generally support CPOL in that there was only one case in these 29 where CPOL flagged a service that all three of the Mentors judged should not be in the care plan, and in the majority of cases the two less conservative Mentors agree with CPOL.

Table 1 summarizes the experimental findings for the Pneumococcal Vaccination and Dietician services. Note that the Mentors varied considerably in their degree of conservatism about the sufficiency of the decision information on the initial medical assessment form (this is interesting in light of the fact that these same specialists helped design the form).

This initial investigation has indicated a few areas for enhancement of both the system, and possibly of the guidelines and procedures in HealthPlus generally. A less sensitive bone density triggering function is being investigated to reduce what some Mentors saw as false positives (Bone Density Studies received a "?" flag for all females). The use of fuzzy logic for the calculation of bone density risk score appears appropriate and is currently being investigated. The study also indicates the need for more definite criteria in the IMA to indicate the Physiotherapy service, which Mentors judged largely on the basis of free text in the P&G statement (fuzzy logic may once again be relevant).

With respect to evaluation of the SA HealthPlus trial of coordinated care, in general, official results are not yet available. However, preliminary findings indicate that there is benefit in terms of cost saving and improved patient outcomes for some groups, chiefly at the higher severity levels. The Commonwealth Government barred the release of findings of its coordinated care trials until after the end of 1999.

Informal observation of Care Coordinators and SA HealthPlus staff has shown that different users approach the interface in different ways. Supporting staff (nurse Service Coordinators and central office staff) are likely to log on for a specific maintenance task, to update the patient record based on a fact that has been observed via receipt of a paper form, visit to the patient, or as the result of a phone call. One day the majority of observations may

Table 1: Comparison of Specialist (Mentor) Decisions, CPOL Alerts, GP Care Coordinator (CC) Actions for Pneumoccocal Vaccination and Dietician Service Assignments to Care Plans of 21 Chronic Respiratory Patients.

Pneumo Vacc.

		Mentor 1			Mentor 2			Mentor 3		
		Yes	No	Insufficient	Yes	No	Insufficient	Yes	No	Insufficient
CPOL	Alert (! or ?)	1	-	19	20	-	-	9	2	8
	No Alert	-	1	-	-	1	-	-	1	-
CC	Yes	1	1	12	13	1	-	5	3	6
	No	-	-	7	7	-	-	4	-	2

Dietician

		Mentor 1			Mentor 2			Mentor 3		
		Yes	No	Insufficient	Yes	No	Insufficient	Yes	No	Insufficient
CPOL	Alert (! or ?)	5	-	3	5	3	-	6	1	1
	No Alert	1	-	12	2	10	1	3	4	5
CC	Yes	1	-	-	1	-	-	1	-	-
	No	5	-	15	6	13	1	8	5	6

be entered immediately using mobile (and possibly pen or voice-based) computing, but at present paper still plays a major role. The staff log on, open the appropriate patient record, move directly to the appropriate tab, enter data and log off (or close the patient and move on to the next patient to update as part of an end-of-day process). Such transactions are common for recording Problem and Goal progress, updating the medication record, recording ongoing clinical observations, and adjusting the detailed schedule of appointments. One surprise was to find some staff using the guideline index (a la the left-hand section of Figure 5) rather than the service tab (as in Figure 4) to enter and update service levels when multiple services were being modified. This illustrates a degree of success in the CPOL design in that the boundary between guideline and patient data is sufficiently blurred that users are spontaneously crossing where we believed that boundary to be.

With GP (Care Coordinator) users, the pattern of use is less directed since they are making an overall judgement of the patient's condition and establishing a new (or modified) care plan. It is for this purpose that the interface is intended to provide its range of decision support. The GP will generally review the key patient information at the top of the screen and then move left-to-right through the tabs, possibly updating clinical observations based on newer pathology data (in a fully integrated electronic healthcare system this would be automatic, but was not in the scope of our trial). The GP may pop over to the service tab out of the left-to-right sequence if struck by the significance of a co-morbidity (secondary diagnosis), clinical observation (with or without alert flag), or a problem the patient has reported. Eventually the GP works his/her way over to the service tab (the next-to-last tab in the left-to-right sequence) and will invariable review the complete list of services to decide if any further services should be added to the patient's care plan. Since the list is rather long, we believe our alert flags play an important role here to focus GP attention. To establish a detailed schedule for a given service, the GP opens the service Status (the main section of Figure 5) and operates the timeline control. Users find this control intuitive for directly positioning services within the year or "spinning" up a number of consistently spaced repeats of a service (e.g., six GP visits, two months apart). A surprise is that the GPs, like the support staff, are frequently drawn to the left-hand index. The physicians tend to review the set of key guidelines grouped under the patient's disease-specific project area (rather than the comprehensive listing which mirrors the service tab). This behavior is very promising for ultimate care plan quality since the project-specific services represent exactly those services the Care Mentors felt should be emphasized to the Care Coordinators.

A chief goal for the remainder of 1999 is systematic observation of CPOL usage, notably to log GP usage patterns and test hypotheses concerning the way users react to the decision support information, as well as examining the overall effect on care plan quality.

FUTURE TRENDS

There is little question that the trend to use Web-based architectures to support health information systems will continue. From the early days of Mosaic the technology was well-suited to distribution of information like patient data and clinical guidelines due to its platform-independence, inherit wide-area distribution and the ability to embed graphics with text. Issues of security and confidentiality of patient data have plagued such Web applications from the start. Their resolution, however, will require more than technology—only when we can arrive at a well-defined policy of who should have access to our information, and under what circumstances, can we hope to formulate a technical solution that suits the societal requirements. Until then the obvious utility of the Web will drive rampant implementation with haphazard attempts at security.

A more interesting question about the future of Web-based health information systems is that of their precise form. How structured should they be? Should they be comprehensive or purpose-built solutions? How integrated should the record be with decision support? And how abstract should the system designs be? With respect to this, the CPOL architecture is structured, purpose-built, tightly integrates records with decision support, and is moderately abstract (and thus flexible)—however, these are not the only defensible choices.

If we simply want to "coordinate" (i.e., share information), then the key element is that all healthcare providers know how to access the same information. If the information is readily available, comprehensive (within the scope of relevance of the given providers), and legible then it is well-suited to the task. Brooks (1999) describes an intranet-based system in New York State that provides extensible patient folders with this character. The information need not be rigorously structured to satisfy this coordination. One can imagine a virtual "whiteboard" (Coiera, 1999), essentially a patient's individual Web page, that can take entries from any authorized provider, as a technically simple but adequate solution to many needs.

If we do elect to have structure beyond free text in our health information systems, there are ample sources of recommendations on what those structures may be. At one end of the spectrum, clinical coding schemes, such as the Read Clinical Codes (notably version 3), provide the mechanism to record symptoms, diagnoses, pathology tests, etc. by selection of concepts and qualifiers from a well-defined (albeit enormous) set. Health Level 7 (HL7) defines a standard structure for messages between health information systems (HL7 is the official recommendation of Standards Australia for clinical messaging). While structure in the messages between systems, does not specifically require any particular structure within a system, the forming HL7 version 3 proposal includes a domain information model (Rishel, 1996). More advanced on this front is the EU-based Good Electronic Health Record (GEHR) proposal that describes the conceptual data architecture for high-quality and standardised clinical health information representation in terms of a hierarchy of objects (Lloyd, 1997). There also clinical guideline structures, such as the Guideline Interchange Format (GLIF; Patel et al., 1998). The Extensible Markup Language (XML) is intended to be a vehicle for structure across the range of Web content. This includes, for instance, HL7 messages, for which there is an SGML/XML working group.

Most proposals and mechanisms for structure in health information content attempt to encompass the entire range of clinical activity, such as the aforementioned Read Clinical Codes, or ICD10, which encompasses the full range of medical diagnoses. However, there may be some benefit in fitting solutions to more specific targets. For instance, the International Classification for Primary Care (ICPC, Lamberts & Woods, 1987) is a clinical coding scheme set to the coarser granularity appropriate in general practice medicine. As such it is much simpler and more compact than Read or ICD10. In this vane, CPOL does not attempt to be a general-purpose electronic patient record or guidance system; it restricts its scope to care coordination in the focus diseases of SA HealthPlus (although the architecture can expand to suit further diseases).

We have already reviewed the significant benefits that can be achieved through automatic alert and reminder systems. These decision aids can only be implemented if the key concepts are represented in the system in a structured fashion. It is not, however, necessary (or always sufficient!) to have a comprehensive clinical coding structure for all information in the database. The key is to have the necessary decision information coded to the level required for alerts and reminders. Without this, decision support must be passive in the sense that the physician seeks out the DSS features. A notable attempt to refine passive DSS is the Stanford Health Information Network for Education (SHINE, Godin et al., 1999). SHINE uses an SGML (progenitor to XML and HTML) structure to decision information to aid searching. The SHINE team is also exploring use of the massive U.S. National Institute of Health's Unified Medical Language System (UMLS) meta thesaurus to expand physician search queries to take in related terms. Furthermore, SHINE offers an innovative solution to the problem of rewarding physicians for time spent in consulting DSSs—award them continuing medical education (CME) credit for using the system.

The typical health information system today is not flexible. Decisions about data, clinical knowledge, the model of care and modes of presentation are inextricably inter-twined in program code and screen designs. CPOL achieves a degree of flexibility via its separation of forms (including guidelines), data, and the client presentation software. The ideal system will have explicit, and largely independent, models of data, knowledge, "business process" and presentation (see Figure 7). With respect to hypertension, for instance:

- The data model would contain the patient's history of blood pressure levels, weight, diet, history of heart disease and other relevant factors.
- The knowledge model would represent recommended blood pressure levels, and known therapies, including their indications, contraindications and side-effects, as well as reference to supporting studies.
- The "business process" model would determine roles and responsibilities in terms of monitoring, treatment and follow-up.
- The presentation model would determine what a certain urgency of hypertension alert might look like, as well as defining how to render the relevant data and knowledge (e.g., in a three-tabbed status, checklist, evidence structure as CPOL does).

In such an ideal architecture, the client workstation code is an abstract framework and the particular screen presentation is not explicitly programmed, but just happens as an interaction of the models. In this way it can be highly flexible if different evidence, healthcare roles, or decision support paradigms (perhaps one making more use of sound!) are introduced.

While our ideal model may not turn out to be the exact shape of the future, the move to greater modularity and flexibility is essential to achieve a coherent best-practice clinical workstation environment for all of the many healthcare roles and processes in the world. Internet technology, portable languages like Java, and structure standards like XML support such innovation. The CPOL team is making its own small steps in this direction by exploring a next-generation architecture that employs *decorator patterns* (Gamma et al., 1995). A decorator is a class of object that provides a transparent interface for another object, while also adding some additional functions (e.g., a border or scrollbar may be a decorator on a text-control object). Currently the CPOL client knows about a dozen fixed types of presentation control (e.g., free text, numeric entry, etc.). The capability to work with these controls is hard-coded into the client. In the next generation CPOL we will be able to apply a decorator to any of various ActiveX controls produced in popular visual programming environments. The decorator will provide the management methods needed by the CPOL framework to provide its database storage and DSS integration functions. In this way it will

Figure 7: An ideal health information system architecture where the clinical workstation interface is a dynamic result of model interaction, not a hard-coded construct.

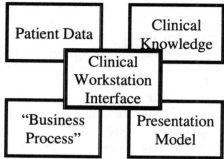

be possible to dynamically load new types of visual controls for clinical observations without redesigning (and recompiling and redistributing) the CPOL client.

CONCLUSIONS

In this chapter we have discussed the context and architecture of the Care Plan On-Line (CPOL) system. This web-based (intranet-based) system provides a single coherent source whereby the GP can review the available information on an SA HealthPlus Coordinated Care patient in the context of devising a proactive and holistic Care Plan. In the same application environment where the GP specifies the Care Plan, CPOL provides access to clinical practice guidelines tailored for SA HealthPlus. Moreover, the GP is signaled to investigate guidelines that may be relevant to the case at hand and finds problem-specific patient status information integrated with the guideline display. The guidelines are layered to promote understanding and to encourage the GP to buy into the reasoning of the Care Mentor groups that have devised them, rather than merely to dictate a decision.

CPOL exemplifies an approach to IT-enabled healthcare where a specific — and in this case proactive and patient-centred — model of care is integrated with the patient record and customised decision support. The use of Web/intranet architecture is a natural fit to enable this sort of ubiquitous wide-area IT infrastructure across a virtual community of Care Coordinators. As well as providing up-to-the-minute patient data from sources statewide, the guidelines and data collection forms can be centrally reconfigured at any time, in many places using conventional HTML technology.

We do not assert that the SA HealthPlus model is ideal for all places and all patient circumstances. In HealthPlus the GP (in partnership with the patient) is given ultimate control of a 12-month proactive Care Plan. In other circumstances, different controllers and different time-scales may be warranted. For instance, establishing the focus of control at hospitals, district nursing services, or with social workers may be more appropriate for cancer patients, the frail elderly and the homeless, respectively. However, the CPOL/HealthPlus experience illustrates the mechanism by which computing can be used to channel control, data and decision knowledge to specific controlling entities to undertake care by a specific model in ways quite at variance to (and more coherent than) the surrounding healthcare system. The flexibility of the IT architecture means that minimal lead time is required for a health authority to trial and ultimately establish a healthcare model that best serves a segment of its citizenry.

ACKNOWLEDGMENTS

The authors gratefully acknowledge the financial support of the Australian Research Council and The Queen Elizabeth Hospital Thoracic Medicine Unit, as well as the advice of Prof. Dick Ruffin, Dr. Brian Smith and Dr. Peter Frith, the cooperation of the SA HealthPlus Unit of the South Australian Department of Human Service, and the expertise of Dr. Gleb Beliakov and Heath Frankel in implementation of the CPOL software.

REFERENCES

Adams, R., Ruffin, R., Smith B., Campbell, D. & Dippy, S. (1997). Problems and some solutions in adapting clinical practice guidelines for Asthma patient management into a computerised management system. The Western Region asthma project (Wrapp). In, *Proc. Asia Pacific Assoc. of Med. Informatics / Health Informatics Soc. of Australia (APAMI-HIC97) Joint Conf.* Brunswick East, Victoria: Health Informatics Society of Australia.

Barnes, M. & Barnett, G. (1995). An architecture for a distributed guideline server, JAMIA, *Symposium Suppl.*, 233-237.

Barnett, G., Cimino, J., Hupp, J., Hoffer, E. (1987). DXplain. An evolving diagnostic decision-support system, *JAMA 258*, 67-74.

Bates, D., Leape, L., Cullen, D., Laird, N., Petersen, L., Teich, J., Burdick, E., Hickey, M., Kleefield, S., Shea, B., Vander Vliet, M., Seger, D. (1998). Effect of computerised physician order entry and a team intervention on prevention of serious medication errors, *JAMA 280*, 1311-1316.

Bolton, P., Usher, H., Mira, M., Prior, G. & Harding, L. (1996). Description of and results from a computerised data collection in primary care. In, (McGuiness, B. & Leeder, T., Eds.) *Proceedings of the Fourth National Health Informatics Conference.* Health Informatics Society of Australia, Melbourne.

Bomba, D. (1997). Australian General Practitioners and electronic patient records (EPRs). In, *Proc. Asia Pacific Assoc. of Med. Informatics / Health Informatics Soc. of Australia (APAMI-HIC97) Joint Conf.* Brunswick East, Victoria: Health Informatics Society of Australia.

Bouhaddou, O., Frucci, L., Cofrin, K., Larsen, D., Warner, H., Huber, P., Sorenson, D., Turner, C. & Warner, H. (1994). Implementation of practice guidelines in a clinical setting using a computerised knowledge base (Iliad), *JAMIA, Symposium Suppl.*, 258-263.

Braund, W., Dippy, S., Schloeffel, P., Sickles, D. & Dalidowicz, L. (1997). A specialised electronic network to coordinate expert care of diabetes. In, *Proc. Asia Pacific Assoc. of Med. Informatics / Health Informatics Soc. of Australia (APAMI-HIC97) Joint Conf.* Brunswick East, Victoria: Health Informatics Society of Australia.

Brooks, R. (1999). Using an intranet for physician desk top data consolidation. In, *Proc. 32nd Hawai'i International Conference on Systems Sciences (HICSS-32)*, IEEE Computer Society Press.

Cimino, J., Sengupta, S., Clayton, P., Patel, V., Kushniruk, A. & Huang, X. (1998). Architecture for a Web-based clinical information system that keeps the design open and access closed, *JAMIA Symposium Suppl.*, 121-125.

Cimino, J., Socratous, S. & Clayton, P. (1995). Internet as clinical information system:

application development using the World Wide Web, *JAMIA 2*, 273-284.

Coiera, E. (1999). Personal communications, University of New South Wales, 13 April.

Cox K. & Walker D. (1993). *User Interface Design*, 2nd ed., Prentice Hall.

Eddy, D. (1990). Clinical decision making: from theory to practice, *JAMA 270*, 520-6

Einsenberg, D. (1986). Clinical decision making: from theory to practice, *Practice Policies - Guidelines for Methods 263*, 1839-41.

Foulston, J. (1997). *Care Net Illawarra: A Coordinated Care Trial.* Dapto, NSW, Australia: Care Net Illawarra.

Gamma, E., Helm, R., Johnson, R. & Vlissides, J. (1995). *Design Patters: Elements of Reusable Object Oriented Software*. Reading Massachusetts: Addison Wesley.

Godin, P., Hubbs, R., Woods, B., Tsai, M., Nag, D., Rindfleish, T., Dev, P. & Melmon, K. (1999). A new instrument for medical decision support and education: the Stanford health information network for education. In, *Proc. 32nd Hawai'i International Conference on Systems Sciences (HICSS-32)*, IEEE Computer Society Press.

Gordon, C., Johnson, P., Waite, C., Veloso, M. (1997). Algorithm and care pathway: clinical guidelines and healthcare process. In, *Proc. AIME Conf*, pp. 66-69.

Grimshaw, J. & Russell, I. (1993). Effect of clinical guidelines on medical practice: a systematic review of rigorous evaluations, *Lancet 324*, 1317-1322.

Hunt, D., Haynes, R., Hanna, S., & Smith, K. (1998). Effects of computer-based clinical decision support systems on physician performance and patient outcomes, *JAMA 280*, 1339-1346.

Jenders, R., Hripcsak, G., Sideli, R., DuMouchel, W., Zhang, H., Cimino, J., Johnson, S., Shareman, E. & Clayton, P. (1995). Medical decision support: experience with implementing the Arden syntax at the Columbia-Presbyterian medical center, *JAMIA, Symposium Suppl.*, 169-173.

Johnson, M., Langton, K., Haynes, R. (1994). Effects of computer-based clinical decision support systems on clinician performance and patient outcomes, *Ann. Intern. Med. 120*, 135-142.

Klein, M. & Methlie, L. (1995). *Knowledge-Based Decision Support Systems*, Wiley.

Kosecoff J, Kanouse D, Rogers W, McCloskey L, Winslow C, & Brook R. (1987) Effects of National Institutes of Health Consensus Development Program on Physician practice, *JAMA, 258*, 2708-2713.

Lamberts, H. & Woods, M. (1987). ICPC, *International Classification of Primary Care*. Oxford: Oxford University Press.

Leape L. (1990). Practice guidelines and standards: An overview, *Quarterly Review Bulletin 16*, 42-49.

Liem, E., Obeid, J., Shareck, E., Sato, L. & Greenes, R. (1995). Representation of clinical practice guidelines through an interactive World-Wide-Web interface. *JAMIA, Symposium Suppl.*, 223-227.

Lindberg, D. & Humphreys, B. (1998). Medicine and health on the Internet, *JAMA 280*, 1303-1304.

Lloyd, D. (1997). The Good European Health Record Project. Centre for Health Informatics & Multiprofessional Education (CHIME). URL: http://www.chime.ucl.ac.uk/HealthI/GEHR/

Lobach, D. (1995). A model for adapting clinical guidelines for electronic implementation in primary care, *JAMIA, Symposium Suppl.*, 581-585.

Lobach, D. & Hammond, W. (1994). Development and evaluation of a computer-assisted management protocol (CAMP): Improved compliance with care guidelines for diabetes mellitus. In, *Proc. SCAMC '94*, pp. 787-791.

Lomas J, Anderson G, Domnick-Pierre K, Vayda E, Enkin M, & Hannah W. (1989) Do practice guidelines guide practice? The effect of a consensus statement on the practice of physicians. *New England Journal of Medicine, 321*, 1306-1311.

Lomas J, Enkin M, Anderson G, Hannah W, Vayda E, & Singer J. (1991) Opinion leaders vs audit and feedback to implement practice guidelines. *JAMA, 265*(17), 2202-2207.

Pierre K. (1991) Obstetrical attitudes and practices before and after the Canadian consensus statement on cesarean birth, *Soc. Sci. Med., 32*, 1283-1289.

Lam, S. (1994). Implementation and evaluation of practice guidelines, *JAMIA, Symposium Suppl.*, 253-263.

Miller, R. & Maserie, F. (1990). The demise of the 'Greek Oracle' model for medical diagnostic systems, *Methods of Information in Medicine 29*, 1-2.

Patient InfoSYSTEMS. (1997). Patient Infosystems announces agreement for Diabetes and Asthma Disease management programs. 16 June, URL: http://www.pathfinder.com

Pew, R. (1988). Human factors issues in expert systems. In (Helander, M., ed.), *Handbook of Human-Computer Interaction*. Elsevier / North-Holland.

Quaglini, S., Saracco, R., Stefanelli, M. & Fassino, C. (1997). Supporting tools for guideline development and dissemination. In, *Proc. 6th Conf. On Artificial Intelligence in Medicine Europe*, pp. 39-50.

Raschke, R., Gollihare, B., Wunderlich, T., Guidry, J., Leibowitz, A., Peirce, J., Lemelson, L., Heisler, M., Susong, C. (1998). A computer alert system to prevent injury from adverse drug events, *JAMA 280*, 1317-1320.

Rigby, M & Robins, S. (1996). Practical success of an electronic patient record system in community care - a manifestation of the vision and discussion of the issues, *Int. J. Bio-Med. Comp 42*, 117-122.

Rishel, W. (1996) HL7 Version 3: Overview. URL: http://nelle.mc.duke.edu/standards/HL7/pubs/version3/version-3-intro/index.htm, accessed 13 May, 1999.

Shiffman, R. (1997). Representation of clinical practice guidelines in conventional and augmented decision tables, *JAMIA 4*, 382-393.

Shortliffe, E. (1987). Computer programs to support clinical decision making, *JAMA 258*, 61-66.

Silverman, B. (1997). Computer reminders and alerts, *Computer*, Jan., 42-49.

Sullivan F, Mitchell E. (1995) Has general practitioner computing made a difference to patient care? A systematic review of published reports. *BMJ 311*, 848-52.

Wall, E. (1993). Practice Guidelines: promise or panacea? *J. Fam. Prac. 37*(1), 17-29.

Weed, L. (1969) *Medical Records, Medical Education and Patient Care*, Case Western Reserve: Cleveland.

Wooldridge M. (1996). *Coordinated care gets the green light*. Commonwealth Department of Health and Family Services, Media Release, 20 Sept. URL: http://www.health.gov.au/hfs/mediarel/ mw7396.htm

Zielstorff R. (1998). Online practice guidelines, *JAMIA 5*, 227-236.

Chapter XII

Using Web-Enabled Technology to Promote the Adoption of Practice Guidelines

James G. Anderson
Purdue University

Linda L. Casebeer, Robert E. Kristofco and Angela S. Carillo
University of Alabama School of Medicine

The rapid expansion of scientific knowledge brings increased physician uncertainty in clinical decisionmaking. Clinical practice guidelines have been developed to reduce physician uncertainty. The broad movement to develop and disseminate clinical practice guidelines is rooted in evidence-based medicine. Although the development and dissemination of evidence-based guidelines has increased dramatically over the past decade, studies indicate serious deficiencies in the adoption of guidelines into practice. Developments such as client/server networks, the Internet, and the World Wide Web are rapidly expanding potential educational applications for information and communications technologies and the capacity for introducing strategies to promote guideline adoption. Web-enabled computer technology can enhance the capability of healthcare information systems to reduce variation in clinical decisionmaking.

Healthcare information systems contain various types of information and data that contribute to clinical decisions made by physicians and other healthcare providers. Some data are patient specific; other types of information and data provide general parameters or frameworks for decisionmaking. Sophisticated links within some systems provide specific guidance at the time a decision is being made, such as the contraindication of a drug by a recent laboratory test for a hospitalized patient. Healthcare organizations, whatever the status of their information systems, wish to reduce variation such as the variation in clinical decisionmaking. Many approaches have been tried to reduce variation including the development of clinical practice guidelines, audit and feedback of information, educational courses, opinion leaders, academic detailing, and computerized reminder systems, but variation remains widespread (Anderson, 1994; Davis, Thomson, Oxman and Haynes, 1992, 1995; Davis and Taylor-Vaisey, 1997; Oxman, Thomson, Davis and Haynes, 1995).

The Internet is an increasingly popular medical information resource for consumers (Classen, 1998). In a 1997 survey 43% of about 40.6 million U.S. adults 18 or older who had accessed the Web did so to obtain health information (Classen, 1998). At least 10,000 health and medical sites are on the World Wide Web (Ferguson, 1998). Physicians cannot only use the Web for patient management tasks, personal and professional learning but are able to offer their patients high quality resources online that can be personalized for them (Ferguson, 1998). Relatively recent developments such as client/server networks, the Internet, and the World Wide Web are rapidly expanding potential educational applications for information and communications technologies and the capacity for introducing secondary strategies to promote guideline adoption (Chodorow, 1996; Masys, 1998; Sebaldt, 1997; Yolton, 1992). Evolving computer and instructional technologies are increasing the use of hypermedia, virtual reality, teleconferencing, and distance education (Dunnington and DaRosa, 1994). Use of hypermedia publications through the Internet is now common. Hypermedia is based on HTML format and can be easily developed and distributed by a Web server (Schulz, Schrader and Klar, 1997). The Internet provides access to a wide range of literature, educational materials, resources, and communication opportunities. The Internet can be used for self-guided education and collaboration. Internet-based continuing medical education modules incorporate multimedia and can be utilized at the physician's convenience (Davis, Wythe, Rozum and Gore, 1997; Jaffe and Lynch, 1995; Jewett, Holsinger, Kuppersmith and Buenting, 1998; Qayumi, 1997; Henry, 1990; Klar and Bayer, 1990).

The purpose of this chapter is to present a Web-enabled technology which will enhance the capability of healthcare information systems to reduce variation in clinical decision-making. The objectives of this chapter are to: 1) describe an electronic strategy designed to promote clinical practice guideline adoption; 2) provide a template for those who wish to develop a Web-enabled strategy to promote clinical practice guideline adoption; and 3) present preliminary data on the effectiveness of a Web-enabled strategy in influencing clinical decisionmaking.

DISSEMINATION OF PRACTICE GUIDELINES

The rapid expansion of scientific knowledge leads to increased physician uncertainty in clinical decisionmaking (Gerrity, Earp, DeVellis & Light, 1992; Kassirer, 1989; Peterson & Pitz, 1988). Ambiguity can be introduced into clinical decisionmaking by the presence of conflicting evidence or by a lack of evidence about the probability of outcomes (Curley, Young & Yates, 1989). In a large study of physician uncertainty, most physicians worried they could not keep up with the medical literature, and most felt they had not been fully aware of the degree of uncertainty medicine entailed when they chose it as a career (Marks, 1997). One study found that the stress physicians experience in dealing with uncertainty has a negative effect on their clinical performance (Anderson, Jay, Weng & Anderson, 1995).

In an attempt to reduce clinical uncertainty and resultant practice variation, numerous clinical practice guidelines have been developed over the past 15 years and distributed in various formats by the Agency for Health Care Policy and Research, medical specialty societies, health maintenance organizations, and third-party payers (Institute of Medicine, 1990). The widening role of practice guidelines represents a significant innovation in the decision making process. These guidelines provide clinicians with information about the benefits of treatment and management strategies for specific conditions (e.g., stroke prevention in atrial fibrillation patients). Their purpose is to encourage more cost-effective care and to improve clinical outcomes.

The broad movement to develop and disseminate clinical practice guidelines is rooted in evidence-based medicine (Guyatt, Sackett and Cook, 1994). Although the development and dissemination of evidence-based guidelines have increased dramatically over the past decade, studies indicate serious deficiencies in the adoption of guidelines into practice (Davis & Taylor-Vaisey, 1997). Results of multiple studies and reviews have noted that the development and dissemination of evidence-based guidelines do not guarantee their use. Evidence-based guidelines have been more effective in raising physician awareness than they have been in improving physician performance (Davis and Taylor-Vaisey, 1997; Kaiser Foundation, 1998; Gorton, Cranford, Golden, Walls and Pawelak, 1995; Grilli and Lomas, 1994).

The problems inherent in reducing variation by promotion of guideline adoption are many. While healthcare systems have incentives for reducing variation in practice, individual physicians have fewer incentives to adopt guidelines. Lack of adequate resources is the largest barrier to guideline adoption, particularly lack of physician and staff time and lack of adequate reimbursement for many aspects of guideline recommendations. Primary care physicians are responsible for a broad knowledge base. Often, the focus of one medical specialty competes with that of others for the primary care physician's time and attention. For example, evidence-based guidelines for preventive health measures such as smoking cessation may compete with guidelines for complex chronic diseases such as congestive heart failure. Resources available to implement recommendations have been severely restricted in many managed care environments. Patient variables also serve as barriers to guideline adoption. Personal attributes of physicians such as levels of experience, knowledge, attitudes and skills may serve as barriers to adoption.

Several factors affect the adoption of guidelines, including incentives, available resources, regulations, patient factors, and the quality of evidence presented (Davis & Taylor-Vaisey, 1997; Kaiser Foundation, 1998). In addition to these factors, current models suggest that physicians may be more influenced by personal attributes (i.e., attitudes, habits, values, competence, and experience) than by other factors in decisions to adopt evidence-based guideline recommendations (Kaiser Foundation, 1998). Researchers studying the diffusion and adoption of HIV evidence-based guidelines have recently noted that the complex influence of physician attributes on guideline adherence demonstrates the need for specific and innovative implementation strategies (Kaiser Foundation, 1998). Experience and the hypothetical construct of physician reaction to uncertainty are key attributes of particular interest in the search for innovative guideline implementation strategies.

There are many issues related to implementing strategies designed to reduce variation in clinical decisionmaking. The explosion of medical knowledge during the past decade, as well as the large increase in the number of evidence-based clinical practice guidelines are symptoms of a growing dilemma. While the increase in medical knowledge is increasing uncertainty, many healthcare systems are attempting to reduce uncertainty and variation by providing practitioners with clinical practice guidelines and other tools designed to provide a framework for decisionmaking. At the same time, the Web has made a vast array of knowledge available to practitioners without efficient means of accessing knowledge at the point of use. Clinical practice guidelines are often posted on the Web, but physicians are not given opportunities to apply the knowledge to specific cases.

An issue of major concern to healthcare systems is finding effective and efficient strategies to reduce variation in practice in order to increase quality of care and reduce costs. While many evidence-based guidelines have been carefully developed for the purpose of using synthesized medical knowledge to reduce variation, a huge gap exists in the adoption of these guidelines into practice. A methodology for the analysis and synthesis of medical evidence into appropriate guidelines has emerged over the past decade, allowing evidence to be appropriately quantified into practice recommendations, although in some cases the available evidence may be weak. For the most part, the synthesis of evidence has provided strong consensus statements of use to practitioners.

Traditional guideline dissemination strategies have included primary and secondary strategies (Davis & Taylor-Vaisey, 1997). Primary strategies are those used first to disseminate evidence-based guidelines, including direct mail, publications in scientific journals and newsletters, Web-postings and electronic data bases, press conferences, and announcements at professional conferences. The purpose of using primary strategies is to develop a consensus on evidence available to practitioners, patients, and other interested parties.

Primary dissemination strategies such as publication and mailing have not demonstrated significant impact on adoption of guidelines into practice. Governmental agencies and specialty societies have committed large amounts of financial resources to publish and mail evidence-based guidelines they have developed. The financial resources dedicated to such strategies, however, have created controversies since they have not been highly effective.

Since primary strategies have been insufficient to ensure guideline adoption, a number of secondary strategies have been developed and implemented with varying success. Physicians report they attend continuing education activities, most often formally organized CME conferences, to maintain and improve professional knowledge and skills in order to provide the best possible care (Putnam & Campbell, 1989). Live traditional CME programs,—sometimes supplemented by video—and case presentations, have been the most frequently used secondary strategy; large amounts of resources have been dedicated to this format even though evidence demonstrates the effects to be weak. However, didactic, traditional CME conferences have had weak effects in facilitating guideline adoption or in changing physician behavior where agendas other than guideline diffusion have been the focus (Bero et al., 1998; Davis, Thomson, Oxman & Haynes, 1992, 1995; Davis & Taylor-Vaisey, 1997; Oxman, 1993, 1995).

Little attention has been paid to enabling strategies which have been demonstrated to enhance adoption of guidelines, strategies such as audit and feedback, reminder systems, academic detailing, multiple interventions, and the largely untested Internet and computer-assisted instruction. Academic detailing, and the use of multiple interventions have been relatively strong in facilitating guideline adoption (Avorn, Chen and Hartley, 1982; Avorn and Soumerai, 1983; Davis and Taylor-Vaisey, 1997; Soumerai and Avorn, 1990; Soumerai et al, 1998). Computerized reminder systems have also been relatively strong in changing physician behavior and in facilitating guideline development (Davis and Taylor-Vaisey, 1997; McDonald, Wilson and McCabe, 1980; McDonald, Hui & Smith, 1984; McDonald, Hui and Tierney, 1992; Overhage, Tierney and McDonald, 1996). More recent strategies have included computer-based strategies and the use of the Internet (Kaiser Foundation, 1998). These strategies have yet to be fully evaluated (Davis, Thomson, Oxman and Haynes, 1995).

The first uses of the World Wide Web in promoting guideline adoption have been at sites where specialty societies and governmental agencies have posted guidelines. This posting of guidelines on the World Wide Web has simulated publishing and allows access at the physician's convenience. This strategy has yet to be rigorously evaluated, but since it is similar to other primary dissemination strategies, the posting of guidelines on the World Wide Web is unlikely to be significantly more effective in ensuring guideline adoption. In the next section we present a template for the development of a more effective Web-enabled strategy for the dissemination of practice guidelines.

TEMPLATE FOR WEB-BASED PRACTICE GUIDELINES

While Web-based technologies have demonstrated potential for use in the development of secondary strategies designed to promote guideline development, little rigorous evaluation has been conducted or published to demonstrate effectiveness. The following is a secondary, Web-enabled strategy developed to facilitate the adoption of clinical practice guidelines with preliminary evaluation data, demonstrating its potential for influencing physician behavior.

This Web-enabled strategy has three components:
- Baseline survey
- Web course with audit and feedback data
- Post survey

The prototype for this strategy was developed in 1995 to promote the adoption of evidence-based guidelines on stroke prevention by the Agency for Health Care Policy and Research (AHCPR, 1995). In order to facilitate adoption of clinical practice guidelines, we have first developed a case-based survey to determine what practicing physicians are doing and what barriers exist to the adoption of a specific clinical practice guideline. In response to a case, the physician selects a course of treatment for the described patient. The physician's answer is then compared to the treatment recommended by the clinical practice guideline being studied. Surveys have been conducted by mail, by fax, and on the Web to determine baseline patterns.

Once baseline patterns are determined, a Web-based course for physicians is developed. If physicians complete the Web-based continuing medical education course, they are awarded a certificate of Category 1 CME credit that is needed by most for licensure and/or board certification. A prototype for a Web-based CME course was developed in 1995 to promote the adoption of 1995 clinical practice guidelines on stroke prevention in atrial fibrillation patients; guidelines were developed by the Agency for Health Care Policy and Research. The guidelines include the following key recommendations for patients with atrial fibrillation:
- Prescribe warfarin unless risk of stroke is low or use is contraindicated.
- Aspirin may be used if warfarin is contraindicated, unless aspirin is also contraindicated.
- Use appropriate anticoagulation monitoring techniques.

The guidelines include the following key recommendations for patients with transient

ischemic attack/minor stroke:
- Consider carotid endarterectomy (CE) if carotid disease is confirmed.
- Treat non-surgical candidates with aspirin or ticlopidine unless contraindicated.
- Monitor neutrophil counts of patients on ticlopidine.

Baseline survey

Using the key recommendations of the guidelines, a baseline case-based survey is developed. The purpose of this survey is to determine practice patterns of physicians compared to guidelines and to assess barriers to guideline adoption. Since audit and feedback have been identified as a relatively effective method for promotion of guideline adoption, these data are then used as a mechanism of feedback to physicians within the Web course so they can compare their responses to those of their peers. Key guideline recommendations are transformed into case-based questions. An example follows.

Guideline recommendation:
Prescribe warfarin unless contraindicated for patients with atrial fibrillation.
Baseline survey case-based question:
Based on your assessment of this patient (a 65-year-old male with a 15-year history of asymptomatic atrial fibrillation, a family history of stroke, normal blood pressure and cholesterol) and your assessment of his risk of stroke, would you prescribe:
  a. no additional treatment
  b. aspirin
  c. warfarin

Web Course with Audit and Feedback Data

Following data collection with the baseline case-based survey instrument and the compilation of data, a Web course is developed. Cases are also used as the basis for the Web course. The Web course uses a pattern for each case, which includes three components:
- A case which describes a clinical problem; each case is derived from a key guideline recommendation.
- Presentation in graph form of how peers in the baseline survey responded to the case, as a mechanism of audit and feedback.
- Comments on the baseline survey results for this case and how they compare to what is recommended in the guideline.

The example is based on the same recommendation cited above, the prescription of warfarin (unless contraindicated) for patients with atrial fibrillation.

The template of the course follows.
1) A description of the clinical problem:

Case Study 1

To answer questions related to the following case, please select the answer which best represents your opinion from the multiple choice answers provided and click on your answer.

In managing the care of a 65-year-old male with a 15-year history of asymptomatic atrial fibrillation, a family history of stroke, normal blood pressure and cholesterol, how would you describe this patient's risk of stroke?
○ low
○ moderate
○ high

Based on your assessment of this patient (a 65-year-old male with a 15 year history of asymptomatic atrial fibrillation, a family history of stroke, normal blood pressure and cholesterol) and your assessment of his risk of stroke, would you prescribe:
○ no additional treatment
○ aspirin
○ warfarin

http://www-cme.erep.uab.edu/onlineCourses/stroke/stroke.htm

2) Presentation in graph form of how peers in the baseline survey responded to the case as feedback:

Before going on to a discussion of this case, you may want to see how other physicians responded to this case. Here are the responses of the first 100 Alabama primary care physicians who responded to this case:

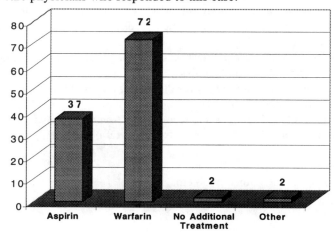

Your approach to this patient, as well as the variation in the responses above may be explained by how you assessed the patient's risk for stroke.

http://www-cme.erep.uab.edu/onlineCourses/stroke/stroke.htm

3) Comments on the baseline survey results and how they compare to what is recommended in the clinical practice guidelines:

> While this patient is not at high risk for stroke, according to the 1995 Stroke Prevention Recommendations from the Patient Outcomes Research Team funded by the Agency for Health Care Policy and Research, anticoagulation treatment is particularly effective for patients with atrial fibrillation and any one of the following additional risk factors: over age 60, prior stroke, diabetes, hypertension, and heart disease.
>
> Additional meta-analyses in this area, however, demonstrate this patient's annual risk of stroke is 1.6% which is in the intermediate zone. In patients without high risk, benefit of treatment other than aspirin is uncertain. If aspirin is prescribed, warfarin should be considered if risk factors develop including hypertension, diabetes, heart failure, coronary artery disease, or prior TIA/CVA. In patients without prior stroke or additional risk factors, meta-analyses of studies indicate an aspirin may be adequate.
>
> http://www-cme.erep.uab.edu/onlineCourses/stroke/stroke.htm

This pattern is then repeated with each additional case study from the baseline survey; usually 8-10 cases are included. Each case covers one major element of the clinical practice guideline.

The purpose of this template is two-fold. First, the use of cases is meant to engage the physician in cases that resemble patients seen in practice. By doing so, the cases engage the physician in the issues which the guideline addresses. Second, the template is meant to provide feedback to the physician on how his/her practice compares to peers and to the guidelines. Audit and feedback have been demonstrated to be more useful in changing physician practice than simply providing information in a lecture format.

The prototype of this electronic strategy may be viewed at the following Web address: www-cme.erep.uab.edu. The course is entitled Stroke Prevention.

EVALUATION

A preliminary evaluation has been conducted on this prototype. Baseline evaluation data were collected from a 1995 survey of a sample of 300 Alabama primary care physicians to determine their practice patterns related to stroke prevention. Ninety-six physicians responded to the survey. Eighty-five percent ranked the most important factor in stroke prevention in patients with atrial fibrillation as risk factors and lifestyle modification, with only 1% ranking warfarin as the most important factor. Sixty-three percent of physicians in responding to presented cases reported they would prescribe warfarin in patients where it was not contraindicated. In patients where aspirin was appropriate and warfarin contraindicated, 46% chose to use aspirin according to guidelines (Casebeer, Kristofco, Carillo, Renkl and Ryan, Unpublished).

Table 1 shows preliminary evaluation data obtained from users of the stroke prevention Web course during the period of May 1997-April 1999. Thousands of hits to the pages representing the stroke prevention program have been recorded during this period. However, data is only reported for physicians who completed and submitted the stroke prevention test for CME credit, a total of 129 physicians.

Table 1: Preliminary Evaluation Data (N = 129)

Recommendation	Correct Answer
Recognition of level of risk for stroke	58%
Prescription of warfarin unless contraindicated	91%
Recognition of contraindications for warfarin	19%
Use of appropriate anticoagulation monitoring	57%
Recognition of side effects of warfarin	87%
Management of stenosis with aspirin or ticlopidine	94%
Monitoring for ticlopidine	95%

Two areas can be compared with the baseline data described above. Prescription of warfarin unless contraindicated increased from 63% to 91% following completion of the course. On the other hand, while participants in the course focused on the Agency for Health Care Policy and Research recommendations for the use of warfarin, the course was less successful in emphasizing recognition of contraindications for warfarin and prescription of aspirin instead of warfarin, which decreased from 46% to 19%.

FUTURE TRENDS

Evidence is growing that computer-based decision support systems can enhance clinical performance (Hunt et al., 1998). Demand for well-designed Web-enabled continuing medical education will increase as practitioners rely more and more on Internet-based systems for medical information, patient records, and other decision support tools.

While our multiple component educational strategy has been a stand-alone initiative up to now, the future will allow us to explore partnerships with various decision support providers to offer integrated educational strategies that use these multiple methods to enhance compliance and reduce variations in patient care. What is necessary is additional research to measure the impact these kinds of Web-enabling strategies can have on the diffusion and adoption of advances in medicine. The partnership referred to earlier will permit pilot projects in selected disease management areas and begin to refine our practice in ways that will sharpen the focus of the interventions and link them to the mainstream of patient management.

In the intervening years since this pilot was designed and implemented, information technology, especially Web-based technology, has changed dramatically. There is now little question about the preferred electronic medium for reaching physicians with interactive education. While CD-ROM will continue to have utility in archival ways, the future of delivering care will increasingly rely on the Web. Not only has e-commerce become a factor in the overall economy, but also use of the Internet as a network to gain health information has expanded dramatically (Lindberg & Humphreys, 1998). Decision support systems are moving to Web-based platforms and standard setting. "Canopy computing," as it has been described by McDonald and his colleagues, becomes a compelling argument for electing to design and deliver CME on the Web (McDonald et al., 1998).

Finally, our extension of this work into the future will have these features: it will be Web-enabled, and it will be featured on decision support systems delivered to the desktop via intranet in health systems. It will alternatively be accessible to a global audience through the Web. The content will continue to be evidence-based and presented in case formats. The cases will be built using aggregated health systems data about gaps between actual practice and the ideal. The practitioner will move freely and instantaneously in and out of pertinent information channels including patient records, medical literature, and other relevant data that are important for reference and for learning. The participation of the practitioner will be recorded and compared with previous performance in this new system.

The challenges for the future then are how to integrate this work into decision support and other Web developments, improving the measurement of its impact and validity, and refining the protocol to take advantage of other developments in systems design and telecommunications to incorporate it into the mainstream of information management in the future.

CONCLUSIONS

While innovative Web-enabled strategies have begun to appear, little rigorous evaluation has been conducted. A template for a Web-enabled strategy incorporating audit and feedback, and designed to promote guideline adoption has been presented in this chapter along with preliminary evaluation data.

Information technology, medical knowledge and medical practice are on a collision course according to Faughnan and Elson (1998). In the future, the way physicians work, the way medical knowledge is processed, packaged and distributed, and the way patients obtain medical care and information will be influenced by the coming together of these forces.

Internet use is growing rapidly in the U.S. health arena and in the population at large (Lindberg & Humphreys, 1998). The challenges and opportunities for the future of Web-based technology include the technology itself, medical information management, and patient care issues. Federal Reserve Board Chairman Alan Greenspan recently speculated that the impact of information technology on business productivity may be the "x factor" responsible for the continuing growth of the U.S. economy. The chairman of Intel Corporation, Andrew Grove (1998), writing in the Journal of the American Medical Association, points out that "it must be only a matter of time before the x-factor comes to the practice of medicine" (Grove, 1998).

According to Lindberg and Humphreys (1998), increased commercial use of the Internet is encouraging the development of more sophisticated, multimedia Web sites. The functionality of Web sites continues to improve because of platform-independent computing languages like "Java." Web interfaces to patient data systems are becoming more common and improving prospects for the effective integration of patient data and relevant published information also available on the Web.

Computer-based clinical decision support systems can enhance clinical performance for drug dosing, preventive care and other aspects of medical care (Hunt, Haynes, Hanna and Smith, 1998). More widespread use of clinical support systems will characterize the future of medical care. The potential of these systems employing Web technologies is enormous (Classen, 1998).

The Web has had a historically profound and qualitative effect on the cost of distributing information. According to Faughnan and Elson (1998) we can expect radical changes in other aspects of information technology. The authors predict that the Web will be the infrastructure for clinical work. It will be networked, mostly wireless, and include special purpose tools for selected applications.

In a commentary concerning the use of the Web in clinical practice, Clement McDonald, MD (1998) suggested that what physicians need are tools that can easily join all of the separate sources of clinical information into one canopy where they can reach all the information pertinent to a particular patient. The Web offers most of the tools to create this ideal of an electronic medical record. In fact, Health Level Seven (HL7), a nonprofit standards development organization, is working to address the issues of coding and Web browser standards. Web-based clinical system development is well underway in various parts of the country (Masys and Baker, 1997; Cimino, Socratous & Clayton, 1995; Willard, Allgren and Connelly, 1994; McDonald et al., 1998), and are examples of what the future will hold for information management.

The same Web-based technology will enable educational interventions to be delivered at the point of care or based on analyses of errors occurring during medical care. Medical education will increasingly be tied to medical practice (Faughnan and Elson, 1998).

The Institute of Medicine National Roundtable on Health Care Quality recently observed that "serious and widespread quality problems exist throughout American medicine." Current efforts to improve will not succeed, they continue, unless we undertake a major systematic effort to overhaul how we deliver healthcare services, educate and train clinicians, and assess and improve quality (Chassin & Galvin, 1998).

Clearly a continuous quality improvement agenda is necessary. The success of any improvement effort will depend on the ability to aggregate relevant data and improve data quality. More adequate information systems will facilitate better research only if they contain the information that is needed to address current deficiencies in knowledge. The imperative to develop standards for the electronic medical record is seen as key to addressing the need for clinically relevant data (Starfield, 1998).

In his text, *Designing the User Interface*, Ben Shneiderman (1992) states, "the computer revolution will be judged not by the complexity or power of technology but rather by the service to human needs. More human interfaces will create challenges for technology in the future including continuing concerns about ethical and legal implications of a Web-based patient physician relationship (Spielberg, 1998). Safeguards will be refined and the shifting technology will be accompanied by vigilance in this area.

New technologies provide extraordinary powers to those who master them (Shneiderman, 1992). Cooperation across the spectrum of users, vendors, practitioners, and others will determine whether the technologies we create can conquer avoidable ignorance (Hubbs, Rindfleisch, Godin & Melmon, 1998).

REFERENCES

Agency for Health Care Policy and Research (AHCPR) & Duke University Center for Health Policy Research and Education. (1995). *Secondary and Tertiary Prevention of Stroke Patient Outcomes Research Team: Seventh Progress Report: March 31, 1995*. Silver Spring: AHCPR Publications Clearinghouse.

Anderson, J.G. (1994). Computer-based patient records and changing physicians' practice patterns. *Topics in Health Information Management, 15*, 10-23.

Anderson, J.G., Jay, S.J., Weng, H.C., & Anderson, M.M. (1995). Studying the effect of clinical uncertainty on physicians' decision-making using ILIAD. *Medinfo, 8*, 869-872.

Avorn, J., Chen, M., & Hartley, R. (1982). Scientific versus commercial sources of influence on the prescribing behavior of physicians. *American Journal of Medicine, 73,* 4-8.

Avorn, J., & Soumerai, S.B. (1983). Improving drug-therapy decisions through educational outreach. A randomized controlled trial of academically based "detailing." *New England Journal of Medicine, 308,* 1457-1463.

Bero, L.A., Grilli, R., Grimshaw, J.M., Harvey, E., Oxman, A.D., & Thomson, M.A. (1998). Closing the gap between research and practice: an overview of systematic reviews of interventions to promote the implementation of research findings. The Cochrane Effective Practice and Organization of Care Review Group. *British Medical Journal, 317,* 465-468.

Casebeer, L.L., Kristofco, R., Carillo, A., Renkl, L., & Ryan, F. (Unpublished). Evaluating the effectiveness of feedback to promote the adoption of stroke prevention guidelines.

Chassin, M.R., & Galvin, R.W. (1998). The urgent need to improve health care quality: Institute of Medicine National Roundtable on Health Care Quality. *Journal of the American Medical Association, 280,* 1000-1005.

Classen, D.C. (1998). Clinical decision support systems to improve clinical practice and quality of care. *Journal of the American Medical Association, 280,* 1360-1361.

Chodorow, S. (1996). Educators must take the electronic revolution seriously. *Academic Medicine, 71,* 221-226.

Cimino, J.J., Socratous, S.A., & Clayton, P.D. (1995). Internet as clinical information system: application development using the world wide Web. *Journal of the American Medical Information Association, 2,* 273-284.

Curley, S.P., Young, M.J., & Yates, J.F. (1989). Characterizing physicians' perceptions of ambiguity. *Medical Decision Making, 9,* 116-124.

Davis, D.A., & Taylor-Vaisey, A. (1997). Translating guidelines into practice. *Canadian Medical Association Journal, 157,* 408-416.

Davis, D.A., Thomson, M.A., Oxman, A.D., & Haynes, R.B. (1995). Changing physician performance: a systematic review of the effect of continuing medical education strategies. *Journal of the American Medical Association, 274,* 700-705.

Davis, D.A., Thomson, M.A., Oxman, A.D., & Haynes, R.B. (1992). Evidence for the effectiveness of CME: a review of 50 randomized controlled trials. *Journal of the American Medical Association, 268,* 1111-1117.

Davis, M.J., Wythe, J., Rozum, J.S., & Gore, R.W. (1997). Use of world wide Web server and browser software to support a first-year medical physiology course. *American Journal of Physiology, 272,* S1-14.

Dunnington, G.L., & DaRosa, D.A. (1994). Changing surgical education strategies in an environment of changing health care delivery systems. *World Journal of Surgery, 18,* 734-737.

Faughnan, J.G., & Elson, M.D. (1998). Information technology and the clinical curriculum: some predictions and their implications for the class of 2003. *Academic Medicine, 73,* 766-769.

Ferguson, T. (1998). Digital doctoring—opportunities and challenges in electronic patient-physician communication. *Journal of the American Medical Association, 280,* 1361-1362.

Gerrity, M.S., Earp, J.A., DeVellis, R.F., & Light, D.W. (1992). Uncertainty and professional work: perceptions of physicians in clinical practice. *American Journal of Sociology, 97*, 1022-1051.

Gorton, T.A., Cranford, C.O., Golden, W.E., Walls, R.C., & Pawelak, J.E. (1995). Primary care physicians' responses to dissemination of practice guidelines. *Archives of Family Medicine, 4*, 135-142.

Grilli, R., & Lomas, J. (1994). Evaluating the message: the relationship between compliance and the subject of a practice guideline. *Medical Care, 32*, 202-213.

Grove A.S. (1998). The x factor. *Journal of the American Medical Association, 280*, 1294.

Guyatt, G.H., Sackett, D.L., & Cook, D.J. (1994). Users' guides to the medical literature: how to use an article about therapy or prevention. *Journal of the American Medical Association, 271*, 389-391.

Henry, J.B. (1990). Computers in medical education: information and knowledge management, understanding, and learning. *Human Pathology, 21*, 998-1002.

Hubbs, P.R., Rindfleisch, T.C., Godin, P., & Melmon, K.L. (1998). Medical information on the internet. *Journal of the American Medical Association, 280*, 1363.

Hunt, D.L., Haynes, R.B., Hanna, S.E., & Smith, K. (1998). Effects of computer-based clinical decision support systems on physician performance and patient outcomes. *Journal of the American Medical Association, 280*, 1339-1346.

Institute of Medicine. (1990). *Clinical practice guidelines: Directions for a new program.* Washington, DC: National Academy Press.

Jaffe, C.C., & Lynch, P.J. (1995). Computer-aided instruction in radiology: opportunities for more effective learning. *American Journal of Roentgenology, 164*, 463-467.

Jewett, B.S., Holsinger, F.C., Kuppersmith, R.B., & Buenting, J.E. (1998). Computer-based physician education. *Comput Otolaryngology, 31*, 301-307.

Henry J. Kaiser Family Foundation Forum for Collaborative HIV Research. (1998). *Dissemination and Evaluation of Clinical Practice Guidelines for HIV Disease, June 1998.* Washington: The George Washington University Medical Center, Center for Health Policy Research.

Kassirer, J.P. (1989). Our stubborn quest for diagnostic certainty: A cause of excessive testing. *New England Journal of Medicine, 320*, 1489-1491.

Klar R., & Bayer, U. (1990). Computer-assisted teaching and learning in medicine. *International Journal of Biomedical Computing, 26*, 7-27.

Lindberg, D.A.B., & Humphreys, B.L. (1998). Medicine and health on the internet: the good, the bad, and the ugly. *Journal of the American Medical Association, 280*, 1303-1304

Marks, R. (1997). Indecision. (Editorial). *Focus, 12*, 2.

Masys, D.R. (1998). Advances in information technology: implications for medical education. *Western Journal of Medicine, 168*, 341-347.

Masys, D.R., & Baker, D.B. (1997). Patient-centered access to secure systems online (PCASSO): a secure approach to clinical data access via the World Wide Web. *Proceedings of the AMIA Annual Fall Synposium, 97*, 340-343.

McDonald, C.J., Hui, S.L., Smith, D.M. (1984). Reminders to physicians from an introspective computer medical record. *Annals of Internal Medicine, 100*, 130-138.

McDonald, C.J., Hui, S.L., & Tierney, W.M. (1992). Effects of computer reminders for influenza vaccination on morbidity during influenza epidemics. *MD Computing, 9*, 304-12.

McDonald, C.J., Overhage, J.M., Dexter, P.R., Blevins, L., Meeks-Johnson, J., Suico, J.G., Tucker, M.C., & Schadow, G. (1998). Canopy computing: using the Web in clinical practice. *Journal of the American Medical Association, 280,* 1325-1329.

McDonald, C.J., Wilson, G.A., & McCabe, G.P. Jr. (1980). Physician response to computer reminders. *Journal of the American Medical Association, 244,* 1579-1581.

Overhage, J.M., Tierney, W.M., & McDonald, C.J. (1996). Computer reminders to implement preventive care guidelines for hospitalized patients. *Archives of Internal Medicine, 156,* 1551-1556.

Oxman, A.D., Sackett, D.L., & Guyatt, G.H. (1993). User's guide to the medical literature: how to get started. *Journal of the American Medical Association, 270,* 2093-2095.

Oxman, A.D., Thomson, M.A., Davis, D.A., & Haynes, R.B. (1995). No magic bullets: a systematic review of 102 trials of interventions to improve professional practice. *Canadian Medical Association Journal, 153,* 1423-1431.

Peterson, D.K., & Pitz, G.F. (1988). Confidence, uncertainty, and the use of information. *Journal of Experimental Psychology, 14,* 85-92.

Putnam, R.W., & Campbell, M.D. (1989). Competence. In: Fox RD, Mazmanian PE, Putnam RW (Eds.). *Changing and Learning in the Lives of Physicians* (pp. 79-97). New York, NY: Praeger Publishers.

Qayumi T. (1997). Computers and medical education. *Journal of Investigative Surgery,* 10, vii-ix.

Schulz, S., Schrader, U., & Klar, R. (1997). Computer-based training and electronic publishing in the health sector: tools and trends. *Methods of Information in Medicine, 36,* 149-153.

Sebaldt, R.J. (1997). Information technology and the future of medical education. *Clinical and Investigative Medicine, 20,* 419-421.

Shneiderman, B. (1992). *Designing the user interface: strategies for effective human-computer interaction.* Reading: Addison-Wesley.

Soumerai, S.B., McLaughlin, T.J., Gurwitz, J.H., Guadagnoli, E., Hauptman, P.J., Borbas, C. (1998). Effect of local medical opinion leaders on quality of care for acute myocardial infraction: a randomzed controlled trial. *Journal of the American Medical Association, 279,* 358-63.

Soumerai, S.B., & Avorn, J. (1990). Principles of educational outreach ('academic detailing') to improve clinical decision making. *Journal of the American Medical Association, 263,* 549-556.

Spielberg, J.D. (1998). On call and online: sociohistorical, legal, and ethical implications of email for the patient-physician relationship. *Journal of the American Medical Association, 280,* 1353-1359.

Starfield, B. (1998). Quality of care research: internal elegance and external relevance. *Journal of the American Medical Association, 280,* 1006-1008.

Willard, K.E., Allgren, J.H., & Connelly, D.P. (1994). W-3 based medical information systems vs custom client server applications. *Proceedings of the 2nd International WWW Conference, "Mosaic and the Web,* 641-651.

Yolton, R.L., (1992). Tools of the trade: enhancing teaching with computers. *Optometry and Vision Science, 69,* 496-498.

Section IV: Web-Empowering Health Practitioners and Patients

There is no doubt that new ways of communicating are evolving as a result of the explosive growth of the Internet and the development of the World Wide Web. While the previous sections of this book focused on the transformation of inter- and intra-organizational communications in the healthcare industry, the chapters presented in this section consider the impact of Web technology on individuals and their health. Specifically, physician-patient communications and the Internet as a vehicle for empowering the individual are explored. The first two chapters in this section describe patient-centered applications designed to enhance communications with physicians and to improve patient self-care. The third chapter examines the Internet as a healthcare education and peer-support communications medium. In the final chapter a Web-based application is designed to meet the needs of disabled individuals by providing building architects and managers with an on-line tool for assessing building and facilities accessibility.

Weinberg, Klein, Anderson, Banerjee, Klepper, Waxman, and Yu discuss the design and implementation of a Web-enabled application that improves the intercommunications between physicians and patients by providing individualized information for each patient and physician relationship. Specifically, they describe the Hypertension Decision Aide (HDA), a Web-based system designed to provide chronic hypertension patients and their doctors with up-to-date data reporting, monitoring, and decision support tools. The authors discuss the design process of HDA in detail, emphasizing the importance of understanding both types of users' needs and expectations. In addition to the system benefits, the authors discuss challenges associated with the system implementation, including data integrity, patient confidentiality, and socioeconomic issues such as Internet access. The authors conclude with an outlook for the further development and expansion of the HDA system.

Soderlund, Reijonen, and Brannback describe the potential for an interactive Web-enabled system that allows individuals with diabetes to improve self-care. Through a Web browser or mobile phone, diabetic patients can conveniently record and access medical data related to their condition. The authors begin by providing readers with background information on diabetes. Next, "Wellmate," an experimental telecare service system in Finland supporting diabetics' self-management, is illustrated in detail. The authors contrast the old, manual way of patient self-care and physician communications with the newly developed electronic system. Preliminary findings from the first four months of implementation suggest that "Wellmate" can improve communication and patient self-care by providing the patients and physicians with a more rapid turnaround of up-to-date information. The authors discuss the future of the application, including technological enhancements and highlight the importance of user commitment.

In the previous two chapters, the use of the Internet for patient self-care was demonstrated by enhancing the physician-patient relationship to include the electronic transfer of digitized medical information. Lemaire's chapter demonstrates from a slightly different perspective, how the Internet is impacting the way patients manage their own care. Lemaire suggests that the open architecture of the Internet and its global accessibility empower individuals with a medium to provide peer support as well as to share medical knowledge and experiences. She further suggests that the extensive amount of medical information available on the Web enables patients to further their own involvement in their healthcare, changing the nature of the physician-patient relationship from a paternalistic to a partnership relationship. In her discussion, Lemaire cautiously points out the limitations of this relatively new medium, including issues associated with information reliability. Lemaire also stresses the importance of correcting the "digital divide", the widening gap between those with online access and those without.

In recent years there has been a greater recognition that people with disabilities share the same rights as others, thanks to changes in legislation such as the Americans with Disabilities Act Accessibilities Guidelines. Bridge and Simoff have developed a model for a Web-enabled, computer-assisted access evaluation system in Australia that can aid in the identification and removal of architectural barriers affecting persons with disabilities. The authors present a detailed analysis of the accessibility audit process, followed by a well-organized discussion on how to best represent accessibility knowledge in a database. They also develop a strategy for integrating a Web-based interface to the system. The authors describe the development of the application with Microsoft Access, including illustrated tables, queries, and reporting features, and discuss its interoperability with other data resources. Additionally, they describe how the system itself is accessible to individuals with disabilities. Based on their preliminary work, Bridge and Simoff conclude that building such a system on a wide scale is feasible, and that it could greatly contribute to reducing the risks and liabilities associated with architectural barriers in building and facilities.

Chapter XIII

Patient-Doctor Interconnectivity: Improving Healthcare Management and Patient Compliance with Web Technology

Jerry B. Weinberg, Steven P. Klein, Robert Klepper,
Bernard Waxman and Xudong Yu
Southern Illinois University-Edwardsville

Daniel K. Anderson
Grinnell Regional Medical Center

Effective physicians must listen to their patient's concerns, take accurate and complete medical histories, and earn patient trust and confidence. Physicians must help patients better understand their problems, and clearly communicate treatment recommendations and medical advice. Communication is a cornerstone of medical practice, while poor communication is a major cause of misdiagnosis, poor compliance of therapy, and malpractice claims (Mechanic, 1998).

Telecommunication technology has created new lines of communication for patient-physician interaction. Most recently, the global computer network of the Internet has provided electronic mail (email) and the World Wide Web (Web). Email allows for a direct one-to-one communication, and the Web is used mainly as a broadcast medium for dissemination of information in a one-to-many form. Just like the Internet's predecessor, the telephone, application and research must be done to determine how this new technology can best be used to enhance the patient-physician relationship (Mandl, 1998).

The Internet provides an unprecedented level of near instantaneous lines of intercommunication. Web browser technologies provide an interface to the Internet that makes this communication accessible even to novice computer users. The combination of communication and interface technology is an opportunity to explore ways of improving patient healthcare by breaking down current barriers to quality healthcare management. Web-based communications enable a continuous interaction between physician and patients where patients can freely enter data and concerns, and physicians can address these asynchronously. With the resulting additional patient data, physicians get a more complete clinical picture, and, with the aid of trending and decision support tools, the computer can help organize and present data in meaningful ways. Patients gain a sense of partnership in their healthcare through the continuous reporting of data and more immediate feedback.

This chapter discusses the design and implementation of a working healthcare management system called "Hypertension Decision Aide" or "HDA". HDA is a World Wide Web system that provides chronic hypertension patients with data reporting, monitoring, decision support tools, and educational material. HDA provides physicians with the ability to monitor a patient's progress between visits, view summary data, and review suggestions from decision support tools. Issues of system design, data integrity, patient confidentiality, and security will be discussed in the context of HDA.

BACKGROUND

Successful healthcare management requires that a number of elements come together for each patient. These include access to healthcare, patient compliance and motivation, and sufficient patient monitoring. A variety of barriers exist that can cause a breakdown in these requirements and reduce the quality of care. Examples of such barriers include:

1. Distances that reduce contact between patient and physician, particularly in rural areas where contact requires some means of transportation and costs patients missed work time.
2. Physician shortages that reduce access to healthcare.
3. Patient's lack of understanding of their condition or their treatments.
4. Patient's loss of self-determination in managing their own care resulting in noncompliance to treatment and lack of motivation to monitor health status indicators.
5. Physician's lack of data about a patient's condition or response to a treatment.

Telecommunication technologies and Internet technologies are a useful tool for the dissemination of medical information, the sharing of medical records, and physician intercommunication (Mandl, 1998). To overcome some of the barriers listed above, recent work applies these new technologies to patient-physician intercommunication (Balas, 1997, Bader, 1998). For example, there has been some exploration into the use of e-mail as a way of linking patients to physicians and clinicians (Neill, 1994). E-mail is a "push medium"; the only activity required by the message receiver is to check his/her e-mail account. In this sense it is much like voice mail. Yet, it differs from telephone and voice mail technology in ways that require special considerations of its use in communicating messages that may be critical, such as treatment changes or sensitive messages (Mandl, 1998). Policy statements are being drafted to address the proper use of e-mail communication with patients in the clinical setting (Kane, 1998). The Web is a "pull medium"; the message receiver must actively send a request for the message. The use of the Web as a mass communication tool for the delivery of medical information is an ongoing topic (Glowniak, 1994, Gentile, 1998, LaPerri'ere, 1998). The Web provides the ability to deliver up-to-date information to patients on medical conditions, treatments, and research results. Web systems have also been developed to provide educational opportunities to patients. These can improve patients' understanding and, subsequently, their compliance to treatment (Consoli, 1995).

The Web can also be exploited well beyond simple information delivery to provide a significant increase in the connectivity between the patient and the physician (Kassirer, 1995; Riva, 1996). Web programming provides the ability to dynamically generate Web page content. By combining this ability with recent technology that allows such programs direct connection to database systems, Web-based systems can be created to deliver individualized content to each patient. Such systems can also allow patients to report changes in their conditions, report effects of treatments, and record monitored vital signs giving physicians more timely data. Further, patients could receive timely feedback concerning their condition or changes to their treatment regimen. Patients become a more integral part of their care, thereby improving their compliance to treatments and increasing awareness of their own health status (Binstock, 1988).

Providing physicians with large amounts of additional data could result in information overload. Web systems that provide a high level of interaction must be able to summarize and organize the data in meaningful ways. These systems can incorporate trending and decision support tools to identify the most relevant information with regards to the patient's specific history, organize it accordingly, and potentially, make suggestions (Kassirer, 1995).

In designing an application to enhance the intercommunication between patients and physicians, it is important that we understand the expectation of each of these groups on how the application fits within the healthcare management relationship. The ability for computer technology to enhance our quality of life rests squarely on how well the application fits our conceptual understanding of how things work (Landauer, 1995; Norman, 1988; Sachs, 1995). The application should fit the users conception of the process, "the user-task model", while the inner mechanisms, "the engineer model", should be as transparent as possible (Gentner, 1996, p. 28-35). Just as most automobile drivers know very little of how a car actually works and yet find the task of driving natural, similarly we want to design computer applications that are natural to use with little worry or concern about how they are being accomplished. In the area of HCI research, a number of approaches have evolved to meet this challenge. These include User-Centered Design (Landauer, 1995), Human-Centered Systems (Flanagan, 1997), Participatory Design (Muller, 1993), and Contextual Design (Beyer, 1997). Though they differ in their techniques, these approaches have a general common vision of seeing "the interplay between human activity and technological systems as inextricably linked and equally important aspects of analysis, design, and evaluation" (Flanangan, 1997, p. 3). These different techniques find ways to interject the designer in the user's world and the user in the designer's world in order to develop a shared conceptual model of the task and the context in which it is being done (Muller, 1993). It is in this spirit that HDA is being developed.

WEB-BASED PATIENT-PHYSICIAN COMMUNICATION: DESIGN AND IMPLEMENTATION OF HDA

Design of HDA

HDA focuses on the management of patients with primary hypertension. Primary hypertension is a chronic condition that requires a high level of compliance and awareness by the patient for successful management. Hypertension is one of the top reasons that patients in the United States seek healthcare. Uncontrolled hypertension can result in serious and life-threatening vascular disorders. Even mild elevations in blood pressure are linked to increased chances of stroke, myocardial infarction, heart failure, and other cardiovascular diseases. Successful management often requires extended drug therapy and lifestyle changes. Compliance with these treatments is frequently poor (Consoli, 1995). For these reasons, the healthcare management of patients with primary hypertension is an excellent example of how systems can be designed to improve the quality of care.

In a typical practice, patients are prescribed a medication and told to return in a month to have their blood pressure checked. At that time, efficacy and side effects are assessed, changes made, and the loop repeats. Patients are urged to call if they are having problems, although in practice they often do not, because they think the physician is too busy, or they think their problem can wait until the next visit. Furthermore, decisions about treatment effectiveness are often made on a few or even one office blood pressure measurement. Many patients have "white coat" elevations in their blood pressure, due to anxiety over doctor visits, and can be shown to have lower pressures at home. To get around these problems, some doctors have their patients obtain their own blood pressure measuring devices and keep logs of their pressures. The physician then analyzes a list of values at the next visit. Under this paradigm, it can take up to a year to achieve adequate control of blood pressure, and patients may endure side effects for weeks or even months before the problem is recognized and rectified.

HDA enables a continuous interaction where patients can freely enter data and concerns, and physicians can address these asynchronously. With the help of trending and decision support tools, the system organizes and summarizes the data and provides suggestions for treatment changes. HDA updates a database that stores patient's observations, which creates a data rich environment for hypertension management. Patients gain a "plugged in" feeling because of their constant access to the database in entering and viewing their data, and continued contact with their physician through the system. As such, they become more motivated to monitor their progress, more inclined to share concerns about their management, and more likely to comply with their treatments. The tighter feedback loop allows faster response to changes and tighter long-term control, which can translate into better quality of life for patients while saving precious healthcare dollars.

With any system, to maximize its usability, the design of the system should fit the user's conceptualization of the task(s) it is meant to perform or supplement. Early in the design process, the designer engages in analysis activities that provide insights into the user's mental model of the tasks for the system (Liddle, 1996). Mental models are cognitive artifacts created as we interact with our environment and are used as a representation of our world (Johnson-Laird, 1989). These models "provide predictive and explanatory power for understanding the interaction" (Norman, 1983). If the designer can devise the conceptual model in ways that reflect a user's mental model, then the application designed from a conceptual model will be more easily understood and more naturally fit into the user's activities (Norman, 1988). This "user-centered" approach to design first considers the interface definition, and then constructs the underlying system to fit the interface. The approach used for this project is a "task-analysis" method (Lewis, 1993). Task-analysis requires the creation of a specific list of concrete tasks the user is expected to perform with the system such as those listed in Figure 1. Specifying the list of tasks has the advantage of improving completeness of the design and providing a test-bed of activities for system testing.

Figure 1: Example User Tasks from a Task-Analysis of HDA

Patient Tasks	Physician Tasks
• Stacy M enters her blood pressure readings for the past 3 days. • Stacy M reports symptoms of fatigue and dizziness. • Stacy M views a graph of her blood pressure readings since the last change in her prescription dosage.	• Dr. Q views a graph of Stacy M's blood pressure readings over the past 4 weeks. • Dr. Q reviews recommendations to changes in Stacy M's treatment regimen generated by the decision module. • Dr. Q updates changes to Stacy M's treatment.

Patients and physicians have different conceptualizations of tasks and differ on the set of tasks they expect to perform in the communication process between them. In very general terms, patients expect to report signs and symptoms to the physician and request and receive information regarding treatments and medical conditions. Physicians expect to record patient data and analyze the data in the context of the patient's history. But, this specification of tasks is too general for our design purposes.

Consider a communication system as a spectrum from free-format to personalized-structure. E-mail can be considered free-format communication. At this end of the spectrum the patient may freely input text indicating observations, questions, or requests. While this system has the specified functionality, lacking the proper medical knowledge, patients are likely to omit important information and include irrelevant information. The physician must go through the labor-intensive process of carefully scanning and parsing out the relevant information, separating the patient's observations from their requests for information.

In the middle of the communication spectrum is a generic questionnaire, much like a history sheet, which can provide lists of questions that structure the communication. From the patient's perspective, it can be unclear which questions pertain to them, and they may answer questions that have no relevance. The physician again is faced with having to discern relevant and irrelevant information.

At the other end of the communication spectrum is a structured interaction that is personalized for each patient, much like a face-to-face interview where the physician guides the conversation based on his knowledge of the patient's history and medical knowledge. From the patient's perspective, this is the kind of intercommunication with their physician that they have come to expect. The physician directs the interview through a series of questions that are relevant to the patient's particular condition and history. The patient may recall events or observations that may have otherwise been forgotten or ignored. From the physician's perspective, the data gathered is immediately available and directly relevant. The ability of a system to personalize the communication would require it to have knowledge of medical conditions, treatments, and patient histories. To identify the knowledge necessary for this, the task analysis must be much more specific than the general task description given above. The design of HDA follows this model of communication.

The system is viewed from the perspective of the two types of users: patients and physicians. These views are shown in Figures 2 and 3. HDA has four major functional components. First, the system has an information area that supplies patients with educational material regarding hypertension and various possible treatments. Second, a front-end

Figure 2: Patient System Perspective

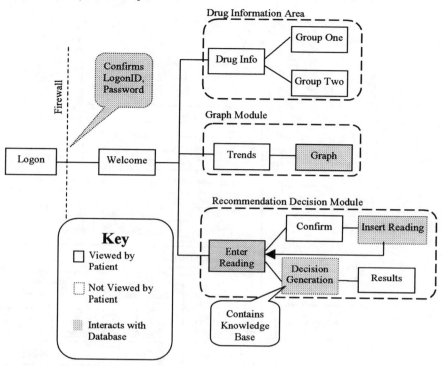

allows patients to record their vital statistics and other relevant health indicators. This front-end is dynamically created to organize the information presented based on the patient's treatment regimen. It also contains a free text entry field that allows the patient to report anything of interest that is not directly represented in the interface, for example, a particularly stressful event that could have affected the patient's vital statistics.

The third component is a graphing module that visually displays trends over time of a patient's vital statistics (diastolic & systolic blood pressure and pulse). This graph module can be altered to show different levels of detail and can indicate time-points when different treatments started, ended, or changed. The final major component is a rule-based decision support system that follows current standards on the treatment of hypertension. The system is designed to send an e-mail log of a patient's activity to the physician along with any generated treatment suggestions. Physicians have access to additional functionality that allows them to maintain the educational information, update information on treatments, and edit the rules of the decision support module.

Implementation of HDA

HDA is implemented as an Active Server Pages (ASP) Web application, which connects to a Microsoft Access database. The ASP technology creates dynamic HTML (hypertext mark-up language) pages. These pages provide the front-end to a database that stores historic data of patients' reported signs and symptoms, vital statistics, and past and current treatments. ASP also maintains session variables that store information about users while they are logged into the system. These variables are created when a user logs on, thus

Figure 3: Physician System Perspective

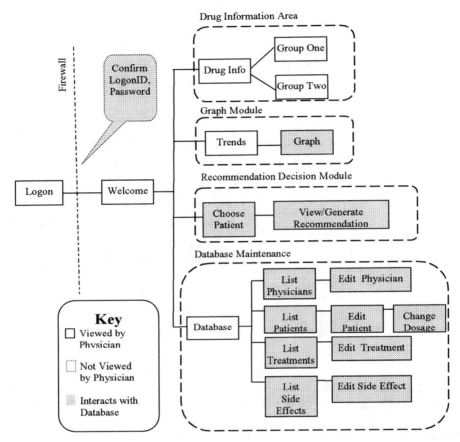

creating a session, and are removed when a user logs off or their session times out due to inactivity. All the Web documents that comprise HDA components (small rectangles in Figures 2 and 3) are implemented as ASP pages. The chart module is a Java applet modified with ASP scripting. Also, a small amount of JavaScript is used to enhance the usability of data entry pages. As the keys in Figures 2 and 3 indicate, some documents are viewed by users, some are hidden, and some interact with the system's database. The five main components of the system are the: Firewall, Drug Information Module, Graph Module, Recommendation Decision Module, and Database Maintenance.

Active Server Pages, delineated from HTML files by their ".asp" extension, are handled by the Active Server portion of a Microsoft Internet Information Server. The Active Server resides on the Web server and previews all requests for Web documents. If a requested file includes the .asp extension, then the Active Server processes the file before delivering it to the Web server. During the processing of the file, the Active Server compiles and executes all ASP scripting in the file. The Active Server also adds any Server Side Includes, and creates and maintains session objects.

An Active Server Page is a combination of HTML and ASP script. The scripting language used in HDA is VBScript, but other scripting languages, such as JavaScript, are also viable. Special tags delimit ASP scripts: <% %> (see Figure 4). All output generated by the execution of an ASP is delivered to the Web server as HTML. By integrating ASP script with HTML, it is possible to create dynamic Web documents. Server Side Includes (SSI) allow the insertion of information stored in text files into an ASP. When the Active Server encounters the code for a SSI while processing an ASP, it replaces the code with the text of the file referred to by the SSI (see Figure 4). In this manner, common routines or page features can be stored in a single location and included in many pages.

Whenever a user first accesses a page in HDA, the Active Server creates a session object for the user. As the user moves from page to page through the system, the Active Server checks to see if the user has a current session object. In this way, the Active Server tracks the progress of a user. The session object is initialized during the *Session_OnStart* event. This event occurs when a user accessing a system page has no current session object. When this event occurs, a subroutine is run that creates a session object and initializes session variables. The session variables are stored for the duration of the existence of the session object. The session object is destroyed when the *Session_OnEnd* event occurs. This event occurs when the session's method, *abandon,* is activated, or the session times out. In the HDA, a session's *abandon* method is called whenever a user logs off of the system, or after 15 minutes of inactivity. A special file, 'global.asa', stores the *OnStart* and *OnEnd* subroutines.

Figure 4: Example ASP File

```
<!--#INCLUDE FILE="FileName.asp"-->        Server
<html>                                       Side
<head>                                       Include
<title>Patients</title>
</head>
<body background="../images/bg.jpg">
<h2><center>Patient Page</center></h2>      HTML
<%
Set dbCon = Server.CreateObject("ADODB.Connection")
dbCon.Open Session("Db_ConnectionString")
sQuery = "SELECT * FROM Patient"
Set rs = dbCon.Execute(sQuery,,1)            ASP
If NOT(rs.BOF and rs.EOF) then               Scripting
%>
        <h4><br>No records returned.</h4>
<%
        Do While Not rs.EOF
%>
          <%=rs("PatientName")%> <%
              rs.MoveNext
        Loop
End If
%>
</body>                                       Variable
</html>                                       Display
```

Database Structure and Interactivity

The database, shown in Figure 5, is implemented in Microsoft Access. Primary keys for each table are shown in boldface. The Physician, Patient, Treatment, and SideEffect tables hold relevant data concerning the entities that their titles refer to, respectively. The TreatmentSideEffect table associates treatments with their common side effects. The PatientTreatment table holds patients' treatment histories. The Reading table stores a patient's vital statistics measured at a given time. The 'Comments' field allows a patient to report any unusual circumstance(s) that occurred at or near the measurement time. The ReadingSideEffect table associates a common treatment side effect with a specific reading. Entries are made into this table when a patient indicates that a listed, common side effect occurred at or near the time of a reading. The Recommendation table stores recommendations generated for patients and the time of recommendation generation.

The relations shown in Figure 5 reflect the following assumptions:
- A physician may be associated with one or more patients.
- A patient must be associated with one and only one physician.

Figure 5: Database Relational Table Structure

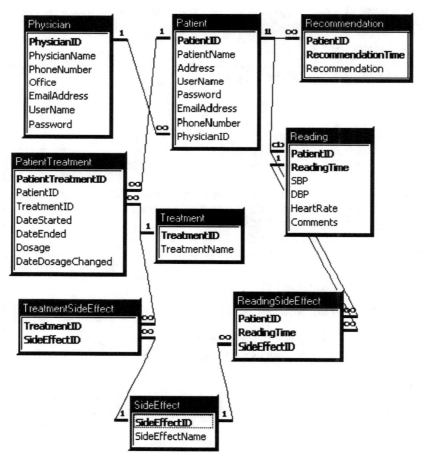

- A patient may be associated with one or more treatments concurrently.
- A patient's treatment dosage may vary over time.
- A patient's treatment may stop, then be renewed at a later time.
- A patient may be associated with one or more readings.
- A patient may be associated with one or more recommendations.
- A reading, recommendation, and/or patient treatment must be associated with one and only one patient.
- A reading may be associated with one or more reading side effects.
- A reading side effect must be associated with one and only one reading.
- A treatment may be associated with one or more side effects.
- A side effect may be associated with one or more treatments.

In order to make the database available to HDA, it is registered as an Open Database Connectivity (ODBC) system datasource on the server. The ASP pages in HDA that connect to the database do so by creating the ActiveX Database Objects (ADO) '*Connection*' and '*Recordset*'. These objects interface with the database via ODBC. By doing so, they can interact with the database using Structured Query Language (SQL) statements. The *Connection* object is used to establish a communication link with the database. Once a link is established, any number or type of SQL queries can be issued. If the query requests information from the database, the results are returned in a *Recordset* object which can be used to display the returned information.

SQL queries are sent from the Active Server to the ODBC driver as text strings. These strings can be dynamically constructed in an ASP page. This is accomplished by inserting variable values into the query's string. For example, if you wanted to select all patients associated with a given doctor, you could edit the *where* clause of the query to check for the desired physician's ID number.

Firewall

The Firewall is designed to provide authentication and system security. It is comprised of the Logon page that accepts information in the form of a username and password, and a hidden file that verifies the entered information and either approves or denies the logon attempt. If the entered information does not represent a legitimate user, the failed attempt is noted and control is redirected back to the Logon page. Once a user has successfully logged on, a session variable, called *logon* is set and the user is transferred to the Welcome page.

All internal HDA pages begin with a small piece of script code that checks the logon variable. Whenever a page is requested, this code is executed before any other portion of the page. If the user's *logon* variable is set, the rest of the page is processed. If the user is not logged on, the code redirects the user to the Logon page. This activity prevents unauthorized users from accessing internal pages by using the page's exact URL.

For each user type, the user interface is composed of all pages that can be viewed according to the key in their respective figures. This means that all visible pages, except Welcome, are simultaneously part of the user interface and their respective system component. This is possible because of the ability of ASP pages to act as both processing and output units.

The Welcome page, shown in Figure 6, contains a short greeting and links to the components of HDA. For all users, it displays links to three components: the Drug Information Area, the Graph Module, and the Recommendation Decision Module. If the current user is a physician, it adds a link to the Database Maintenance component.

Figure 6: Welcome Page: Physician View

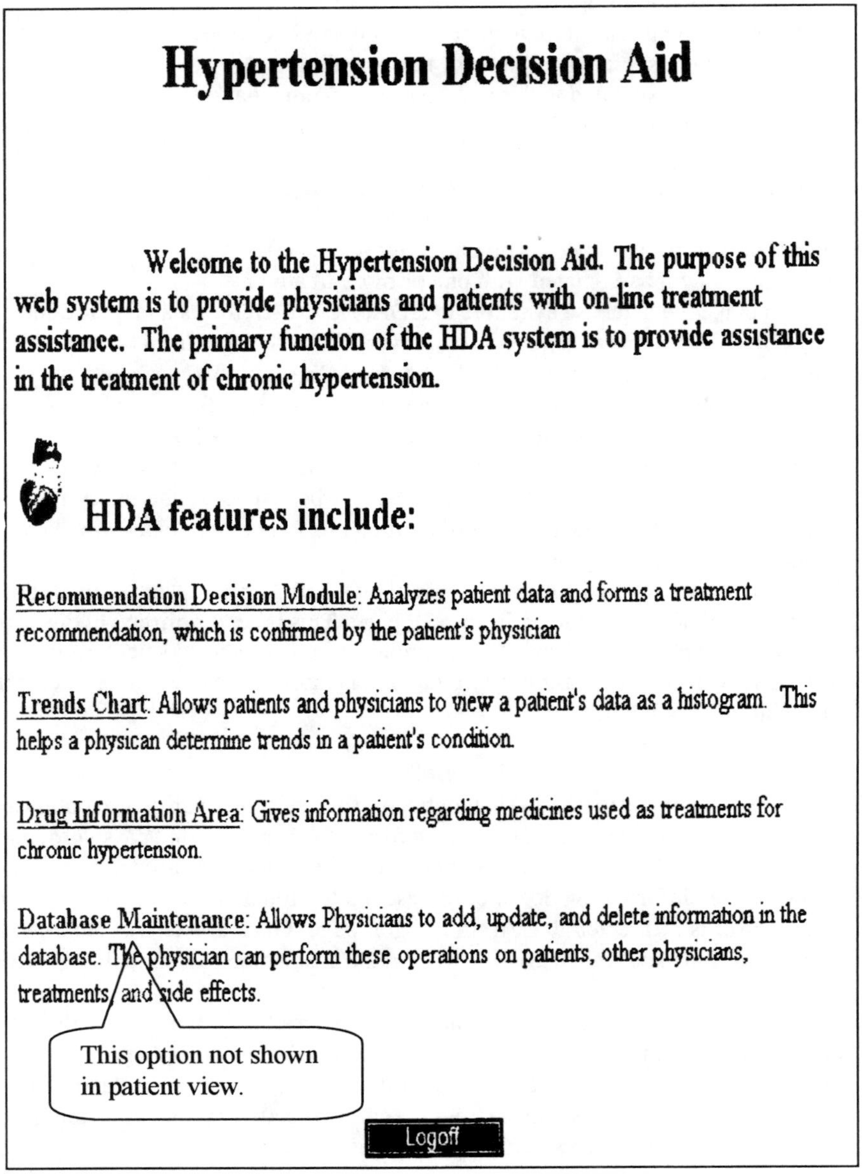

Hypertension Decision Aid

Welcome to the Hypertension Decision Aid. The purpose of this web system is to provide physicians and patients with on-line treatment assistance. The primary function of the HDA system is to provide assistance in the treatment of chronic hypertension.

 HDA features include:

Recommendation Decision Module: Analyzes patient data and forms a treatment recommendation, which is confirmed by the patient's physician

Trends Chart: Allows patients and physicians to view a patient's data as a histogram. This helps a physican determine trends in a patient's condition.

Drug Information Area: Gives information regarding medicines used as treatments for chronic hypertension.

Database Maintenance: Allows Physicians to add, update, and delete information in the database. The physician can perform these operations on patients, other physicians, treatments, and side effects.

This option not shown in patient view.

Logoff

Graph Module

The Graph Module generates graphs displaying trends over time concerning blood pressure and pulse. It also displays treatment events such as treatment or dosage changes. The Graph Module contains two pages, Trends and Graph. For a patient, the Trends page acts as a gateway to the Graph page. This is important because the Graph page contains a

Figure 7: Graph Page

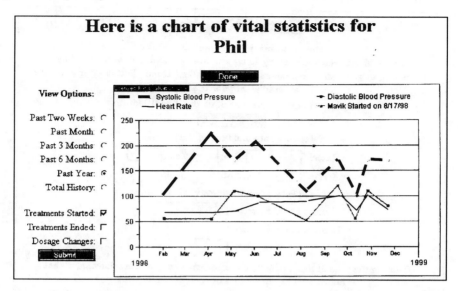

Java applet that displays the Patient's chart. This applet is 80k in size and may take time to download. While users wanting to view a Graph must move through an extra page, users who enter the Graph Module by accident or out of curiosity do not have to wait through a long download. For a physician, the Trends page lists his/her registered patients. By choosing a patient, the physician can view that person's chart. The Graph page, shown in Figure 7, also contains radio buttons and check boxes that allow for customization of the displayed chart.

Recommendation Decision Module

The Recommendation Decision Module performs different tasks for patients than for physicians. For patients, it uses the Enter Reading page (shown in Figure 8) to collect individual readings of patient vital statistics. HTML 'select' fields allow for entry of the date and time of the reading and the measured values. The values listed as options for selecting vital sign measurements are based on the expertise of hypertension physicians. The exact items listed as checkbox fields are created dynamically according to the needs of the patient filling out the form. The Enter Reading page checks the database and notes the treatments being used by the currently logged-on patient. It then displays a checkbox list of known potential side effects for any treatments used by the patient. The final field in the form is a text field that allows the patient to report other symptoms or unusual events that occurred on or around the time of the reading. For the sake of data integrity, certain fields are required and data validity checks are made. For example, in order to add the reading time, all the date and time fields must contain data. If any required fields are missing or invalid, HDA informs the patient and allows for data reentry.

Once all required fields are filled, control is moved to the Confirm page. This page displays the form entries for review, enabling for correction of data entry error. The Confirm page has two buttons, the *Change* button, which passes control back to the Enter Reading page, and the *Confirm* button which delivers the entered form values, and control, to the

Figure 8: Enter Reading Page

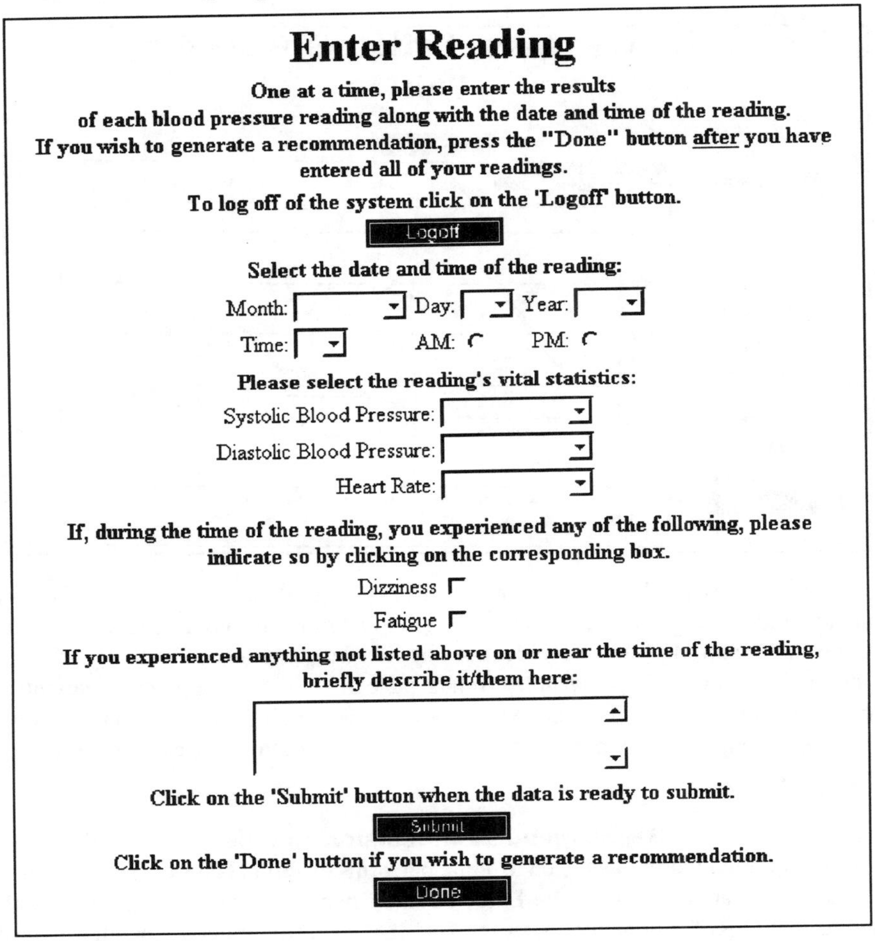

Enter Reading

One at a time, please enter the results
of each blood pressure reading along with the date and time of the reading.
If you wish to generate a recommendation, press the "Done" button <u>after</u> you have
entered all of your readings.

To log off of the system click on the 'Logoff' button.

[Logoff]

Select the date and time of the reading:

Month: [▼] Day: [▼] Year: [▼]

Time: [▼]   AM: ○   PM: ○

Please select the reading's vital statistics:

Systolic Blood Pressure: [▼]

Diastolic Blood Pressure: [▼]

Heart Rate: [▼]

If, during the time of the reading, you experienced any of the following, please
indicate so by clicking on the corresponding box.

Dizziness ☐

Fatigue ☐

If you experienced anything not listed above on or near the time of the reading,
briefly describe it/them here:

[▲]
[▼]

Click on the 'Submit' button when the data is ready to submit.

[Submit]

Click on the 'Done' button if you wish to generate a recommendation.

[Done]

Insert Reading page. The Insert Reading page inserts the form values into the database and moves control back to the Enter Reading page to allow for more readings to be entered.

Upon request, a patient also receives a *notification* from the Recommendation Decision Module. Currently, this notification takes one of two forms: the patient is directed to seek medical assistance if warranted, or the patient is notified the information has been forwarded to the physician. If a patient enters readings into the database and does not activate the decision module, a recommendation is automatically generated when the user's session ends.

The decision module contains the system's knowledge base that the Decision Generation page, not viewed by users, accesses. The knowledge base is a rule-based expert system that uses the current hypertension treatment standards outlined in *The Sixth Report of the Joint National Committee on Prevention, Detection, Evaluation, and Treatment of High Blood Pressure* to generate suggestions for treatment continuance or modification. These rules are accessible by physicians to allow for customization, enabling physicians to modify the system's recommendation generation to more accurately reflect their own professional decisions. It is important to note that this expert system is not designed to replace the decisions of an actual physician. It is simply a tool to enhance the decision-making process.

When a physician enters the Recommendation Decision Module, a list of the physician's patients is displayed as in Figure 9. By clicking on a patient's name, the physician can view a list of recommendations generated by that patient in descending chronological order.

Database Maintenance

The Database Maintenance component provides database connectivity to physicians for routine maintenance. This component is only visible to physicians. The pages in this component are protected from patient access by a small routine similar to the one described in the Firewall.

The initial page in the Database Maintenance component, shown in Figure 10, presents the physician with links to four list pages: Physician, Patient, Treatment, and Side Effect. These pages display an HTML table containing the contents of their corresponding tables in the database. The List Physician, Treatment, and Side Effect pages show the entire table. Each of the list pages allows the physician to move to the respective edit or process page and either create a new item, or edit an existing one. Clicking on the Create New button on a list page moves to the corresponding edit page with all the fields blank, while clicking on the name of an item listed will move to the edit page with the fields filled with the chosen item's data from the database.

FUTURE WORK

One of the issues yet to be addressed is accessibility to the Internet. There are some concerns that socio-economic factors will determine a patient's access to the Web thereby increasing the gap regarding access to quality healthcare (Mandl, 1998). The potential usage of public access points such as public libraries, clinics, and public schools is currently under investigation. If systems like HDA become mainstream tools for physicians and patients, pharmacy chains and pharmaceutical companies may consider placing Internet access

Figure 9: Recommendation Decision Module: Physician View

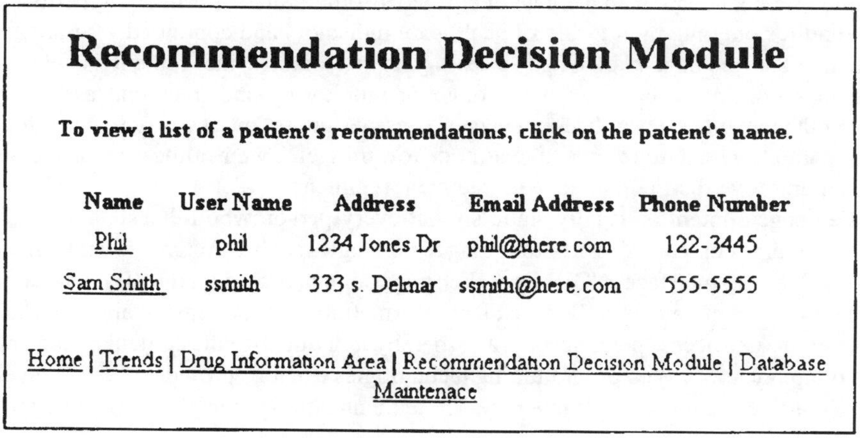

Recommendation Decision Module

To view a list of a patient's recommendations, click on the patient's name.

Name	User Name	Address	Email Address	Phone Number
Phil	phil	1234 Jones Dr	phil@there.com	122-3445
Sam Smith	ssmith	333 s. Delmar	ssmith@here.com	555-5555

Home | Trends | Drug Information Area | Recommendation Decision Module | Database Maintenace

Figure 10. Database Maintenance

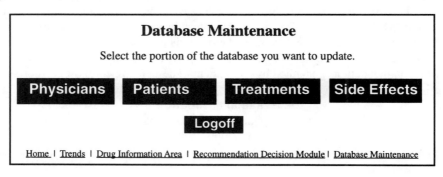

terminals at local pharmacies to attract business. Further, if clinical studies uphold the expectation of reducing the cost of healthcare through better control of medical conditions, then insurance companies could be persuaded to provide funds for Internet access.

Another concern is the population of the Drug Information Area in the system. Currently the project is relying on freely distributed information. This material is insufficient to provide a complete picture of available treatments. A relationship with major pharmaceutical companies is being explored to provide access to relevant up-to-date material. In addition, methods of formatting and organizing this information must be developed that make it readily searchable by patients and physicians so they can easily locate the information that is most relevant to their questions.

HDA is currently being tested with a small group of patients and physicians, after which the system will go through redesign and further development. Plans are being developed for a larger deployment with numerous physicians and patients. Patients will be recruited to study the system's effects on compliance, hypertension control, treatment management, and overall satisfaction.

CONCLUSION

The approach of personalizing the content of the communication of the Web page is well suited for healthcare management of chronic disorders such as primary hypertension, which requires ongoing monitoring of healthcare indicators and continued assessment of treatments. The medical knowledge necessary to personalize the content is relatively limited in scope. Also, because of the ongoing monitoring and treatment assessment, including the patient as a healthcare manager, becomes important. As an active healthcare partner, patients gain a more proactive attitude toward their own healthcare management, which can improve their compliance to treatment regimens.

Web page content is usually static so that every person who requests a Web page receives the same content. Web programming technologies such as Active Server Pages and Common Gateway Interface (CGI) allow Web page content to be dynamic. By maintaining a database of patient data as well as medical information on hypertension and treatments, Web programs can access personal data and thereby individualize the content of each page in the communication. Web programming technologies can also provide a certain level of security, confidentiality, and data integrity. The authentication provides security by limiting access to only Web users who are registered users with valid passwords, and by limiting access to data in the system specific to them. Further, the Web programming can use page dating and user authentication to ensure that pages cannot be accessed from a Web browser's cache or that unauthorized users can access parts of the system by getting past the password entry screen by guessing the Web address of a page. The Web programming validates the data patients enter, thus maintaining the integrity of data. Also, Web page dating disallows patients from back paging and changing previously entered data stored.

Web programming techniques and technologies like those used in HDA have the potential for facilitating and structuring intercommunication between patients and physicians for managing specific medical conditions. An important aspect in the development of these systems is to employ a user-centered approach to design. The user-centered design approach helps to ensure that the application fits the user's needs in performing tasks. It provides the necessary modeling of information so that it can be organized and presented in a manner that is most relevant to the user. Further, this design approach can help identify the necessary medical knowledge needed to include in the system so that message content can be individualized and structured based on the patient's history and current treatment regimen, and the patient data can be analyzed and summarized appropriately.

Evidence already exists that telecommunication technologies can have a positive impact on healthcare management (Balas, 1997). With the successful application of Web-based systems for managing major medical conditions such as primary hypertension, it can be anticipated that systems that address other conditions will follow.

REFERENCES

Bader, S. A., R. M. Braude. (1998). Patient Informatics: Creating New Partnerships in Medical Decision Making, *Academy of Medicine, 73*(4), 408-411.

Balas, E. A., F. Jaffrey, G. Kuperman, S. A. Boren, G. D. Brown, F. Pinciroli, J. A. Mitchell. (1997). Electronic Communication With Patients, *Journal of American Medicine, 278*, 152-159.

Beyer, H., & Holztblatt, K. (1997). *Contextual Design: A Customer-Centered Approach to Systems Designs*. San Francisco, CA: Morgan Kaufman Publishers.

Binstock, M. L., & K. L. Franklin, (1988). A Comparison of Compliance Techniques on the Control of High Blood Pressure, *American Journal of Hypertension*, 192-194.

Consoli, S. M., M. B. Said, J. Jean, J. Menard, P. Plouin, & G. Chatellier, (1995). Benefits of a Computer-Assisted Education Program for Hypertensive Patients Compared with Standard Education Tools, *Patient Education and Counseling, 26*, 343-347.

Flanagan, J., Huang, T., Jones, P., & Kasif, S., eds. (1997). NSF Workshop on Human-Centered Systems: Information, Interactivity, and Intelligence, Final Report. (http://www.ifp.uiuc.edu/nsfhcs).

Gentile, JA. Jr. (1998). Databases, Websites, and the Internet, *Oncology, 12*(11A), 356-359.

Gentner, D. & Grudin, J. (1996). Design Models for Computer-Human Interfaces, *IEEE Computer, 29*(6), 28-35.

Glowniak, J.V., M.K. Bushway (1994). Computer Networks as a Medical Resource. Accessing and using the Internet, *Journal of American Medicine, 271*, 1934-1939.

Johnson-Laird, P. (1989) Mental Models, In M. Posner, Ed., *Foundations of Cognitive Science* (Ch. 12). Cambridge, MA: MIT Press.

Kane, B., DZ. Sands. (1998). Guidelines for the Clinical Use of Electronic Mail With Patients. The AMIA Internet Working Group, Task Force on Guidelines for the Use of Clinical-Patient Electronic Mail, *Journal of American Medical Informatics Association, 5*, 104-111.

Kassirer, J. P., (1995). The Next Transformation in the Delivery of Healthcare, *The New England Journal of Medicine, 332*(4), 52-53.

Landauer, T. K. (1995) *The Trouble with Computers: Usefulness, Usability, and Productivity*, Cambridge, MA: The MIT Press.

LaPerri'ere B., P. Edwards, JM. Romeder, L. Maxwell-Young. (1998). Using the Internet to Support Self-Care, *Canadian Nurse, 94*(5), 47-48.

Lewis, C., J. Rieman. (1993). *Task-Centered User Interface Design*. Boulder, CO: Shareware, Clayton Lewis and John Rieman.

Liddle, D. (1996) Design of the Conceptual Model. In T. Winogard, Ed., *Bringing Design to Software* (pp. 17-31), New York, NY: ACM Press.

Mandl, K. D., I. S. Kohane, A. Brandt. (1998). Electronic Patient-Physician Communication: Problems and Promise, *Annals of Internal Medicine, 129*(6), 495-500.

Mechanic, D. (1998). Public Trust and Initiatives for New Healthcare Partnerships, *Milbank Quarterly. 76*(2), 281-302.

Muller, J., & Kuhn, S. (1993) Participatory Design, *Communications of the ACM, 36*(6), 24-28.

Neill, R.A., A.G. Mainous, JR. Clark, M.D Hagen. (1994). The Utility of Electronic Mail as a Medium for Patient-Physician Communication, *Archives of Family Medicine, 3*, 268-271.

Norman, D. (1983) Some Observations on Mental Models, In D. Gentner & A. Stevens, Eds., *Mental Models* (Ch. 1). Hillsdale, NJ: Lawrence Erlbaum Assoc.

Norman, D. (1988) The Psychopathology of Everyday Things, In D.Norman, *The Psychology of Everyday Things* (Ch. 1), New York, NY: Basic Books.

Riva, A., (1996). A Web-Based Architecture for the Intelligent Management of Chronic Patients, *Journal of the American Medical Informatics Association*, 179 - 183.

Sachs, P. (1995) Transforming Work: Collaboration, Learning, and Design, *Communications of the ACM, 38*(9), pp. 36-44.

Chapter XIV

A Web-Based Solution for Enhancing Diabetic Well-Being

Riitta Söderlund and Pekka Reijonen
University of Turku/Laboris

Malin Brännback
Turku School of Economics and Business Administration/Innomarket Unit

INTRODUCTION

In most Western countries, healthcare systems are in economic crisis. It is not possible to increase available resources, but at the same time, there is a growing demand for publicly funded healthcare services, e.g., because the number of aged people is rising. To solve this problem, countries can either increase the effectiveness and efficiency of their present healthcare activities and/or decrease public demand. Public demand can be controlled by raising user charges for publicly funded services, redefining those services, encouraging self-care, and/or subsidizing services that are privately financed. However, so far there are not many countries that encourage self-care in order to control demand, but it is considered one possibility with strong future potential (Moore, 1996). Self-care means shared responsibility in healthcare. The formal system is no longer the only institution that is responsible for individuals' health status; individuals must also take care of their own health. One of the most widely used methods for encouraging self-care is providing and sharing knowledge (Smee, 1997).

One way to enhance knowledge sharing and thus one possible way to increase the efficiency of activities in healthcare is the exploitation of information technology (IT). As Tapscott (1996) has envisioned, healthcare may be one of the primary beneficiaries from the new information technology-based networked economy. However, so far IT has provided only the infrastructure for telemedicine, expert systems, and multimedia, which have supported doctors in making diagnoses, and for databases, which have been efficient platforms for patient records, and thus, IT has mainly supported healthcare personnel and governmental institutions (e.g., Griep et al., 1996; Iakovidis, 1998; Kalra, 1996). Apart from improving the infrastructure enabling the integration of the various stakeholders within healthcare, we need IT-based tools to support and activate the individual patient. These tools specifically aim at empowering the patient, at the same time resulting in reductions in the healthcare demand, and thus the need for public funds. To make this happen, as pointed out by Moore (1996), there must be many social changes in healthcare, besides these technical innovations.

In this chapter, we describe an interactive Web-based system which is aimed at encouraging and aiding a diabetic in self-care by offering a convenient way to record and access essential data related to diabetes using a Web browser or a mobile phone. The system also gives healthcare personnel access to a more detailed and up-to-date data of the status of their diabetic patients and a possibility to give immediate feedback via a mobile phone or the Web. As a logical and technical construction, the system is rather straightforward and its potential benefits can clearly be seen. However, the system's benefits are only potential as long as the system is implemented properly. The implementation of the system calls for changes in the daily routines both by the diabetics and the healthcare personnel: the diabetics must record their data carefully using the new technology and the healthcare personnel must change their working habits and division of labor. Putting these changes into effect requires acceptance of the system by all parties. Initial training must be given to all participants in order to gain acceptance, but the future use is dependent on the perceived long-term benefits of the system.

The remainder of this chapter is organized as follows. The next section offers background information on the prevalence of diabetes and the current trends in diabetes care and management. Then a schematic description of the Web-based system in an experimental phase in Finland is given, and the differences between the old and the new care procedures are highlighted. The following section presents results from the first phase of the field experiment, in which about 100 diabetics used the system. The final section includes a summary of the results and discusses the implications of the system from the point of view of self-care, clinical diabetes care and healthcare management.

DIABETES: PREVALENCE AND CURRENT TREATMENT APPROACHES

Diabetes is one of the main chronic diseases in the world. There are two main types of diabetes: Type I diabetes and Type II diabetes. Type 1 diabetes (previously called insulin-dependent diabetes mellitus IDDM or juvenile diabetes) is considered an auto-immune disease, in which the pancreas produces little or no insulin. Thus a person with Type I diabetes needs daily injections of insulin to live. Type II diabetes (non-insulin-dependent diabetes mellitus NIDDM) usually develops in adults over the age of 40 and is most common among adults over age 55. In Type II diabetes, the pancreas usually produces insulin, but for some reason the body cannot use the insulin effectively. Approximately 40% of diabetics with Type II diabetes require insulin. (e.g., NIDDK, 1999)

The prevalence of diabetes is increasing globally. It has been estimated (King et al., 1998) that there are at present over 100 million diabetics in the world, and by the year 2025, there will be about 300 million adults with diabetes. The reasons why prevalence of diabetes is increasing are related to the fact that people live longer, have unwholesome diets, are overweight, and do not take physical exercise. Type 1 diabetes accounts for about 5 to 10% of diagnosed diabetes in the United States, but the figure is much higher in Finland. There the figure is about 18% (Diabetesliitto, 1998). There is also a tremendous geographic variation in the incidence of Type I diabetes. The incidence is lowest (0,7/100000 persons) in Shanghai, China, and in Finland the incidence is more than 50 times greater (35,3/100,000 persons) (AMA, 1996).

Diabetes is for most people associated with several restrictions and burdens and too high levels of blood glucose for a longer period of time may lead to severe complications such as retinopathy, neuropathy, and nephropathy. It has been estimated that the costs related to diabetes care are between 5-10 % of national health budgets. In Finland, this means approximately 300 million USD (Kangas, 1995). More than 80% of these costs have been estimated to be inpatient care costs, which are mainly related to treating acute and long-term complications of diabetes (Kangas, 1993).

Internationally, the economic situation is much the same. In the USA, when the yearly medical care cost for diabetics (n = 85209) and age and sex matched non-diabetic control subjects (n = 85209) were compared, it was estimated that healthcare expenditures per person for diabetics were 2.4 times higher (Selby et al., 1997). The largest proportion of total excess costs was spent on inpatient care and nearly 38% on treating the long-term complications of diabetes.

During the 1970s and 1980s, the therapeutic strategy of managing Type I diabetes changed dramatically. In the 1990s, the results of the effect of self-management from the Diabetes Control and Complications Trial (DCCT) were published (DCCT, 1993; 1995; 1996). These developments concerned mainly insulin therapy and are characterized by the following three factors: (i) self-monitoring of blood glucose has become a routine practice, (ii) patient self-management and flexibility in lifestyle are the most central ideas in the philosophy of diabetes management, and (iii) it has been proved that meticulous glycemic control reduces the risk of chronic complications (Skyler, 1997). So, the background philosophy of diabetes treatment has changed and the meticulous glycemic control has become the primary therapeutic goal (DCCT, 1995). Despite increased patient well-being, the new diabetes treatment approach is supposed to have important economical consequences. When using conventional therapy, approximately half of the expenditures of the medical care for diabetes are hidden in the treatment of the metabolic condition and the other half in the treatment of chronic complications. Intensive diabetic therapy uses more outpatient resources than conventional therapy and is a more expensive option, in this respect. However, because intensive therapy is associated with a lower incidence of chronic complications, it has been demonstrated that intensive diabetes therapy is cost-effective (Herman et al., 1997). It has been estimated that a 10 percent reduction in the long-term blood glucose level diminishes the diabetes-related healthcare costs by approximately 40 percent (DCCT, 1993; 1996).

Intensive therapy and keeping blood glucose level low are accompanied by an increased risk of hypoglycemia. Therefore, the adjustment of blood glucose level is crucial to intensive treatment and this calls for frequent testing and interpretation of data. As a consequence, diabetics must take the key role in the day-to-day management of diabetes and the responsibility for their own health, i.e., self-management must be encouraged. The role of healthcare personnel is to ensure that diabetics are adequately prepared for this challenge and the course of action in healthcare is changing towards teamwork. Besides different healthcare professionals, patients are becoming partners of these teams. This requires effective collaboration and communication between team partners. Patients must also possess the necessary information and knowledge for making decisions concerning their own health. In the case of diabetes, this means, for example, that patients must be able to interpret the patterns of glycemic response and adjust the therapeutic regimen accordingly.

Blood glucose level can be adjusted to an appropriate level by following a diet and by administering diabetes drugs correctly. Insulin, the most important drug in diabetes treatment, is very difficult to administer because reactions to insulin are individual. Also other factors, like physical activity and other diseases, have an effect on the blood glucose level (Rönnemaa, 1999). In accordance with current diabetes regimens, insulin treatment can be customized so that it suits every diabetic's eating habits and rhythm of life. The goal is that after a learning process the diabetic has enough knowledge to purposefully change the insulin doses by herself (Saraheimo & Ilanne-Parikka, 1999).

To sum up, in order to keep the long-term blood glucose level appropriate and diminish the likelihood of complications, blood glucose level must be controlled regularly. This calls for frequent blood glucose self-measurement, recording of the measuring results and other relevant factors, recurring interpretation of the data both by healthcare personnel and diabetics themselves, and fluent communication between diabetics and healthcare personnel. On the other hand, data storing, processing, and transfer are exactly the basic functions of computer-based information technology, and thus, this kind of technology should be applicable in diabetes management processes. Actually, many new solutions for supporting diabetes self-care using IT are under development (Albisser et al., 1996; Gomez et al., 1996; Lehmann, 1998; Piette & Mah, 1997; Riva et al., 1997). An example of how to use the telephone in a new way for enhancing communication between diabetics and physicians is the VISTA 350, telephone[1] combined with the Home Monitoring Module (Cytryn & Patel, 1998; Edmonds et al., 1998). The system consists of a central database, which the subjects can enter data via fixed telephone lines by using a certain type of telephone. The data consists of blood glucose levels, insulin doses, changes in diet, activity, stress, and hypoglycemic reactions. The system can provide feedback to diabetics in the form of averages and ranges of glucose levels entered. The system has proved considerably easy to use, but results of its long-term effects have not yet been reported.

Most of the research on diabetes self-management using traditional self-care methods has focused on (i) patterns and levels of self-management, (ii) correlates of self-management, and (iii) interventions designed to improve self-management (Ruggiero et al., 1997). However, major published studies involve small samples, focus solely on people with one type of diabetes (IDDM or NIDDM), and use a variety of different methods of measuring self-management. That is why many basic questions concerning self-management in diabetes remain unanswered. In the following sections we describe a Web-based system aimed at enhancing patient self-management and blood glucose control and report the results from its implementation phase.

A WEB-BASED SOLUTION FOR INFORMATION GATHERING AND ACCESS

This chapter describes a telecare service system for supporting diabetics' self-management that is in an experimental phase under the name WellMate[2] in Finland. This interactive service system consists of a central database which the diabetics and the healthcare personnel access using a Web browser or a mobile phone (Figure 1). The service provider is responsible for the database, and a diabetic who wants to use the service must make a contract to license the provider to gather and file her diabetes data. The diabetic also

Figure 1: A Schematic Diagram of the Telecare Service System for Diabetics

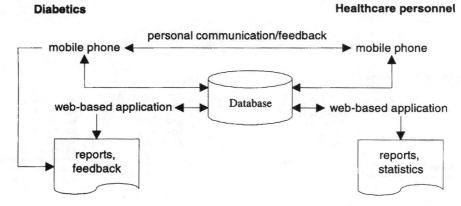

authorizes the healthcare personnel of the diabetes clinic, or some of the personnel to use the gathered data.

From the diabetic's perspective, the primary component of this system is a mobile phone. The mobile phone makes the system quite flexible and independent of time and place, because phone owners usually always carry the phone with them. In Finland, the coverage of mobile phone nets is practically total, and nearly 60 percent of the population have a mobile phone (Mobile communications statistics, 1999). Accessing the Internet is not very difficult in Finland. The use of the Internet has increased rapidly during the last few years, and the latest statistics show that about 47 percent of 15-to-74-year-old Finns have used the Internet sometime and about 17 percent use it weekly at home (Taloustutkimus, 1999). A considerable matter in this context is that at least in Finland it has become normal to use the Internet at home, even so normal that home is now in the first place from which to access the Internet.

The mobile phone used in this diabetes system is a GSM (the Global System for Mobile Communications) mobile phone. One of the advantages of the GSM system is that the same handset can be used widely: a mobile phone registered to a GSM network in Finland can be used on a GSM network in Australia for example. Besides, the GSM system provides users with several digital channels. The channels are either synchronous or asynchronous, and because the system encrypts the data over the channels, the system is relatively secure. The synchronous channels enable voice and data communications, and the asynchronous packet data channel provides a form of e-mail for GSM users. The asynchronous channel is also known as the short-message service (SMS). In the system depicted here, the most important channel is the asynchronous channel, which is most often used for communication between diabetics and healthcare personnel. It is the channel diabetics use for sending data and retrieving reports.

Before the GSM phone with the special diabetes module can be used for the service, special settings must be made. Namely, a diabetic must set the server number of the service provider and the personal password in the memory of the phone. These settings enable automatic secure messaging from point to point, and the server number identifies the database and the personal password identifies the diabetic. In order to further increase the

Figure 2. Sending a Blood Glucose Value Using a Mobile Phone with the Special Diabetes Module

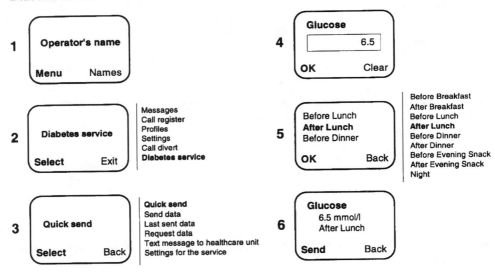

security of the phone and the service, it is recommended that the following general security settings are also done: the PIN (Personal Identity Number) code request is set on, and both the PIN code and the security code set in the factory are changed.

The diabetes module of the mobile phone offers tailored diabetes functions which appear to the user as a special diabetes menu. The diabetes menu is under the main menu. Using a function keypad to scroll the menu, the different options of the main menu can be seen in the display of the phone one by one. The special diabetes functions under the diabetes menu can be found in an analogous way. There are six functions in the diabetes menu: 1) *Quick send*, 2) *Send data*, 3) *Last sent data*, 4) *Request data*, 5) *Text message to healthcare unit*, and 6) *Settings for the service*. The use of the functions is quite easy. The diabetic uses function keypads for choosing the functions and numeric/alphabetic keypads for data input (Figure 2).

Quick send is the fastest way to send a blood glucose value and the relation of the measuring moment to a meal, e.g., before breakfast, after evening snack, night. This function automatically inserts the date and time to the data to be sent. So, this function is applicable when the data are sent in real-time and when there is no need to send more detailed information. *Send data* includes options for sending different combinations of diabetes-related information (blood glucose value, insulin, size of meal, exercise), entering the date and time, and adding free-form comments to data. *Last sent data* shows the last sent message and provides options for editing, erasing and re-sending the data. *Request data* makes it possible to view one's own data stored in the diabetes database, e.g. one can get reports on mean glucose values of different measuring periods or reports on the glucose profile. By using the function *Text message to healthcare unit*, ordinary text messages (SMS) can be written and sent to the healthcare unit. The *settings for the service* menu includes, among other things, the option to choose the language used and the option to make a glossary of comments which can then be used in combination with the *Send data* function. The data sending described above proceeds via the asynchronous channel, but naturally the mobile phone can also be used for traditional personal communication between the diabetics and the healthcare personnel via the synchronous voice channel.

The other possibility to use the system is via the Internet. There are separate versions of the Web-based application for the diabetics and the healthcare personnel. Both of the versions use the SSL (the Secure Socket Layer) system for providing the security of data and require a Web browser that must be either Netscape Navigator or Internet Explorer. Further, both the personnel and the diabetics must have user IDs and passwords to use the WWW service.

The Web-based application of the diabetics offers both a personal and a general service. On the personal user page, a diabetic can, e.g., examine the long-term reports of her own blood glucose levels either in graphic or in verbal form (Figure 3). The pages common to all of the users of the service offer e.g. general information of diabetes and the possibility to send e-mail to the provider of the service. The personnel's application is typically used to examine the reports of the data sent by a diabetic, to write treatment prescriptions, and to send messages to the diabetics. Thus, the healthcare personnel can benefit from the system both during the regular face-to-face checks or telephone consultations and between the checks and telephone consultations, e.g., by sending treatment prescriptions or other advice to the diabetics. Besides supporting data management on the level of an individual diabetic, the application supports data management and reporting on an aggregate level.

Figure 3. A diabetic can examine the long-term report of her blood glucose values in graphic and verbal form on the personal user page

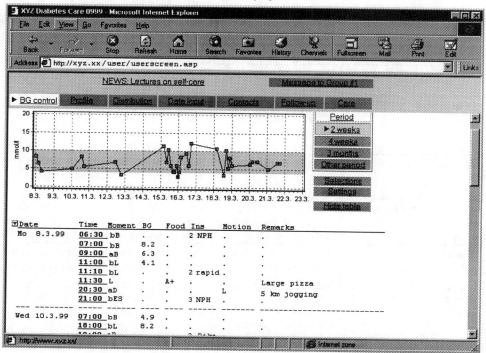

The system has several effects both for diabetics and healthcare personnel (see Table 1). The data, which have earlier been available in diabetics' handwritten notebooks, are now stored in the database. This changes the possibilities of data usage tremendously: the diabetics can send data via a mobile phone or the Web quite irrespective of their actual location, and the healthcare personnel has real-time access to the data. Reliable, real-time data increase the possibilities for accurate adjustment of blood glucose level for each diabetic either on her own or with the help of experts.

The data do not, however, appear in the database without the diabetics' activity. In other words, the implementation phase of the system is crucial for its future success, and diabetics must be motivated to use the system. Training has an important role in the initial phase, but perceived benefits (better health) become crucial after the introductory period. Also the healthcare personnel must accept their new role as personal coaches and tighten their contact with the diabetics.

It is expected that the diabetics are motivated to take more responsibility for their health, i.e., input their data so frequently that reliable interpretations can be made. This would mean fewer complications and a better quality of life for the diabetics. It would also bring about considerable cost savings especially with respect to inpatient care.

Table 1. The Differences Between the Old and the New Web-Based Diabetes Telecare System

Affected variable	Old system	New system
Data gathering media	Manual: diabetic's notebook and pencil	Electronic: database accessed via mobile phone or Web browser
Data access	Local and delayed: presence of diabetic's notebook is necessary	Global and real-time: via the Web or mobile phone
Data analysis	Difficult: requires re-inputting of the handwritten data (hence not done)	Easy: reports, statistics etc. can be produced both for individuals and groups using a computer
Diabetic's skill requirements	Low: hand writing	Moderate/high: use of mobile phone or Web-browser for sending or retrieving data
Healthcare personnel's role	General advisor: care is based on general medical knowledge and tacit knowledge of diabetic	Personal coach: individual data enable accurate interpretation and adjustment
Diabetic's role	Passive self-care: diabetic follows the instructions (e.g. notifies data in the notebook)	Active self-care: diabetic takes responsibility for one's own treatment
Contact between diabetic and healthcare personnel	Discontinuous: face-to-face check every three months and when severe problems or complications	Continuous: direct access to up-to-date data and possibility to immediate contact and feedback

RESULTS FROM THE IMPLEMENTATION PHASE

A field experiment is being carried out in order to gain knowledge of the use of the system in a real-life situation. A randomly selected group of diabetics is using the system and their experiences as the log data are collected and evaluated. In the next section, we report the results of the first four months after the implementation.

Research Design and Procedures

The experimental group was formed by drawing a random sample from the patient database of a Finnish diabetes clinic. The criteria for acceptance into the study were that the person must be insulin-dependent and willing to participate in the experiment. Patients with severe handicaps hampering use of a mobile phone, e.g., serious neuropathy in fingers or problems with sight, were excluded from the sample. By these means 102 diabetics entered the experimental group.

At the beginning of the experiment, all the subjects were given a mobile phone augmented with the tailored diabetes telecare functions. For the subjects, the mobile phone and its use for the service are free of charge during the experiment. The subjects participated in a combined introductory and training session in order to learn how to use the system. Training was arranged individually for each subject by two trainers, who both trained an equal amount of the subjects. After the training, the skills of the subjects were tested using representative tasks. The sessions lasted from 15 minutes to two-and-a-half hours with the mean of one and a half hours. The large variation is explained by the goals of the training: each subject should get used to the system and be able to use at least the basic functions of the system, i.e. to send the measuring data. Younger subjects who had mobile phones of their own needed very little training. The other main goal of the training was to motivate the subjects to use the system by informing them about the importance of the patient's own active role in the treatment, of which measuring and interpreting blood glucose levels form a fundamental part. All the subjects received detailed manuals and were encouraged to practice the use of the system and to contact either the personnel of the clinic or the technical

Table 2. Descriptive Data of the Experimental Group (absolute figures).

Variable	Women	Men	Total
N	43	59	102
Mean age	43	43	43
Length of time with diabetes	18	17	17
Complications	12	14	26
Blood glucose measures per week	11	9	10
Always writes down measuring result	16	17	33
Never writes down measuring result	7	11	18
Owns a mobile phone (before experiment)	17	38	55
Never used a mobile phone	14	14	28
Never sent text messages (phone owners)	3	14	17
Never sent text messages (all subjects)	25	30	55
Never uses a computer (at work or home)	27	33	60
I will increase my measuring frequency	33	45	78
Self-care will get better with the new diabetes telecare system	39	57	96

support person if any help was needed.

At the end of the training session, the subjects filled in a questionnaire concerning descriptive information and some diabetes-related issues. Sixty-two percent of the subjects have at least part-time work and 14 percent are unemployed. Their age varies from 21 to 66 years with the mean of 43 years (see Table 2). Their mean diabetes duration is 17 years and about 1/4 of the subjects have at least one complication. According to their own report they have been measuring their blood glucose level about 10 times a week, which is the common recommendation of their clinic under normal circumstances. About one third have always written down the measuring results and 1/6 have never written down the results. Half of the subjects owned a mobile phone before the experiment and 40 percent have used a computer (home or work). The subjects feel positive about the new system: nearly all believe that their self-care will get better and 76 percent believe that they will increase their blood glucose measuring frequency while using the system.

All data traffic between the mobile phones and the database, i.e. sending the measuring data, detailed data, and text messages and receiving reports, is automatically saved into the log file of the server, hence exact use statistics are available.

Results

After the training session, only three subjects were unable to send the measuring data (the quick send function) without mistakes and almost all the subjects felt that they had received enough training. There were, however, considerable differences between the learning results across the functions: 90 percent of those who took the test on the quick send

Figure 4: Number of blood glucose measurements per week before (Earlier) and after the implementation of the new diabetes telecare system (New system) (t = 2.78, df = 96, p = 0.007). Earlier (self-reported) data are used as constant comparison values and they come from the questionnaires and with the new system data (log data) from the log file of the diabetes telecare database.

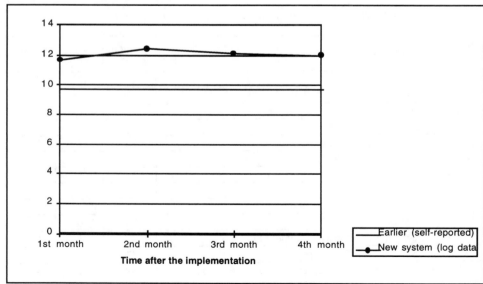

function $(n = 88)^3$ passed the task but only 47 percent $(n = 73)$ managed the request data function which also requires interpretation of the data. The send data function test was passed by 80 percent $(n = 85)$ and the text message function test by 71 percent $(n = 76)$. It seemed, however, that the subjects who did not pass the tests quickly learned to use the system by practicing on their own with help from the manuals. This is confirmed by the fact that there are no statistically significant differences between the passed and non-passed subjects in their average use of different functions.

On average, the subjects have used the system very actively and only two subjects never started to use it. The total number of contacts (any of the four functions) the subjects made during the 17-week period varied from 9 to 917 and the mean number of contacts was 208, i.e. about 12 contacts per week. Practically all contacts were data sending: either pure measuring data (72 percent quick send) or measuring data augmented with more detailed information (24 percent send data). Data requests (1 percent) and text messages (2 percent) were used only occasionally.

According to the questionnaire answers, the subjects had been measuring their blood glucose level on average about ten times a week before the implementation of the new diabetes telecare system. As seen in Figure 4, after the implementation the mean number of measurements per week is about 12, i.e. an increase of 23 percent $(t = 2.78, df = 96, p = 0.007)$. The increase of measuring frequency does not, naturally, concern all the subjects, but 61 percent of the subjects have increased their measuring frequency after the implementation of the system. This means, however, that 63 percent of the subjects measure and send blood glucose levels at least eight times a week and 52 percent at least ten times a week.

The measuring frequency does not seem to be significantly associated with gender, basic education level, earlier mobile phone usage, diabetes duration, or existence of

Figure 5: Number of blood glucose measurements per week after the implementation of the new diabetes telecare system for age groups 34 and under (n = 27) and 55 and over (n = 18). Except for the 2nd month, the difference between the age groups is statistically significant (ANOVA, p = 0.035 or less).

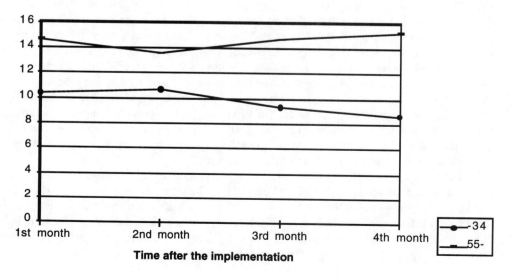

complications. Interestingly, however, it is connected to two variables: the anticipated effect of the system and the age of the subjects. Two thirds of the subjects (n = 74) who anticipated an increase in their measuring frequency have actually increased their measuring frequency but they still measure their blood glucose levels more seldomly (10 times/week) than the subjects who did not anticipate any change (17 times/week). These statistically significant (ANOVA: F = 4.71, df = 4, p = 0.002) differences are readily understood when the self-reported earlier measuring frequencies are compared: those who anticipated an increase in their measuring frequency have earlier measured six to seven times per week while others have done it 14-15 times per week.

The mean age of the subjects who have increased their measuring frequency is 46 years, while it is 39 years for the subjects who have kept their measuring frequency constant or decreased it (ANOVA: F= 8.54, df = 1, p = 0.004). In other words, the older subjects have both learned to use the system and become more active in their self-care.

The increase in measuring frequency is not only a relative change, but the older diabetics have also been controlling their blood glucose more often than the younger diabetics have. The difference between the age groups is depicted in Figure 5, which shows that while using the new system, diabetics under 35 have been measuring their blood glucose 9-10 times a week whereas diabetics over 54 have done it 14-15 times a week. It is noteworthy that the baselines for the two groups, i.e., the self-reported measuring frequencies before the implementation of the telecare system, were practically the same ('- 34 years' 9.1 and '55- years' 8.7).

DISCUSSION AND FUTURE TRENDS

The results from the implementation phase of the interactive information service system, which is integrated into the diabetes management and self-management processes, were very encouraging. The system made the communication between the diabetics and the healthcare personnel easier and faster than before. A diabetic could send the diabetes data immediately after the measurements, and the personnel was able to examine the data whenever they wanted and were free from face-to-face checks with other patients. A diabetic could also get information or advice quite rapidly from the personnel via text messages, whereas before it was almost impossible to communicate with the physician between the regular visits. Also, the physician could examine the blood glucose information of a diabetic whenever needed; before this was possible only during the face-to-face checks. However, it is not the best practice that only the physician authorized by the diabetic can examine the information. Secrecy and privacy are very important issues, but the kind of authorizing used may induce problematic situations: a diabetic has acute complications and the physician authorized is not working, i.e. there is information, but nobody can use it. Thus, there should be some solutions to give the physician the right to read and write information in an emergency in the system's database.

The mobile phone proved to be easy to use and practically all the subjects were able to use the basic function after a couple of hours of introductory training session. The results from the first 17 weeks after the implementation show that the subjects have been using the system very actively and had on average 12 contacts per week via mobile phone. Nearly all contacts were data entering (*Quick send* or *Send data* functions) and data requests and text messages were used only marginally. For data requests this result could be expected, because the subjects automatically receive printed reports by mail twice a month and are able to examine reports via the Internet, and reports requested on the phone display are not as visual as the other two forms of reports. This is the situation because the display of the mobile phone is quite small, and it does not enable the use of graphic presentation. However, the *Request data* function is not useless, because it enables a diabetic to get reports when paper-based reports are not available, or it is not possible to use the Internet, e.g. when travelling. The use of GSM technology is possible almost everywhere outside very sparsely populated areas, in which the GSM coverage is not dense enough. So, the GSM technology is not a solution for telecare in these areas. However, it is possible to benefit from mobile phones, but in those circumstances satellite-based mobile phone systems are needed.

When blood glucose level measuring frequencies were compared to the earlier self-reported ones, it was found that the measuring frequencies had increased on average by 23 percent after the implementation of the new diabetes telecare system. What is more important is that the mean measuring frequency stayed at this higher level during the first four months after the implementation period. The measuring frequency seems to have increased quite independently of the earlier measuring frequency, i.e. even those who had been measuring 14 times per week have increased their measuring frequencies. This might be partly connected to the fact that sending measuring data can be done quite independently of time and place while using a mobile phone. It is interesting to perceive that the measuring frequencies have increased most and are the highest among the older subjects. This is a positive indication of the possibilities of the system and shows that when motivated, older people are ready to change their habits, prove new approaches, and take advantage of new technology.

The data do not, so far, allow us to interpret if the measuring frequencies are at an appropriate level. The need for blood glucose measurements depends on many factors: the type of diabetes, treatment type, goals of treatment, and current condition of health. When beginning or changing the treatment type, there is always a greater need for frequent measurements than at other times. Some recommend for Type I diabetics that it would be wise to measure the level of blood glucose round-the-clock (5-7 tests), e.g., twice a week to get the diurnal changes of blood glucose level (Rönnemaa, 1999). This kind of measurement would make it easier to plan insulin doses in the long run. However, the diurnal variations in glycemia may be too great to be detected by self-monitoring (Bolinder et. al., 1997). The optimal goal could be continuous recording of glucose levels. It may become a clinical reality in the near future, but it probably cannot be used for routine care. However, some kind of automation of the measuring event might be needed for other reasons. Namely, it has been demonstrated that diabetics tend to over-report the number of blood glucose tests and enter lower values in notebooks than the real values given by the blood glucose meter (Strowig & Raskin, 1998). A more automated measuring system would allow a wider use of the system by children and handicapped people, too. In this case, it could be a good solution to combine the functions of the blood glucose meter and the diabetes module of the mobile phone. Thus, the blood glucose value measured would be sent automatically, and the value sent would be the value measured.

Even though the experiences of the implementation of the system are positive, they only depict a part of the whole picture: diabetics have increased their blood glucose testing and the data are stored effectively, but the collected data must also be efficiently exploited before any real benefits can be gained. The implementation of intensified insulin regimens rely heavily on diabetics' self-monitoring and self-management of blood glucose levels.

Hence, self-management education plays a decisive role in the process. Self-management education refers to the process of teaching individuals to manage their diabetes (TFTRTNS, 1995). Self-care and self-management of diabetes does not mean that the diabetic can complete certain activities, but the diabetic must be able to see associations between these activities and to implement appropriate changes in everyday life when necessary.

Although self-management of diabetes would be effective, the importance of face-to-face routine checks must not be underestimated. Those who neglect routine checks often have the most serious complications (Rönnemaa, 1999). Treatment of diabetes is based on two factors. The key factor is the diabetic's knowledge, her abilities and enthusiasm to take care of her illness. In the general opinion, motives for effective self-management of diabetes originate from experiences of success and from feelings that one is able to master diabetes. Also, it is important that one can live quite freely. However, we cannot forget the other key factor, namely the support and professional knowledge of healthcare units. Patient-doctor-nurse relationships of long duration are essential for effective self-management. With the help of the healthcare personnel, the diabetic is able to solve special problematic questions and get support for her efforts. In Finland, routine checks of diabetics take place mostly every third or fourth month, but if necessary, there can be fewer or a greater number of these checks. The objective of the checks is to support the diabetics' self-management abilities and to help keep a good level of blood glucose values. Once every year the state of the patient's health is examined very thoroughly to diagnose any complication at a very early stage and if necessary, begin treatment activities to stop progression of these complications. The use of the new diabetes telecare system does not eliminate the need for these regular meetings of the diabetics and healthcare personnel; indeed quite the contrary: these meetings are an excellent opportunity to train and educate the diabetics in interpreting the collected data. However, in the long term, the new ways to communicate will reduce the need and thus also the frequency of face-to-face visits.

The time elapsed from the onset of the experiment, about half a year, is much too short to get any health economic benefits, and that is why no health economic analyses have been done. We do not know which health effects there will be, if any. The high level of enthusiasm at the beginning of the experiment may give biased evidence of the descending trend of the HbA_{1c} in the long term, for it may be that the effect of the new system on the motivation of diabetics do not survive. The time elapsed is also too short to implement new processes and working practices in diabetes care. It takes time to change traditions in healthcare: who does what, where, when, how and why. So, any cost savings have not yet been realized; on the contrary, the costs have risen. Besides the costs of the old practices, there are the costs of the investment in new technical equipment and applications, the training costs, and the costs of the use of the new system. Cost accounting concerning these matters is quite easy. However, there are some problems also related to this cost accounting, there is especially the question of sunk and common costs. For example, nearly 60 percent of the Finnish population have a mobile phone and the percentage is rising all the time. Is the cost of the mobile phone sunk or not? And in an analogous way, how should the periodical basic fees be handled?

To summarize, information technology is one way of enhancing knowledge sharing and also a possible way to increase the efficiency of activities in healthcare. In actual practice, increasing the effectiveness and efficiency of healthcare with IT and knowledge sharing means that individuals have access to relevant and understandable medical data and they can benefit from it by taking care of their own health. The formal system supports individuals in this process, but the formal system is no longer the only system that is responsible for individuals' health status. The new healthcare strategy presumes that individuals have the ability and the motivation to use new IT facilities, understand the meaning of the information accessed with IT, and can use the information to take care of themselves. Besides, there is the issue of whether everyone can afford to have the necessary IT facilities. Thus, the healthcare sector must be very careful not to participate in the segmentation of our society on the grounds of the use of new IT with its new strategy: 1) to people who can afford and take advantage of new IT, 2) to people who can afford but cannot take advantage, 3) to people who cannot afford but could take advantage, and 4) to people who can neither afford nor take advantage of new IT. The segmentation described does not increase the well-being of any individual, which is the main goal of healthcare. We hope that this segmentation is not going to happen. However, one must realize that this negative development may happen without different forms of support to those who cannot afford and to those who cannot take advantage of new IT.

CONCLUSION

Reliable, valid, and up-to-date data have a central role in all healthcare activities. It can be argued that data form the basis for the patients' self-management, effective and efficient patient care, and, as an aggregate form, for the planning and management of the whole healthcare sector. The centrality of data makes the healthcare sector extremely suitable for the deployment of new information and communications technology.

Our results from the implementation of an interactive information service system for diabetes care show clearly that the new technology can be effectively applied. So, there is obviously a great pull from the healthcare sector to develop new IT solutions. It is not only the IT industry that pushes the new technology to be used in healthcare, as used in other service sectors. It must be remembered, however, that the technology only forms the infrastructure and is a kind of enabler of changes. Hence, even though technology can be effectively used to initialize changes, the realization of the potential benefits of technology require concurrent changes in work processes and in actors' skills and knowledge as well as in attitudes. In the presented case this means that both the diabetics and the healthcare personnel must learn their new roles with new requirements. The implementation of these changes may require, unfortunately, more time and monetary investment than the pure technological infrastructure. So far, the technical solutions must also be improved.

ENDNOTES

1 VISTA 350 is a product of Northern Telecom
2 WellMate is a registered trademark of Nokia Mobile Phones
3 The number of subjects taking part in different tests varies. Some subjects had considerable experience in mobile phones, and testing them seemed inappropriate. Some had no time to take the test, some wanted to practice on their own, some refused to take the test, and some were released from the test by the trainer, because it was obvious that they were unable to pass it.

REFERENCES

Albisser, A. M., Harris, R. I., Sakkal, S., Parson, I. D., & Chao, S. C. (1996). Diabetes intervention in the information age. *Medical Informatics, 21* (4), 297-316.

AMA [American Diabetes Association] (1996). *Diabetes 1996: Vital statistics.* Available at http://www.amylin.com/website/diabfact/diabfact.htm, 10.8.1999. Diabetes Facts. Epidemiology.

Bolinder, J., Hagström-Toft E., Ungerstedt U., & Arner P. (1997). Self-monitoring of blood glucose in type I diabetic patients: comparison with continuous microdialysis measurements of glucose in subcutaneous adipose tissue during ordinary life conditions. *Diabetes Care, 20* (1), 64-70.

Cytryn K. N., & Patel, V. L. (1998). Reasoning about diabetes and its relationship to the use of telecommunication technology by patients and physicians. *International Journal of Medical Informatics, 51*, 137-151.

DCCT [The Diabetes Control and Complications Trials Research Group] (1993). The effect of intensive treatment of diabetes on the development and progression of long-term complications in insulin-dependent diabetes mellitus. *New England Journal of Medicine, 329*, 977-986.

DCCT [The Diabetes Control and Complications Trials Research Group] (1995). Implementation of treatment protocols in the diabetes control and complications trial. *Diabetes Care, 18*, 361-376.

DCCT [The Diabetes Control and Complications Trials Research Group] (1996). The absence of glycemic threshold for the development of long-term complications: the perspectives of Diabetes and Complications Trial. *Diabetes, 45*, 1289-1298.

Diabetesliitto (1998). *Diabetes pähkinänkuoressa.* Diabetestietoa. Available at http://www.diabetes.fi/su/tiedote/pahkina.htm, 15.9.1998. (Diabetes in a nut shell. Information of diabetes, only in Finnish.)

Edmonds, M., Bauer, M., Osborn, S., Lutfiyya, H., Mahon, J., Doig, G., Grundy, P., Gittens, C., Molenkamp, G., & Fenlon, D. (1998). Using the Vista 350 telephone to communicate the results of home monitoring of diabetes mellitus to a central database and to provide feedback. *International Journal of Medical Informatics, 51*, 117-125.

Gomez, E. J., del Pozo, F., & Hernando, M.E. (1996). Telemedicine for diabetes care: the DIABTel approach towards diabetes telecare. *Medical Informatics, 21* (4), 283-295.

Griep, P., van den Berg, N., Doelman, J., & Starrenburg, R. (1996). An epilepsy information system to support routine and research. *International Journal of Bio-Medical Computing, 42*, 135-141.

Herman W. H., Dasbach E. J., Songer T. J., & Eastman R. C. (1997). The cost-effectiveness of intensive therapy for diabetes mellitus. *Endocrinology and Metabolism Clinics of North America, 26* (3), 679-695.

Iakovidis, I. (1998). Towards personal health record: current situation, obstacles and trends in implementation of electronic healthcare record in Europe. *International Journal of Medical Informatics, 52*, 105-115.

Kangas, T. (1993). Diabeetikoiden hoito Suomessa: Avohoito, sairaalahoito ja hoitotasapaino. *Research Reports/National Research and Development Centre for Welfare and Health, 29.* ('Diabetics' healthcare in Finland: Non-institutional care, inpatient care, and treatment balance', only in Finnish.)

Kangas, T. (1995). The FinnDiab report: Healthcare of people with diabetes in Finland. *Research Reports/National Research and Development Centre for Welfare and Health; 58.*

Kalra, D. (1996). Information technology for doctors. *British Journal of Hospital Medicine, 55* (3), 144-146.

King H., Aubert R. E., & Herman, W. (1998). Global burden of diabetes 1995-2025: Prevalence, numerical estimates, and projections. *Diabetes Care, 21* (9), 1414-1431.

Lehmann, E. D. (1998). Preliminary experience with the Internet release of AIDA – an interactive educational diabetes simulator. *Computer Methods and Programs in Biomedicine, 56* (2), 109-132.

Mobile communications statistics (1999). *Number of subscriptions to the mobile telephone networks since 1980.* The Finnish Ministry of Transport and Communications. Available at the http://www.mintc.fi/telecom.htm, 12.5.1999.

Moore, J. F. (1996). *The death of competition: Leadership & strategy in the age of business ecosystems.* Chichester: John Wiley & Sons.

NIIDK [National Diabetes Information Clearinghouse] (1999). *Diabetes statistics.* Available at http://www.niddk.nih.gov/health/diabetes/pubs/dmstats/dmstats.htm, 10.8.1999.

Piette, J. D., & Mah, C. A. (1997): The feasibility of automated voice messaging as an adjunct to diabetes outpatient care. *Diabetes Care, 20* (1), 15-21.

Riva, A., Bellazzi, R., & Stefanelli, M. (1997): A Web-based system for the intelligent management of diabetic patients. *MD Computing, 14* (5), 360-364.

Ruggiero, L., Glasgow, R., Dryfoos, J. M., Rossi, J. S., Prochaska, J. O., Orleans, C. T., Prokhorov, A. V., Rossi, S. R., Greene, G. W., Reed, G. R., Kelly, K., Chobanian, L., & Johnson, S. (1997). Diabetes self-management: self-reported recommendations and patterns in a large population. *Diabetes Care, 20* (4), 568-576.

Rönnemaa, T. (1999). Määräaikaistarkastukset. In P. Ilanne-Parikka, T. Kangas, E. A. Kaprio, & T. Rönnemaa (Eds.), *Diabetes* (pp. 55-57). Jyväskylä: Gummerus Kirjapaino Oy. ('Periodic controls', only in Finnish.)

Saraheimo, M., & Ilanne-Parikka, P. (1999). Mitä diabetes on? In P. Ilanne-Parikka, T. Kangas, E. A. Kaprio, & T. Rönnemaa (Eds.), *Diabetes* (pp. 9-20). Jyväskylä: Gummerus Kirjapaino Oy. ('What is diabetes?', only in Finnish.)

Selby, J. V., Ray, T. G., Zhang, D. & Colby, C. J. (1997). Excess costs of medical care for patients with diabetes in a managed care population. *Diabetes Care, 20*, 1396-1402.

Smee, C. H. (1997). Bridging the gap between public expectations and public willingness to pay. *Health Economics, 6*, 1-9.

Skyler, J. S. (1997). Tactics for type I diabetes. *Endocrinology and Metabolism Clinics of North America, 26* (3), 647-657.

Strowig, S. M., & Raskin P. (1998). Improved glycemic control in intensively treated type I diabetic patients using blood glucose meters with storage capability and computer-assisted analyses. *Diabetes Care, 21* (10), 1694-1698.

Taloustutkimus (1999). *Internetin kotikäyttö tuplaantunut.* Lehdistötiedote 18.3.1999. Available at http://www.toy.fi/uutisiainternetinkotikaytto.html, 19.8.1999. (The use of the Internet at home has doubled, only in Finnish.)

Tapscott, D. (1996). *The digital economy: promises and perils in the age of networked intelligence.* New York: McGraw-Hill.

TFTRTNS [Task Force To Revise The National Standards] (1995). National standards for diabetes self-management education programs. *Diabetes Care, 18* (1), 141-143.

Chapter XV

The Web-Enabled Patient

Michèle Lemaire
Anabase International Corp., USA

The past decade has witnessed major changes in the concepts of health and disease and in the respective role and responsibility of doctors and patients in health maintenance and disease management. These changes were triggered by cost-containment imperatives. Although constraining by nature, these imperatives are also enabling.

The original incentive to engage people in taking larger responsibility in their own care was economic. The strategy used to foster commitment to better health was increasing people's health awareness and making them confident they could modify their behavior, and in so doing reduce their risk for preventable diseases such as cardiovascular diseases (primary prevention) or detect diseases at earlier stages such as cancers (secondary prevention). Only recently, the concept of encouraging people to participate in their own care has been extended to patients with chronic diseases. Here, the objective is to make the patient able to practice self-care in the management of his/her disease, and the incentive is still to reduce the demand for and cost of care. Health promotion, disease prevention and disease self-management all rest on education: systematic education about diseases and risks, practical information on how to adopt appropriate behaviors, and training in self-care skills along with the message that people have the capability to change their behavior and acquire the necessary skills. These changes brought about by economic concerns can be seen as constraining, since they require active self-monitoring and self-discipline. However, as they rely heavily on health information and the development of self-confidence, their unintended consequences, enhanced by the current technology developments, are patient empowerment and a change in the doctor-patient relationship.

The Internet, by offering both unfiltered information resources and powerful communication tools, increases the capacity of the willing patient to take an active role in his/her own care. It allows him/her to do it more extensively and more efficiently. Better-informed patients, building up on real-life experiences exchanged with other patients in disease-specific forums can discuss treatment options with their physician, understand and comply with treatment guidelines, and achieve better clinical outcomes. Besides the growing number of Internet companies and medical institutions offering medical information, we are seeing the growing number of patient-initiated Web sites that provide at once up-to-date disease-specific information, practical advice and emotional support. We are witnessing the organization of the Web-enabled patient community significantly changing the politics of medicine and healthcare. Education and peer support play a primary role in making this revolution possible. By providing the necessary logistical support, the World Wide Web makes it happen.

The purpose of this chapter is to describe an emerging trend, to identify the factors that contributed to its occurrence, and the implications this has for healthcare and the practice of medicine. The emerging trend is that of patients using each other's experiential expertise and the World Wide Web[1] on their own initiative to deepen their understanding and knowledge of their disease(s), so to enable them to team-up with their physician to address their specific care needs and hopefully improve their health outcomes. This emerging trend finds its roots in education promoted by the new medical models of health promotion and disease prevention, as well as in the self-help movement. Because Web-enabled patients do not intend to use the World Wide Web to replace their doctors, and because there is also a need to make these resources accessible to people from all boards, this emerging trend brings both opportunities and challenges to the medical community. There is a need for physicians to contribute their expertise in new ways, but it is conditioned upon their increased participation in the interactive health communication networks.

PATIENT EDUCATION: FROM PASSING DOWN INFORMATION TO EMPOWERMENT AND ITS CONSEQUENCES

The interest in health promotion and disease prevention preceded by about a decade the restructuring of healthcare delivery prompted by cost-containment imperatives. For Becker and Rosenstock (1989), the Lalonde report published in 1974, which assessed the health of Canadians, demarcates the origin of the health promotion movement. This report identified four contributing factors to death and disease, one of them being unhealthy behaviors. The American experts represented in the Surgeon General's report (DHEW or U.S. Department of Health, Education, and Welfare, 1979) showed that about 50% of U.S. mortality in 1976 was due to unhealthy lifestyles and behaviors against 20% due to environmental factors, 20% due to human biological causes and 10% due to healthcare inadequacies. A more recent investigation (McGinnis and Foege, 1993) demonstrates that about half of the deaths that occurred in 1990 could be attributed to unhealthy behaviors, socioeconomic status and access to care. Among these contributors, the leading causes of death in the U.S. in 1990 were still tobacco, diet and physical activity patterns, and alcohol. Rather than concluding that health promotion doesn't work, we need to recognize that in the short term, expectations should be limited to change in behaviors and public attitudes, which is the case regarding smoking. Improved outcomes can be evaluated only on the long term. Therefore, health promotion, a "combination of health education and related organizational, economic and environmental supports for behavior conducive to health" (Green, 1984, p.190), should have beneficial outcomes in terms of disease prevention and represents one promising way of reducing health expenditures. However, it requires expanding the physician's role and redirecting his/her training from solely diagnosing and treating diseases to including risk detection and disease prevention, in addition to making people more involved and responsible for remaining healthy.

Health promotion in its incipiency was conceived within the traditional approach of medicine where education involves passing down knowledge from physician and health professionals to patients, where appropriate behavior is prescribed, and where patients are expected to follow medical orders. Health promotion and disease prevention as described above, and whether primary (aimed at risk reduction) or secondary (aimed at early detection) mainly apply to the healthy population and are used to reduce the demand of care in this particular population. How do we address the increasing burden of chronic diseases on healthcare expenditures?

The responses proposed use the key elements of health promotion, education and behavior change, but replace the traditional paternalistic approach by patient empowerment. One example is Lorig's (1996) chronic disease self-management model that incorporates tertiary prevention objectives. Tertiary prevention addresses the return to maximal function and the prevention of further loss of function for people with chronic diseases. Rehabilitation medicine is an example of tertiary prevention. Maintenance of maximum function for patients with multiple chronic diseases requires that they learn to manage their day-to-day lives to accommodate living with one or more chronic conditions, thus learning how to self-manage their disease. The self-management model assists patients in gaining skills and in gaining the confidence they will apply these skills on a day-to-day basis. Contrary to the traditional model of care, self-management places patients and professionals in partnership, and the key to partnership full success is communication between patient and health professionals. At the education level, peers rather than professionals communicate and relay the information. This type of intervention encouraging patient participation in his/her own care and based on patient empowerment principles has shown significant benefits in terms of patients' well being and utilization of care (Lorig et al., 1999).

Recent definitions of health promotion extend the concept to any population and reflect on the recent shift from the paternalistic to the partnership approach newly advocated in the practice of medicine. For example, Fries, Koop, Sokolov, Beadle, & Wright (1998) propose to use an expanded definition of health promotion to include all activities that educate, guide and motivate the individual to act in a way that increases the likelihood of sustained good health and the use of appropriate medical services. For these authors, the purpose of health promotion is to reduce the need and demand for care at any level of the continuum between healthy and chronic disease states. Achieving this goal requires autonomous and responsible behavior on the part of the individual, and a move from paternalistic attitude to health advocacy on the part of health professionals. Indeed, the key to success is the articulation and integration of medical management and self-management.

Education is central to all initiatives undertaken to increase public health and contain healthcare costs. As the definition and scope of health promotion changed, so did the way education was dispensed. Education meant to increase people's participation in their own care is not passive information. It consists of providing individuals with the means of taking responsibility for remaining healthy and learning how to manage their disease when necessary. More specifically, it necessitates giving them relevant information and timely advice on what to do on their own, when to request outside help, and how to become skillful at living daily with a chronic condition (Steinweg, Killingsworth, Nannini & Spayde, 1998). On the physician's part this requires being an educator, a facilitator, and a partner. On the patient's part, it implies learning, becoming knowledgeable and self-confident. Overall, it marks a sharp turn in the patient-doctor relationship, from paternalistic to partnership (Mechanic, 1999).

The change in the patient-doctor relationship happens at a time when, on average, people are more interested and more knowledgeable regarding medical issues than they used to be (Lowes, 1997). This increased interest in health issues is the direct result of health promotion and disease-prevention campaigns, the popularization of health issues, and the rising education level[2]. Since people today are encouraged to actively take responsibility for their health and care rather than to passively wait for and blindly follow medical advice, they are more genuinely interested in health issues. As they learn, they become more curious, investigative and ready to take initiatives. The Internet provides them with a faster way to satisfy their need of health information and allows them to access more information than what pamphlets, booklets, doctors or nurses would provide. As Desmond Pinkowish writes, "The patient education and self-care trends of the past 20 years have been accelerated by a technology that offers patients and consumers access to nearly all of the same medical information used by physicians" (1999, p. 37).

Today's physicians need to be aware that some of their patients who have access to the Internet and the time to search it might challenge their therapeutic decisions. As suggested by Lowes, there are ways to "manage the relationship with patients educated in cyberspace"(1997, p. 176). A collaborative approach towards on-line research can help doctor as well as patient. The Internet can come to the rescue of physicians who over-whelmed by the demands of both the profession and the healthcare system find less and less time to inform patients about their illness. The use of the Internet along with specific software can also help physicians distribute and customize information to the need of their patients (Gabello, 1997). In any case, the first sound advice to physicians right now is that they get on the Internet if they do not want to be left behind (Ukens, 1998).

Internet access provides the educated and empowered patients with the means to further their involvement in their own care and become real partners of their physicians now expected to guide and advise, not to make the final decision (Lowes, 1997). On-line advice and support provided by others sharing the same disease will better prepare patients to get the most out of their encounter with their physician.

PEER SUPPORT IN SELF-HELP GROUPS: FROM FACE-TO-FACE TO ONLINE SUPPORT, JUST A MATTER OF SCALE.

Contrary to patient education, originally a top-to-bottom initiative, self-help groups represent a grassroots endeavor aimed at meeting collective and individual needs and rest on the resources provided by peers rather than experts and professionals. Self-help is against elitism, hierarchy, and bureaucracy. Self-help values getting help by helping, and recognizes peer power (Humm, 1997). It is perfectly in line with the American culture of voluntary association that amazed, so much, the French aristocrat Alexis de Tocqueville when he visited America in 1831. De Tocqueville explained this distinctive habit of associating as the result of American traditions of limited government and of social egalitarianism that encouraged individuals of all stations to mingle and work together in common endeavors (1951).

The self-help movement was largely used as a response to social upheavals in the 1950s, and continued to assist Americans to their changing society and the antiwar movement in the 1960s and 1970s (Humm, 1997). Self-help groups have been, and are still being extensively used to help people address behavior control problems such as alcohol, drug abuse, and weight control (Humphreys, 1997). They are also widely used to address life crises. The last two decades have witnessed their increasing acceptance among health professionals as a valuable and complementary adjunct to medical care in chronic diseases and cancers (Gartner, 1997), but not as an alternative to professional services. As many as 10 million Americans are estimated to have participated in a self-help group during the year preceding a survey conducted in 1995-1996, compared to 7.5 millions estimated from data collected in 1979 (Kessler, Mickelson and Zhao, 1997).

While the majority of the mutual aid and self-help (MASH) groups continue to provide help through face-to-face groups in meeting rooms, on-line support communities are growing exponentially to meet unfulfilled needs. Group members communicate through message boards, newsgroups, forums, or interactive Web sites. Self-help and support groups known for their ability to pool their members' experience while tapping professional expertise can only thrive in the information age. The on-line encounter being faceless also enhances a key value in self-help, egalitarianism (Madara, 1997).

THE INTERNET PROMISE: UNRESTRICTED ACCESS TO A POWERFUL RESOURCE NETWORK

The Internet, by bringing at once information and support, can enhance the ability of patients with chronic diseases to deal with their condition on a daily basis and dramatically improve their outlook on life. At the other end of the spectrum, people with rare or with "new" conditions not yet well defined or well categorized such as fibromyalgia and chronic fatigue will find information, advice and support more easily and rapidly on the Web than they would by going to the library. In addition, at a touch of a button, they will be able to reach instantly those sharing the same problem. In between, anything related to health and disease can be found on the Internet using the existing search engines. The World Wide Web hosts a wealth of health-related information, and almost half of the content searches performed by U.S. active adult users are in the health and medicine domain. According to Cyber Dialogue Inc. (1999), in 1998, out of the 53.5 millions of U.S. active adults users, 17.3 million were "HealthMed Retrievers". In Cyber Dialogue Inc. language, this represents the adults who look for health and medical information online. Their number is expected to reach 30 million by the year 2000, up from 7.8 million in 1996.

Information technology with its powerful communication tools opens a new era where lay-people can access unrestricted health information, rely on peer support and experiential advice, and tap medical expertise independently of and in addition to their personal network resources. Lay people have this new option and use it quite extensively (Widman & Tong, 1997). Conversely, health professionals interested in improving the medical outcomes of their patients suffering from multiple chronic conditions begin to take advantage of the existing information and support networks to increase the willingness and ability of their patients to take better care of themselves (Deatrick, 1997). Using the new communication tools allows rapid exchange of information between patients, their caregivers and the health professionals. It allows better adjustment of and closer patient compliance to treatment, both leading to better outcomes. The Internet, because of its powerful communication properties allows tailoring health information according to an individual's specific health needs and information processing ability level. Of course, the use of these powerful technologies is conditioned by the ability to access them.

THE INTERNET MAIN LIMITATION: ACCESS

Available survey data shows that penetration of PCs into American homes is progressing at great strides. According to a National Telecommunications and Information Administration report (http://www.ntia.doc.gov/ntiahome/net2/falling.html), between 1994 and 1997, the nationwide telephone penetration has remained unchanged at 98.3%. By contrast, the computer penetration rate has grown substantially in the last three years: PC ownership has increased 51.9% (to 36.6%), modem ownership has grown 139.1% (to 26.3 %), and E-mail access has expanded by 397.1%. However, all segments of the population have not progressed into the information age at the same speed during that period. Although all economic and racial groups now own more computers than they did in 1994, there is a widening gap between those at upper and lower-income levels with Blacks and Hispanics now lagging even further behind Whites in their levels of PC ownership and on-line access.

There is a serious effort made at the national level to correct that "digital divide" in the near future, mostly by using public initiatives to make possible universal on-line access to health information and support (Eng, Maxfield, Patrick, Deering, Ratzan, & Gustafson, 1998). The rationale for this effort is the changing structure of healthcare delivery, primarily driven by consumers, not by the healthcare industry. Nevertheless, if more healthcare services are being shifted from traditional healthcare settings to the home and the community, the prerequisite to make this new organization successful and cost effective is to render access to health information and support virtually universal. Indeed, people do not have to own a computer to access on-line health information and support. Public resources help provide the answer. As reported by the National Telecommunications and Information Administration (NTIA), the federal government supports initiatives developed to wire schools across the nation by encouraging "business leaders to develop public-private partnerships with schools" (http://www.ntia.doc.gov/ntiahome/netday2000.htm). In addition, every public library across the nation is expected to provide Internet access by 2000; 73% of them offered some access to the Internet in 1998. Lack of high-speed equipment and the costs of information technology utilization still limit the access in rural and poor areas. Programs such as the E-rate discounts have been set to ensure that all people will have access to on-line information, especially those in poor and underserved areas (American Libraries Association at http://www.ala.org/news/v4n7/newreport.html).

With the further development of new technologies to improve usability and access, television-based and touch screen systems, as well as the use of programs tailored to different literacy skills levels, the final barriers could be progressively removed. Evidence shows that when access barriers are removed, with appropriate training, people of underserved areas want and can successfully use Internet technology to address health issues (Eng et al., 1998). Access to health information and support can help them achieve better health, improve their clinical outcomes, and promote their more efficient use of healthcare services (Mishra & Chavez, 1998).

THE INTERNET: RISKS AND BENEFITS.

In their comparative analysis of the new information technology—telecommunication and computers—versus old media—radio, TV, pamphlets, and pictures—with regard to health information and the promotion of healthy behaviors, Robinson, Patrick, Eng, & Gustafon (1998) identify main advantages of the new media. They are: access to information tailored to individuals' needs and demands, as well as the possibility to interact and communicate with professionals and peers. In that perspective, the interactive health communication tools can be used to relay information, promote behaviors conducive to health, promote peer information exchange and emotional support, promote self-care, and manage the demand for health services. The same authors warn that this technology that allows people to access health-related information on the World Wide Web may also harm them through misleading claims for medical products, and that misleading information could confuse people or erode their trust in their healthcare professionals.

From the brief description above, it appears that the clear benefit envisioned by the use of the new communication technology is the possibility to increase the efficiency of health promotion and prevention initiatives, and enhance the already recognized power of peer support to emulate health promotion and interventions. The risks identified above infer that misleading information and quack medicine is a new phenomenon specifically associated with the Internet, which it is not. If we assume that less educated people are more likely than the more educated to be harmed by fraudulent claims and low quality health information, we may worry that they might take misinformed decisions that may be damageable to their health. However, we have to recognize that the source of their misinformation is more likely to be another media than the Internet, if not friends or family members. As underlined by Coiera (1998), there is no evidence that the quality of information provided on the Internet is different from that of other media, or influenced different health decisions in the public.

Nevertheless, there are reasons for pinpointing the Internet as a possible source of misinformation and misleading help. It is a fact that health information found on the World Wide Web is highly variable in terms of accuracy, completeness and consistency (Impicciatore, Pandolfini, Casella, & Bonati, 1997). In particular, medical information available on the Internet in discussion groups may come from non-professionals, be unconventional or based on limited evidence (Cuver, Gerr, & Frumkin, 1997). On the other hand, it is difficult to check the credentials of a participant who claims to be or behaves like an authority. The argument, however, that Internet Web sites providing valid, reliable information from a reputable source may be just as useless because lay-people may not be able to understand it completely, doesn't really hold true as will be shown in the next section. In the arena of fraudulent and misleading claims, there are the sites providing quack remedies such as Dr. Hamer –his discovery of cancer healing (http://www.geocities.com/HotSprings/3374/index.htm), or unverified claims for the miracle power of herbal and exotic remedies. Often these sites are mostly appealing to people in real despair such as those with terminal cancer. They mainly cause harm in the fact that they bring false hope.

Rating instruments constitute one way to protect users of health information from relying on poor quality information or not accessing the right information to make informed decisions. However, these instruments can be of help only if the ratings they provide are themselves valid and reliable. Jadad (1998) analyzed 47 of these instruments. Their findings are very discouraging in the sense that only 14 of them described the criteria used to produce the ratings and five provided instructions for their use. None appeared to have been tested for validity and inter-observers reliability. After such findings, the authors' remaining question was whether these instruments should be available, and whether their use might cause harm rather than provide help as expected.

Rather than relying on rating instruments, Eysenbach & Diepgen (1998) argue that methods to help Net users evaluate the quality of the health information they retrieve should focus on developing means to allow users to easily check a site and/or information in terms of its value and trustworthiness. The main goal of these methods should be to minimize the risks of information doing harm to the user. Eysenbach et al. propose several solutions involving filtering and labeling while using both electronic means and "label services" provided by health-literate professionals.

What all these interventions designed to protect the consumers have in common is that they do not take into account the context in which health information is accessed and shared on the Net. They underestimate the discriminatory abilities of those accessing the information and forget that because this information is public and centralized, it is also rated and controlled on a permanent basis by the users themselves as well as by professionals. For example, Quackwatch operated by Stephen Barrett M.D. (http://www.familyinternet.com/quackwatch/index.html) is committed to improve the quality of health information on the Internet by investigating dubious claims, attacking misleading advertising, reporting illegal marketing, providing reliable publications, and making all this information available to the consumer. It also provides consumers with tips and clues so as to help them spot "quackery" when they encounter it. On the other hand, there are the accounts of those having been the victims of quackery such as Bill Ross denouncing People Against Cancer fraud and reporting it on Healthcare Reality Check (http://www.hcrc.org/contrib/ross/pac.html), another anti-quack Web site.

The Internet is a free market of information and therefore is self-regulated. Its dynamic and interactive nature allows constant monitoring and expert input, providing experts use it as much as they should. In the area of health and medicine, we could expect to find more publicized and authoritative Web sites operated by health practitioners with peer review of the material published there. Rather than dismissing the value of the Internet in providing suitable information to their patients as shown in the 1998 survey conducted by Cyber Dialogue Inc, more physicians should be involved in producing this information to ensure its quality. Most physicians' lack of interest and trust in the Internet seem to come from their uneasiness with this media, a direct result of their using it too sparsely. Meanwhile, patients are getting increasingly at ease with the medium, more familiar with the medical jargon, and more knowledgeable about the specific medical issues that interest them personally. This accounts for the "Health Care Interactive Communication Gap" identified by Cyber Dialogue Inc.

THE WEB-ENABLED PATIENT: THE EVIDENCE

In spite of all the difficulties and obstacles to accessing relevant health information on the World Wide Web and using it efficiently, patients are demonstrating how the Web is enabling them. It mainly works by increasing people's ability to get in touch with others sharing the same condition and thereby benefiting from each other's experience. Stipp (1998) reports the case of a 67-year-old man in the U.K. found with a kidney cancer having metastasized in the bones. Because of his age and the advanced stage of his cancer, this man was only offered palliative treatment under the British National Health Services and a six-month survival's perspective. Through the shared experience of another cancer patient, Steve Dunn, who set up his own site on the Web (http://www.cancerguide.org/), this man learned about an experimental therapy that put his cancer into remission. Another example how the Web can help patients improve their care through the help of others is Linda Stone's story (March 29, 1999). After she was diagnosed with a chronic inflammatory disease, she researched the Web and joined an on-line support group to find more about her condition. She eventually discovered that she had been misdiagnosed.

On-line support groups are also instrumental in changing patients' attitudes towards their doctors, from passive obedience to inquisitiveness, and this is to their benefit. On-line support groups help patients increase their self-confidence and sense of control over their life, in spite of their illness. These groups also enable patients to make informed decisions regarding what care they want after having explored the available possibilities, and get access to the type of treatment they want in spite of barriers. Smith (1998) tells the story of a man found with prostate cancer who discovered brachytherapy using radioactive implanted seeds as an alternative to surgery. He also found an on-line group that focused specifically on that therapy. Exchanges with members of that group convinced him that this was the right treatment for him. The first three doctors he consulted tried to convince him to have surgery, which he kept refusing. The fourth one was ready to use brachytherapy but using gold seeds instead of Iodine-125 or palladium-103 as mentioned in online discussion groups. The patient, who used to work as a radioactive waste manager, suspected that gold might not be as good a source of radioactivity. So, he brought the issue before the online group who confirmed that using gold seeds was an outdated therapy. That patient eventually found the right doctor who gave him the treatment he requested. This story illustrates quite well the power of support groups, enhanced by the interactive communication technology environment, to enable patients in very practical ways.

What makes the World Wide Web a more accessible, reliable and valid source of health information for users than what it seems to be at first glance is the mere existence of the on-line community of patients providing peer support and guidance. Peer support, more specifically, the strong desire patients have to let others reap the benefits of their own experience, as commented on by patients on their own Web sites,[3,4] appears to be of primary importance in helping users locate the relevant information tailored to their needs. By making this information understandable, peer support also prepares users to interact more efficiently with their personal physicians or the on-line medical experts. The ever-growing number of sites providing good and reliable health information can help users understand the nature of a disease or a condition, which is an important step in the learning process. However, they are still limited to providing in lay-terms academic-like general type of information about medical conditions. They can rarely provide the information tailored to the particular needs of a patient suffering from the disease. This is true even for the more sophisticated Web sites in terms of search protocols and content quality when prestigious universities supply this information.[5] They also offer limited tips on how to zero-in on relevant information, or on how to move up from simple to more complicated and sophisticated types of information. Although they offer access to medical experts, patients with little understanding of their disease and of the array of available treatments will not take full advantage of this fine resource. By contrast, patients who have learned the hard way seem to be better at understanding the particular needs and learning processes of other patients than people who have a theoretical knowledge of diseases. This is particularly true for chronic and life-threatening diseases. When these patients have the desire and capability to create a Web site to make their experiential knowledge available to other patients, a place where the information is well structured and a place for people to meet and share, it becomes an invaluable tool of empowerment.

How does it work? First, these patients are a living example of successful fight over dreadful diseases such as cancer [2, 3] and heart failure.[6] Second, through the telling of their personal story, they explicit the universal process involved in getting control over the disease. Once the patients are past the denial, despair, and anger stages, they always start by reading as much as possible about their disease. Whatever their education background, they all end up reading medical literature. They become genuine experts in their disease field.[7] Structure and organization are the primary ingredients in making information research successful; this is precisely what these patient initiated Web sites offer and what other Web sites are missing. Contrary to "commercial" Web sites, those operated by patients have links organized thematically. They also have lots of pragmatic information such as low salt recipes or how to apply for Social Security disability.[8] Patient-initiated Web sites have another characteristic in common; they serve as a how-to guide for patients to get involved in clinical trials.[9] Clinical trials mean access to new and potentially more powerful treatments, it also means mandatory free treatment and follow-up (Watanabe, 1996). Finally, because individuals rather than organizations host these sites, their forums appear more like friends' gatherings than public meetings. Many sites emanate a genuine sense of community.

Health-related information and on-line medical experts made available through university medical departments, renowned clinics or hospitals, medical associations, or even health insurance companies become of real interest to self-empowered patients. These are patients who, through the help of their peers and peers' Web sites, have found ways to master medical knowledge. Because they understand quite intimately what their disease is about, what treatments are available, and what specific life style and diet they have to follow, they can ask specific questions to the experts and take full advantage of their advice to make appropriate decisions regarding their care. These are the Web-enabled patients (Ferguson, 1997) who are changing the rules and the philosophy of healthcare.

THE FUTURE OF HEALTH CARE: JOINING IN THE REVOLUTION AND USING INFORMATION TECHNOLOGY MORE EXTENSIVELY.

As observed by Ferguson (1997) and confirmed by the results of the 1998 American Internet User Survey (Cyber Dialogue Inc.), an ever-growing number of people are using the World Wide Web and the new communications technologies to address their healthcare needs. On-line communities facilitate the navigation of the Web and offer customized support to health information consumers. Patients helping other patients in cyberspace constitute a critical resource that enhances their ability to take an active role in their own care often improving their outcomes. There is room for physicians to step in what Ferguson calls "a revolution in healthcare" (1997, p. 29) and close the "Health Care Interactive Communication Gap" (Cyber Dialogue Inc). However, past medical training and current time constraints may hamper physicians' increased participation in the interactive health communication networks.

Physicians can help their patients to start using and navigating the Web by directing them to specific sites while informing them about these sites' particular content and the type of resource they constitute. For example, physicians can guide their patients through the Web maze by sending them to Healthfinder and to Netwellness. Healthfinder (http://www.healthfinder.gov/) was developed by the U.S. Department of Health and Human Services (DHHS) in collaboration with several other federal agencies and is designed to contain links specifically to high-quality health information. NetWellness (http://www.netwellness.org) is a Web-based consumer health information service developed by the University of Cincinnati Medical Center with several university partners to provide the most current and accurate health information (Marine, Guard & Morris, 1998). Physicians can inform their patients about the Health on the Net Foundation (http://www.hon.ch), an organization devoted to monitoring Web sites for information value and credibility which posts links to the most credible ones. This gives patients an easy way to check the sites they found on their own for information quality. The MayoClinic Health Oasis (http://www.mayohealth.org) lets users e-mail questions to Mayo Clinic physicians. RxList (http://www.rxlist.com) allows looking up detailed information on specific drugs, by their brand or generic name. The Web-based pharmacies (http://www.drugstore.com) and the manufacturers' sites help them crosscheck and deepen the information if they need it. WellnessWeb (http://wellweb.com) contains reliable information on alternative medicines, as well as conventional ones. These are just examples of sites of interest. The idea being that once patients have been introduced to some, they quickly start to fly on their own. Providing them with navigation tips and ways to check sites quality while being available to answer their questions will prevent them from being harmed and overwhelmed.

Physicians can also encourage their patients to participate in specific disease forums and to search for patients' initiated Web sites. Once their patients have become more familiar with the Web and wish to access medical literature, PubMed (http://www.ncbi.nlm.nih.gov/PubMed) gives them entry to MedLine. By limiting the number of articles they can bring to a specific visit, physicians will avoid being overwhelmed by Internet and health savvy patients. Although perceived as a threat by most physicians, and certainly requiring some shaping of the communication infrastructure to address issues such as security, confidentiality and medicolegal liability (Mandl, Kohane, & Brandt, 1998), the early adopters of e-mail demonstrated that it is a convenient communication vehicle between patients and their health providers (Borowitz & Wyatt, 1998).

While there are clear individual and societal benefits associated with the new attitude expected from physicians in their practice, there are significant challenges preventing them from teaming up with their patients. First of all, there is the medical training that has not changed enough to accommodate the new cultural context in which medicine is practiced: from a paternalistic and authoritative approach, to a participatory one (Mechanic, 1998). Besides the change in content brought about by the advances of the biomedical science leading to the practice of evidence-based medicine, medical training needs to acknowledge and satisfy the current desire for autonomy and self-determination. The day when patients used to follow medical orders blindly is over. New client-focused models, which recognize the client as the primary care manager, are proposed for the management of chronic diseases. These models promote client choice and educated participation in addressing the client's needs (Suber, 1996). These models are also proved to be cost effective. Whether reflecting a patient's choice or as a designed way to improve the efficiency of care, the participatory approach requires new skills and attitudes on the part of physicians, and the most important is the art of communication. Unfortunately the demands of medical education represented by the continuously growing body of medical knowledge and the need to keep up with new guidelines and discoveries leave little room for training in communication skills.

The good news is that new information tools may offer efficient responses to the challenges of the overwhelming accumulation of evidence-based medical knowledge on the part of physicians on the one hand, and to the need for improved communication between patients and their doctors on the other. For example, knowledge-coupling software that retrieves medical theoretical information and links it with patient data may improve diagnostic accuracy and the physician's ability to make appropriate treatment decisions. The tools would give the evidence for and against each diagnosis and/or treatment management option based on details provided by the patients. Human judgement comes into play to assess trade-offs and ambiguities and extract the real choices. Patients would then input their own preference and goals (Weed, 1997). It is currently difficult to assess the real efficiency of these computer decision support systems (CDSS) because the number of quality CDSS trials is still limited, particularly those assessing these systems as diagnostic aids and in terms of patient outcomes (Hunt, Haynes & Hanna, 1998). However, aside from efficiency issues, to be fully functional, these new tools, by design, require a high level of communication and strong collaboration between patients and physicians. Interestingly, bringing the "machine" to the patient-doctor relationship has the potential to strengthen the relationship and make it more human. Currently, the Internet by allowing direct communication to be established independently of time and space increases the ability of patients and doctors to strengthen their mutual communication and collaboration since it allows both parties to work together at their most convenient time.

CONCLUSION

While poor quality of health information gathered by patients on the World Wide Web may lead to adverse consequences, and while the misunderstanding of the proper relevance of particular treatments might foster demand for inappropriate and/or costly interventions, accurate, relevant and evidence-based information retrieved by patients can enhance the quality and appropriateness of their healthcare (Coulter, 1998). In this perspective, there is a need for physicians and health professionals to shift gears and join both consumers and patients on the Internet. The clinicians' new task will be to contribute their expertise in locating high quality health information, in defining its optimal use, and in making themselves available online to answer consumers and patients' questions.

A collaborative approach toward on-line research that would help patient and physician does not seem to be farfetched (Biermann, Golladay and Greenfield, 1999). The World Wide Web by making available medical and scientific literature to the public allows lay people the opportunity to access the same evidence-based medical resources as practicing doctors. Some avant-garde physicians see patients coming to them with *JAMA* articles as an opportunity to keep abreast on new advances in their field rather than a threat to their authority (Lowes, 1997).

Technology will never replace human intervention as a prerequisite to effective healing and caring. However, as an interactive agent for promoting self-care through education and peer support, the Internet will act as a direct and effective means of achieving health promotion and disease prevention for the healthy and better outcomes for those dealing with chronic diseases. It will also ease and strengthen the communication between Web-enabled patients and their physician-partners.

ENDNOTES

1 I restrict the subject of this paper to initiatives taken by patients to improve their knowledge of medical issues and their ability to participate in their own care by using information available on the Web and the new communications technologies. I am purposely excluding disease-specific programs developed by universities within the denomination of "health information network" —such as CHESS (Comprehensive Health Enhancement Support System) or WHIN (Wisconsin Health Information Network) which are using the Web technologies to educate and help patients and their families to manage their disease (for a full description of these systems, see Brennan et al., 1997). These programs are not public; they are restricted to patients served by medical institutions who acquired that software. Therefore they are not relevant to the subject of this paper.

2 According to the U.S. Bureau of Census, the percentage of 25 year olds and older who completed high school rose from 65.9% in 1978 to 82.8% in 1998, while the percentage of college undergraduates increased from 15.7% to 24.4% during the same period. Data available on the World Wide Web at http://www.census.gov/population/socdemo/education/tablea-02.txt. Accessed on April 22, 1999.

3 "Most patients with advanced kidney cancer in 1989 did not get what I got, and did not have the chance that I had. In general only a few percent of patients ever take part in a clinical trial, and only a small fraction of those actually search for and find the best as I was fortunate enough to have done. I believed my experience put me in a special position to be able to help other patients... After a while, I realized that I could help people more if I developed a Web site. So I converted my FAQ files to HTML and created CancerGuide, which I am still improving and updating. " (Steve Dunn). Available on the World Wide Web at http://www.cancerguide.org/. Accessed on April 19, 1999.

4 "It is my intention to provide the Internet community with a full spectrum of information about prostate cancer and general problems of the prostate. It is not my intention to pass judgment about any information source; all are treated equally. The reader should be careful to note that most introductory remarks were taken from the site and do not represent my views. Remember, I'm just the information provider. It is up to you to carefully weigh the information you find. Good luck in your search." (Gary Huckabay). Available on the World Wide Web at http://rattler.cameron.ehdu/prostate/. Accessed on April 19, 1999.

5 Intelihealth. The trusted source of information. Provided by Aetna/US healthcare to its users with the collaboration of Johns Hopkins University. Available on the World Wide Web at http://www.intelihealth.com. Accessed on April 15, 1999.

6 "Lumber mills were my livelihood and after being a planer jockey (Oliver Strait-O-Planes) for 10 years, I was a moulder man and knife grinder until I got sick....

At the ripe old age of 36, the day after surgery to take out my gallbladder, my entire lower body swelled up like a ballon about to pop—very scary. In the emergency room,

I was found to have congestive heart failure — specifically, idiopathic dilated cardiomy-opathy, with an Ejection Fraction of 13%. At 36, this was a big shock. Also a big shock was the fact that my gallbladder wasn't the problem in the first place — my heart condition should have been diagnosed earlier and wasn't. The misdiagnosis almost killed me. A few types of cardiomyopathy can be "cured" and some cases spontaneously get better but for most of us, the illness is chronic and will eventually be terminal. Needless to say, I am now retired due to disability. Although my EF has risen to 45% by 1999, my exercise tolerance and general quality of life did not go up with it. In mid-1998, my Vo2max was down to 13.5. So it goes." (Jon's Place). Available on the World Wide Web at http://www.geocities.com/Heartland/Hills/2571/bios/jonsplace2.htm. Accessed April 23, 1999.

7 "Educate yourself. Hospital medical libraries are open to patients as well as doctors, and the librarians are very helpful. I provide a page of links to Internet resources like Medline as well as many pages of collected information. Read everything you can get your hands on, and never be afraid to ask your cardiologist if he's heard of this drug or that treatment —a good cardiologist is not upset by this at all. Information about new drug trials can be found here. " (Jon's Place). Available on the World Wide Web at http://www.geocities.com/Heartland/Hills/2571/heartforum.htm. Accessed on April 19, 1999.

8 See Site Index at Jon' Place. Available on the World Wide Web at http://www.geocities.com/Heartland/Hills/2571/index.html. Accessed April 23, 1999.

9 "So I went to the medical library and read books with titles like, *Research Methods in Clinical Oncology* to deepen my knowledge of the clinical trial system, and I found out how to use computer databases, like MedLine, to search the medical literature. With this research, plus my experience, I put together a course on cancer clinical trials for other patients," (Steve Dunn). Available on the World Wide Web at http://www.cancerguide.org. Accessed on April 19, 1999.

REFERENCES

American Libraries Association. New report shows more libraries connect to the Internet; access still limited. Available on the World Wide Web at http://www.ala.org/news/v4n7/newreport.html. Accessed on April 6, 1999.

Becker, M.H. & Rosenstock, I.M. (1989). Health promotion, disease prevention, and program retention. In Freeman & Levine (Eds.) Handbook of medical sociology. (pp. 284-305). (4th ed). New Jersey: Prentice Hall.

Biermann, J.S., Golladay, G.J., Greenfield M.L., Baker L.H. (1999). Evaluation of cancer information on the Internet. *Cancer, 86(3)*, 381-90

Borowitz, S.M. & Wyatt, J.C. (1998). The origin, content, and workload of e-mail consultations. *JAMA, 280(15)*, 1321-1324.

Coiera E. (1998). Information epidemics, economics, and immunity on the Internet. *BMJ, 317(7171)*, 1469-1470.

Coulter A. (1998). Evidence based patient information is important, so there needs to be a national strategy to ensure it. *BMJ, 317(7153)*, 225-226.

Cuver J.D., Gerr F., Frumkin H. (1997). Medical information on the Internet: a study of an electronic bulletin board. *Journal of General Internal Medicine, 12(8)*, 466-470.

Cyber Dialogue Inc. (1999). The healthcare industry in transition: the online mandate to change. (Miller T. & Reents S.). Available on the World Wide Web at http://www.cyberdialogue.com/pdfs/white_papers/intel.pdf. Accessed on April 6, 1999.

Deatrick, D. (1997) Senior-Med: creating a network to help manage medication. *Generations, 21(3)*, 59-60.

Desmond, Pinkowish M. (1999, January 15). The Internet in medicine: An update. *Patient Care, 33(1)*, 30-48.

de Tocqueville, A. (1951). *De la Democratie en Amerique* (Vol 2). Librairie de Medicis, Paris.

DHEW (U.S. Department of Health, Education, and Welfare). (1979). *Healthy People: The Surgeon General's Report on Health promotion and Disease Prevention*. (Publication No.79-55071). Washington, D.C.: U.S. Government Printing Office.

Dr. Hamer - his discovery of cancer healing. Available on the World Wide Web at http://www.geocities.com/HotSprings/3374/index.htm. Accessed on April 8, 1999.

Dunn, S. http://www.cancerguide.org/

Eng, T.R., Maxfield, A., Patrick K, Deering M.J., Ratzan S.C., & Gustafson D.H. (1998). Access to health information and support: A public highway or a private road? *JAMA, 280(15)*, 1371-1375.

Eysenbach G. & Diepgen T. (1998). Towards quality management of medical information on the Internet: evaluation, labelling, and filtering of information. *BMJ, 317(7171)*, 1496-1502.

Ferguson T. (1997). Health care in cyberspace: patients lead a revolution. *The Futurist,* November-December, 29-33.

Fries J. F, Koop E.C., Sokolov J., Beadle C.E., & Wright D. (1998). Beyond health promotion: reducing the demand for medical care. *Health Affairs, 17(3)*, 70-84.

Gabello, & William J. (1997, February 15). How computers enrich patient education. *Patient Care, 31(3)*, 88-113.

Gartner, A. (1997). Professionals and self-help: the uses of creative tension. *Social Policy, Spring*, 47-51.

Green L.W. (1984). Health education models. In Matarazzo et al. (Eds.) *Behavioral Health: A Handbook for Health Enhancement and Disease prevention*. (pp 182-203). New York: John Wiley

Healthcare Reality Check. People Against Cancer: an open letter to anyone dealing with cancer from a son of a cancer victim. June 29, 1998. Available on the World Wide Web at http://www.hcrc.org/contrib/ross/pac.html. Accessed on April 12, 1999.

Humm, A. (1997). Self-help: a movement for changing times. *Social Policy, Spring*, 4-5.

Humphreys, K. (1997). Individual and social benefits of mutual aid self-help groups. *Social Policy,* Spring, 12-19.

Hunt D., Haynes B., Hanna S., Smith K. (1998). Effects of computer-based clinical support systems on physician performance and patient outcomes: a systematic review. *JAMA, 280(15)*,1339-1346.

Impicciatore, P, Pandolfini, C., Casella, N., & Bonati M. (1997). Reliability of health information for the public on the world wide web: systematic survey on managing fever in children at home. *BMJ, 314 (7098)*, 1875-9.

Jadad, A.R.(1998). Rating health information on the Internet: Navigating to knowledge or to Babel? *JAMA, 279(8)*, 611-614.

Kessler ,R.C., Mickelson, K.D. & Zhao, S. (1997). Patterns and correlates of self-help group membership in the United States. *Social Policy, Spring,* 27-46.

Lorig, K.R., Sobel D.S., Stewart, A.L., Brown, B.W. Jr, Bandura, A., Ritter P., Gonzalez V.M., Laurent D.D. & Holman H.R. (1999). Evidence suggesting that a chronic disease self-management program can improve health status while reducing hospitalization: a randomized trial. *Med Care, 37*(1), 5-14.

Lorig, K. (1996). Chronic disease self-management: a model for tertiary prevention. *American Behavioral Scientist, 39*(6), 676-683.

Lowes, R.L (1997, January 27). Here come patients who've "studied" medicine on-line. *Medical Economics, 74*(2), 175-184.

Madara E. (1997).The mutual aid self-help online revolution. *Social Policy, Spring*, 20-26.

Mandl, K.D., Kohane, I.S., & Brandt, A.M. (1998). Electronic patient-physician communication: problem and promise. *Annals of Internal Medicine, 129*(6), 495-500.

Marine, S., Guard R., Morris T., Haag, D., Kaya, B., Riep, J., Schick L., Tsipis G., Shoemaker S. (1998). A model for enhancing worldwide personal health and wellness. *Medinfo, 9*(pt 2), 1265-8.

McGinnis, M., & Foege, W.H. (1993). Actual causes of death in the United States. *JAMA, 270*(19), 2207-2212.

Mechanic, D. (1999). Issues in promoting health. *Social Science and Medicine, 48*(6), 711-718.

Mechanic, D. (1998). Public trust and initiatives for new healthcare partnerships. *The Milbank Quaterly, 76*(2), 281-303.

Mishra, S.I., & Chavez, L.R. (1998). Improving breast cancer control among latinas: evaluation of a theory-based educational program. *Health Education Behavior, 25*(5), 653-670.

National Telecommunications and Information Administration. Information on Net Day 2000. Available on the World Wide Web at http://www.ntia.doc.gov/ntiahome/netday2000.htm. Accessed on April 6, 1999.

National Telecommunications and Information Administration. Falling through the net II: new data on the digital divide. Available on the World Wide Web at http://www.ntia.doc.gov/ntiahome/net2/falling.html. Accessed on April 6, 1999.

Quackwatch: your guide to health fraud, quackery and intelligent decisions. Available on the World Wide Web at http://www.familyinternet.com/quackwatch/index.html Accessed on April 12, 1999.

Robinson, T.N., Patrick, K., Eng, T.R., & Gustafon, D. (1998). An evidence-based approach to interactive health communication. *JAMA, 280*(14), 1264-1269.

Smith, J. (1998)."Internet patients" turn to support groups to guide medical decisions. *Journal of the National Cancer Institute*, (90)22, 1695-1697.

Steinweg, K.K., Killingsworth, R.E., Nannini, R.J., & Spayde, J. (1998). The impact on a healthcare system of a program to facilitate self-care. *Military Medicine, 163*(3), 139-144.

Stipp, D. (1998, January 12).Health help on the Net. *Fortune, 137*(1), 135-136.

Suber, R. (1996). Chronic care in ambulatory setting. *American Behavioral Scientist, 39*(6), 665-675.

Ukens, C. (1998, November 16). Internet access transforming healthcare, says Koop. *Drug Topics, 142*(22), 80-82.

Watanabe, M.E. (1996). Bottom line, culture clash impending cooperation of managed care organizations in clinical trials. June 24, 1996. Available on the World Wide Web at http://165.123.33.33/yr1996/june/hmo_960624.html. Accessed on April 19, 1999.

Weed, L. (1997). New connections between medical knowledge and patient care. *BMJ, 315*(7102), 231-235.

Widman, LA, & Tong, DA (1997). Requests for medical advice from patients and families to healthcare providers who publish on the World Wide Web. *Archives of Internal Medicine, 157*(2), 209-212.

Woody, T. (1999, March 29). Patient heal thyself. *The industry standard*, 42-43

Chapter XVI

Disability Access to the Built Environment: On-Line Evaluation and Information Dissemination

Catherine E. Bridge[1] and Simeon J. Simoff[2,3]
University of Sydney, Australia

Identifying and removing architectural barriers to access for people with disabilities follows community recognition that people with disabilities share the same rights as others. In terms of access to buildings and facilities, it is a question of degree. Examination of the steepness of a gradient, the available circulation space at a doorway, the type, fixation and position of a handrail, the amount of colour contrast and lack of other sensory cues determine degree of compliance. Absence of critical features discriminates against certain users and influences the likelihood of litigation. This chapter presents a methodology for computer-assisted access evaluation, which encapsulates facility features for accessibility auditing, describes a data model representation which capturing relevant information and demonstrates mapping of access audit analysis onto sets of queries via a Web-accessible information system. Thus the Web-accessible information system provides on-line accessibility information, generated from the accessibility database.

In this chapter, the on-line evaluation of accessibility for people with disabilities is explored as a potential enhancement of existing methodologies derived from practical application of data modeling. Initial data modeling was undertaken as a part of a large-scale accessibility audit undertaken for a major Australian University. A systematic outline of on-line approaches is suggested for the entire audit process. To demonstrate this process an object-orientated database and data model is described. This model underpins the collection and analysis of access-related building data and provides the basis for the development of an on-line Web-based interface. Detailed analysis of the audit process itself provides the basis for describing techniques for utilization of other available Web tools to better manage the training, education, data gathering and reporting processes. This is particularly important as many large-scale accessibility audits are commissioned by organizations including major healthcare providers whose facilities are spread across cities, states, and sometimes, whole continents. Implementation of on-line technologies that can facilitate collaboration and teamwork between a variety of locally-based audit teams and across rural and remote sites makes this type of large-scale auditing more feasible.

Any perspective on the issue of accessibility auditing stems from an understanding of how computer applications can assist in evaluation and prediction of human responses to the built environment. Understanding the legislative and social imperatives allows the reader to grasp the issues associated with capturing knowledge needed to develop effective evaluative and predictive on-line tools including appropriate digital representation. Computer technology can impact positively by providing opportunities to present and interact with information in ways previously unseen.

There are thus two major foci that will be addressed in this chapter: (1) how best to represent knowledge required for accessibility auditing, and (2) how best to integrate on-line methodologies into the audit process. Presentation of our data model allows exploration of issues, controversies and problems encountered in accessibility auditing and indicates how on-line methodologies assist in addressing them. Following this, exploration of the stages or steps in accessibility auditing allows us to present a more comprehensive and integrated picture. Finally the authors work in development of on-line tools illustrates the benefits of implementing and enhancing these technologies in creating environments which support all people to achieve their full potential without experiencing secondary disabilities or discrimination.

BACKGROUND

Large numbers of individuals in our community experience functional limitations as a direct outcome of occupational health injuries, home accidents, road trauma, crime, genetic predisposition, and/or the onset of chronic disabling conditions associated with the aging process. Consumers, families and healthcare professionals agree that physical settings are critical in reducing institutionalisation and promoting integrative and inclusive environments (Iwarsson and Isacsson, 1998; Fox, 1995). Indeed in rehabilitation practice, the environment has been conceived of as a prosthetic support for functional independence (Steinfeld and Danford, 1997). In addition, the pressure to identify and remove architectural barriers to access for people with disabilities has markedly increased following community recognition that people with disabilities share the same rights as others (Goldsmith, 1997; McAuley, 1994). Recognition of these rights is reflected in recent changes to federal legislation, such as the Americans with Disabilities Act Accessibility Guidelines (ADAAG-1991). The USA is just one of many industrialized nations to enact this type of legislation; similar legislation exists in Australia and England.

Analysis of recent discrimination complaint trends in Australia indicates that indirect discrimination associated with lack of access to premises demonstrates the greatest area of increased litigation (Human Rights & Equal Opportunity Commission, 1997). The fear of litigation by building owners and operators means that disability action or transition planning based on building evaluation has become essential (Kelly, Deshon, Jones and Fisher, 1996; Government of Western Australia, 1996; Martin, 1997).

In terms of access to buildings and facilities, it is a question of degree. Examination of the steepness of a gradient, the available circulation space at a doorway, the type, fixation and position of a handrail, the amount of colour contrast and lack of other sensory cues determine degree of compliance. Absence of critical features discriminates against certain users and influences the likelihood of litigation. In the same way that eliminating kerbs in the built environment by provision of 'kerb-ramps' or 'curbcuts' creates more accessible environments for wheelchair-dependent users provision of 'electronic curbcuts' makes on-line information more accessible (Campbell & Wadell, 1997).

Because a diverse range of individuals are involved in accessibility auditing including architects, occupational therapists and people with disabilities it is important that any computational system designed to improve access outcomes facilitates universal access both in the built and electronic environments. For many consultants with disabilities, the occupation of accessibility auditing is particularly attractive because it presents a career path, which draws upon personal experiences of disability. Consideration of accessibility in on-line technologies such as Web page navigation is essential because the World Wide Web (WWW) has rapidly advanced from a primarily text-based medium to an increasingly interactive audio-visually enhanced format. Without attention to special coding, graphics are impenetrable to visually impaired users and like the built environment can effectively discriminate against users with disabilities. Producing on-line tools designed to facilitate the creation of accessible environments thus also raises the additional issues associated with ensuring that tools developed can also be delivered in a nondiscriminatory way. Thus our discussion of on-line audit tools will also include references to strategies known to enhance electronic access such as homepage design and software testing.

Measuring and Reporting on Aspects of the Built Environment for People with Disabilities

During the last decade, considerable work has been done in the development of access evaluation methodologies. As a rule they are derived from National and International Standards in the form of a "Yes/No" questionnaire about compliance of different facility components. The structure of included components, the relative significance of included items and the taxonomies created is what gives the evaluation tool content validity and credibility.

Audit validity is concerned with the ability of the audit performance criteria selected to accurately and comprehensively identify and prioritize accessibility issues. Indeed, without a means of articulating performance criteria so they can be objectively and accurate measured, auditors jeopardize recommendations being made, validity in this case being the "overall evaluative judgement of the degree to which empirical evidence and theoretical rationales support interpretations and actions based on assessment" (Linn 1988).

An accessibility evaluation can be a complex undertaking because building attributes and legislative guidelines include an almost unlimited number of variables. Thus valid evaluative judgements in this context means ensuring that performance criterion have clear theoretical rationales and those relevant variables can be empirically measured.

Both logical (face and content) validity and empirical (criterion-related or construct) validity are important. Accessibility audits are intended to compare systematically and rigorously the actual performance of buildings with explicitly stated performance criteria; the difference between the two constitutes the evaluation process. Thus, the structure of the questionnaire defines the algorithm for checking facilities against the requirements of a particular criterion or standard. Evaluation in this context means deriving a conclusion about whether or not a particular facility or parts of that facility comply with the expected performance criterion or standard.

The advantage of the questionnaire methodology is that it is straightforward and produces results "on the spot". However, "on-the -spot" decisionmaking requires extensive knowledge and experience from the evaluation team. The measurement recorded is "discrete" in the sense that it provides answers for each component regarding absolute compliance, but fails to provide an estimate of partial compliance. This limitation is of importance to concerned parties, e.g. facilities management, as knowledge about partial compliance can become crucial for the progressive improvement of facilities audited and can provide a basis for on-line planning of activities to improve facilities.

Providing concerned parties with the actual data rather than only with evaluator judgements assists not only with the specificity of remediation strategies selected, but can also assist later audits of facilities. As long as the building remains the same, the data is never obsolete, even if codes or regulations change. For instance, facilities managers would like to be able to track changes without engaging in costly ongoing auditing programs. Whereas, occupational therapists would like to check the current accessibility of particular facilities, so as to provide appropriate recommendations to 'clients' in the broadest sense. Clients in this broad sense may be facilities managers trying to improve facilities or individuals with disabilities who desire to carry out specific occupational tasks and activities in a particular facility. Access standards are 'living documents' that are socially derived and are thus likely to change over time, so separating standards-based performance criteria from actual facilities data means that as minimum performance criteria change, the associated building elements can be reevaluated without re-auditing actual facilities. This means that further surveying can be restricted to tracking modifications or to elements not initially covered.

The motivation for the original research and development was the inherent limitations and frustrations associated with the available access tools, facing us at the starting point of a large-scale audit procedure. The overall problem came from the absence of a cohesive information model. Consequently, existing tools contained inadequate information to guide evaluator judgments, i.e., deciding when an item should be skipped or checked not applicable. Incorporating the results of previous audits was also impossible without a cohesive information model. In addition, the majority of tools were paper based and managing paper based forms also raised major problem associated with flow, flexibility and the inadequacy of additional comment spaces provided. But by far the most important limitation was the fact that no available tool including checklists or database programs matched the most recent federal or state legislative guidelines on either minimum or desirable access standards.

At the same time researchers in the field of design computing have come up with models, which consider the relations between the functionality of a design artifact and its physical implementation. These models provided the staring point in the development of the conceptual model for representing building facilities in the context of disability access auditing.

Moving Towards a Computational Solution

Facilities and the end use spaces, which they enclose or define can be viewed from at least two distinct aspects: either as 'physical objects', or as 'function' or 'use'. The physical view includes dimensional or topological measurement such as floor area, volume of space, or gross dimensions. These physical characteristics are widely used in the design, production and use of facilities and spaces. The methods and rules for expressing these characteristics are widely known and standard practices are accepted. The facilities management information models usually implement some form of the "Structure-Function" model, which is a reduced derivative of the more general Function-Behavior-Structure model (Gero, 1990). The "Structure-Function" model provides the skeleton for categorization of variables, which describe existing classes of facility structures and the knowledge about the elements that these variables represent, according to the structural properties and a description of the functions performed by the object. For example, following this model, existing rooms and their database representations are categorized into functional groups.

Another viewpoint starts from the intended activity or use of the facility or space (Maher, Simoff and Mitchell, 1997). The intended activity has a critical influence on the design stage of the construction process and, of course, the utilization phase will determine the success of the implementation of the design for the intended use. It is clear that classification must be based on the principle that facilities and spaces can be associated with activities or pattern of usage and that these activities are the distinctive characteristics by which the facilities and spaces are defined. In an access audit project the focus is on the activities, specific requirements and constraints defined by the kind of disability and/or combination of disability characteristics.

A pattern of activities is encapsulated in the building form. The variety can be very large and aggregation can be realized following different criteria —by departments, houses, age groups, social or pastoral care groups, or by grouping together those spaces requiring similar environmental or structural characteristics. Whatever basis is chosen, the decision is permanent but its validity endures only as long as the activity pattern it represents or as long as it is robust enough to accommodate variations in the activity pattern. By formally representing and manipulating the activities and their associated spaces in a building, we have the opportunity to accommodate changes in use more effectively.

Checking this validity requires capturing substantial amount of data. The database development, undertaken as part of the audit project, required the identification of the relevant data, understanding the relations between data elements and disability requirements, and demonstrating how we can use this data for facilities' access audit evaluation and management.

To be able to address these questions, we developed a methodology for computer-assisted access audit, described in this chapter.

ARTICULATING AND REPRESENTING KNOWLEDGE CRITICAL TO ACCESSIBILITY AUDITING

When considering the accessibility domain, data and knowledge processing, which includes acquisition, analysis and discovery, and dissemination, draw on many sources of information in diverse forms, such as standards, audit reports, handbooks, and so on, recorded in a variety of media. A major part in a knowledge base design framework is to collect these materials, to develop or to use an already developed information model, which arranges information in an efficient way. Efficient arrangement or grouping of information is the basis for modeling data structures that are suitable for computer implementation. The

Figure 1: Basic Steps in Proposed Computer-Assisted Methodology for Building Evaluation

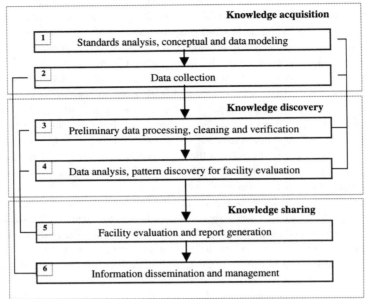

basic stages of our knowledge processing methodology are shown in Figure 1.

We distinguish three major phases: knowledge acquisition, knowledge discovery and knowledge sharing. In each phase, the different procedures are grouped in two stages. The stages are numbered in sequential order. The first stage is in some sense a key prelude. Once the information model is developed and implemented, the audit procedure can rely on it. The procedure itself consists of steps two through five. The result of an audit project can provide feedback for modification of the underlying information model, which in its turn can initiate changes in the collection and analysis stages. In this section, we discuss in detail each of these steps. If the data model determines the underlying information structure, the results of stages 3 and 4 in Figure 1 provide the data and query structures for the computational support of a Web-based access information system. The last two stages in Figure 1 belong to the knowledge-sharing phase: they consider the technologies and procedures for the dissemination and delivery of the results, and putting the knowledge gained through the previous phases in use by concerned parties.

Knowledge Acquisition

Conceptual data modeling is recognized as a tremendously important tool not only for organizing knowledge, but also for domain knowledge analysis and acquisition. Information model building includes the definition of the scope of the subject domain, possible changes in the domain and priority of domain entities, and the ability to accommodate these changes. These factors determine what information is relevant to the information model.

When developing an access audit information mode,l there are at least three strategies to follow:

• development of a stand-alone model, which represents the domain only from an access audit point of view;

- development of an extension to an existing model which adds additional, audit-related features to each entity in the model when preserving the structure and relations in the initial model;
- development of a model with a "docking" concept which allows connection with an existing conceptual model.

Usually in a large organization, whether a university or a large healthcare facility, a data model of existing facilities already exists. As a rule it is developed and used by the facilities management department. Therefore, it is reasonable to establish a connection with that model at the conceptual level. In our initial approach, we started with the analysis of existing standards as the basis for the identification of critical features that approximate the access performance elements. The acquisition of information, construction of a conceptual model and its representation through a particular database schema is an interdisciplinary knowledge engineering exercise, shown in Figure 2. The knowledge engineer combines the information from the domain experts in occupational therapy, facilities management and building design/redesign. The expert from occupational therapy provides interpretation of the standards in the context of disabilities that have to be covered by the model and participates in the conceptual modeling. The facilities management and building design experts provide the necessary information about respective data models to enable compatibility.

The identification of the critical features needs to be based on the most up to date legislative criteria. For example, when involved in auditing the university campuses this required data extraction from numerous sources including the Building Code of Australia (BCA) Guidelines on access to premises published by the Human Rights and Equal

Figure 2: Basic Participants in the Information Modeling Stage

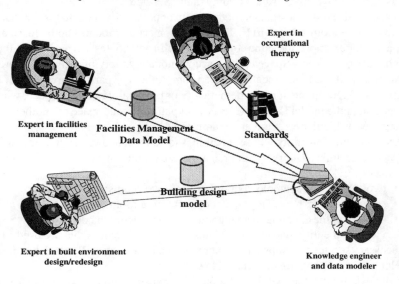

Expert in occupational therapy

Expert in facilities management

Facilities Management Data Model

Standards

Building design model

Expert in built environment design/redesign

Knowledge engineer and data modeler

Opportunity Commission and several Standards Australia publications covering Access and Mobility, Lifts and Parking. Depending on the environmental context i.e. auditing an acute health care setting, differing criteria may apply, but the essential structural elements will remain the same. For instance, requirements for accessible paths for a prone trolley from an operating theatre to a recovery or intensive care area will be determined by the assumptions made about anthropometrics and spatial requirements of users and equipment. Measurements and algorithms to determine the required spatial envelope at an entry point will nevertheless remain the same. In this way, data can be compared to any code requirement.

The variety of extracted features with sometimes-contradictory constraints on their values required the introduction of priority relations. Hierarchical relations in the data model were used to reduce the dimensionality of collected data. To be able to accommodate changes to the model, we developed an open structure where the set of attributes that describes a class of entities is divided into a common group of attributes for that class and specific groups for a particular type of entities in that class.

To be able to address these issues, we developed a data model and designed a database for capturing relevant information. The data model and database schema developed takes into account the existing data models used in the facilities management department for which this database was developed. This approach was beneficial for all participants. On one hand, it provided the audit team with the ability to use directly the data available in the facilities management department. On the other hand, it provides the facilities management department with the potential for direct integration of audit results.

Conceptual Model

The graph representation of the conceptual model is shown in Figure 3. We identified four groups of entities whose common characteristics were united in four basic entities named as "Space"[4], "Link", "Access Point" and "Service":

- Space—a three-dimensional hypothetically or physically bounded space that enables one or more required activities. This definition accommodates both closed and open spaces, for example, the same common modeling attributes can be defined for a room and a car park space. Space entities accommodate variety of activities related to the university life. Lecture theatre, office room, toilet, car park are example of spaces.
- Link—a three-dimensional hypothetically or physically bounded space, whose only function in the model is to provide a travel path from one space to another. Corridor, stairway, vehicular crossing are examples of links.
- Access Point—an entity whose function is to connect and/or provide access between spaces and links. Doorway, door, gate are example of access points. Access can connect:
  - two spaces, for example, a door between two rooms;
  - space and link, for example, a door between a room and a corridor;
  - two links, for example, a change in level between two corridors.
- Services—an entity that accommodates a variety of devices that are used to provide necessary services for supporting major university activities. Rubbish bin, flexi teller, telephone, post box are examples of services.

In the data model accessibility of a particular space with respect to other spaces are considered. A space is accessible by people with disabilities if every link and access in the

Figure 3: Illustration of Conceptual Model

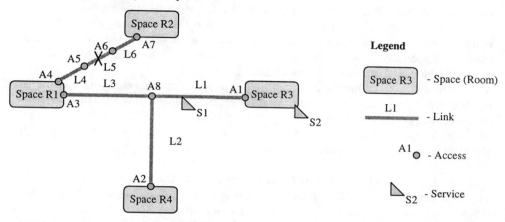

chain of links meets the necessary requirements for that link. For example, space R1 is accessible from space R3 as far as links L1 and L3 satisfy all criteria for disability access. Room R2 cannot be accessed from room R1 because link L5 does not satisfy at least one criterion. Depending on the accessibility criteria, we can have a case of partial accessibility, in the sense we define structural and disability access relations between these entities. Structural relations represent the physical structure when access relations are connected with the disability access criteria. The entity-relationship (ER) diagram in Figure 4, shows the two basic structural relationships used in the model.

Either of the entities "Space", "Link" and "Access Point" can have many services attached to it. Each "Space" may have many access points connected to it. Each "Link" may also have many access points, however, in the current version of the database the cardinality of the "connected-to" between link and access point is restricted to two.

Building facilities and their parts can be represented as a combination of these four

Figure 4: Basic Structural Relations

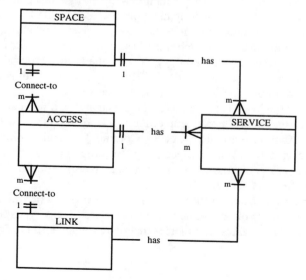

basic entities. A level in a building is a collection of spaces and links with associated access points and services. Whereas a building is a collection of levels and internal links, i.e., a collection of spaces, links and access points forms a building. Car parking bays are represented as individual spaces, the road along them as a link or collection of links, and the entrance to each bay as an access point. Representation in this way thus leads to a model similar to the model of a level within a building.

To be able to represent the variety of rooms, services and other elements from the real environment by one of the above-mentioned categories, we have split the attributes in the data model of each entity into two groups: common and specific. The use of two sets of attributes allows the preservation of the simplicity of our basic model (Figure 4) while allowing us to capture the necessary amount of specific detail.

Data Model and Implementation

The conceptual model has been expressed in terms of an object-relational schema, thus it can be implemented in a database system, which supports this model. For example, in this particular project the schema was implemented in the Microsoft Access database management system. The major factors that influenced the decision making were: (i) the necessity for mobile computing on a low end notebook machine for data acquisition; (ii) ODBC[5] compatibility for transfer and coupling to a backend server database; and (iii) integration with an electronic office suite with data analysis applications. The decision to use notebook computers for direct data entry onsite was necessary to reduce paper management and to increase reliability. The ODBC compliance guaranteed that the database wouldn't remain a stand-alone research exercise. The integration with a popular office suite simplified several aspects of data processing and report generation. In the object-relational schema, each entity is represented by a maximum of n+1 tables, where n is the size of the group that it models, in other words it has a table with the common attributes and n tables with the specific attributes for different entity types. The idea is illustrated in Figure 5. A one-to-one relation of the primary key (entity ID, in this case the rm_id field) connects the "extension".

The record for each instance is split between the common table and the corresponding type table as shown in Figure 5. Type tables were derived from the corresponding Australian standards. These tables provide the details for checking whether that instance meets disability criteria or not. The formulation and formalization of these criteria in terms of queries and the algorithms for criteria check provides the basis for querying the database.

In the final database the common table for each entity has all the records for that entity. Common tables include the Boolean field "criteria". A "Yes" value in the "criteria" field means that the entity has passed the access audit criteria. Thus, for queries about accessibility we can select only the four common tables from the database.

The table-naming convention used is as follows: all tables that describe a particular entity start with the name of that entity. For example, the names of the tables with the common attributes of the four entities are "Access_Common", "Link_Common", "Service_Common" and "Space_Common", respectively. Specific type tables follow similar naming convention. For example, the table, which includes the specific attributes of laboratory spaces is called "Space_Laboratory".

Some entity types do not have specific attributes, thus there are no separate type tables for them. Table 1 shows the number of tables and the list of covered entity types for the current version of the database. The names of the tables that represent an attribute domain

Figure 5: Space Entity in Access Audit Database.

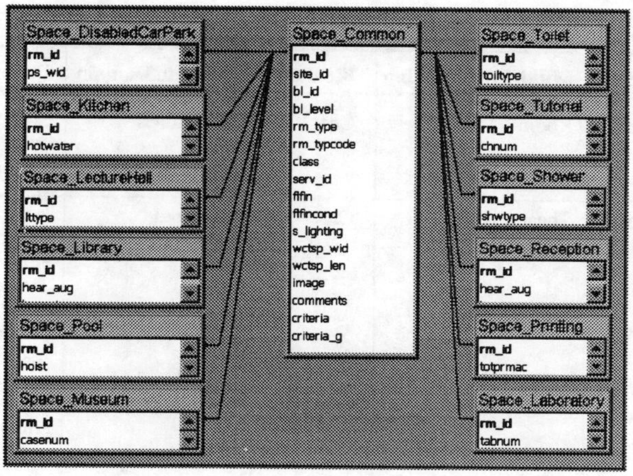

Table 1. Entities and Their Table Descriptions

Entity	Number of tables	Covered entity types
Access	5	Doorway/Gateway, Hinge door, Sliding door, Gate
Link	10	Kerb or Step Ramp, Landing, Lift, Parking isle, Raised median strip, Ramp, Stairway, Vehicular crossing and Walkway.
Service	17	Alarm, Ambulant seat, Doormat, Drinking fountain, Grab rail, Grating, Hand Rail, Kerb/Rail, Post box, Rubbish bin, Signage, Table (plus Counter, Workshop, Desk), Telephone, Traffic Lights, Vending or Ticket Machine, Wheel Chair Space
Space	13	(Dark, Gym, Office, Recreation, Store, Tea/Common room)[6], Disabled car park, Kitchen, Laboratory (Workshop, Refectory, Dining), Lecture hall, Library, Museum/Exhibition Hall, Pool, Printing/duplicating room, Reception (Shop, Medical service), Shower, Toilet, Tutorial room.

begin with the prefix "zSp", for example "zSp_DoorType". A detailed description of each entity with its attribute names, database fields and reference to the relevant legislation and/ or appropriate recommendations has been documented in a database format. An example of the format is presented in Table 2.

Table 2. Example of Entity Type Description

Space: Lecture Hall

Attribute Name	DB field	Multi-Line Heading	Field type	Attribute Domain	Comments
Room ID (PK)	rm_id	Room ID	Char	Code values	Corresponds to field "rm_id" of table "rm" of FM database
Theater type	lttype	Theater type	Char	flat, tiered	Is the Lecture Theatre provided either tiered or flat. Tiered Lecture Theatres should provide wheelchair seating spaces at the level of the main entrance, where flat could provide anywhere (AS1428.1-93, cl 15.1, p. 43).
Number of seats	totseat	Seats	Number integer	Integer numbers	The number of seats provided in the lecture theater.
Number of wheelchair	wcs	Wheel chair spaces	Number integer	Integer numbers	The number of wheelchair seating spaces include only those wheelchair seating spaces which comply with F16, p. 43). If there is a wheelchair seating space but it does not satisfy cl 15, then it is not counted.
Percentage	wcsp	Percentage	wcs/totseat	Computable field (Query in MS Access)	Wheelchair accessible spaces should be provided >= 1% of total (RD 97/01 cl D3.3)
Hearing augmentation	hear_aug	Hearing augmentation	Boolean	Y/N	Y-provided, N - not provided. Hearing augmentation provided (HREOC advisory notes on access to premises-97, 5.12.1) and cover at least 10% of the total area of the enclosed space (AS1428.2-92, cl 21.1, p. 29).

Table 2 continued on next page

Table 2. Example of Entity Type Description (continued).

Hearing augmentation type	h_augtype	Hearing aug	Char	audio frequency induction loop, induction field radio, infrared light transmission, vhs frequency modulated radio, other	Acceptable listening system types are: audio frequency, induction loop, infrared light transmission, induction field radio, vhs frequency modulated radio (AS1428.2-92, cl 21.2, p. 29).
Row clearance	row_cl	Row clearance	Number - integer	in mm	Clearance between rows should be <= 300 mm if the distance to an aisle is <= 3500mm (RD 97/01, cl H1.4ci) or 500mm if greater (RD 97/01, cl H1.4cii)
Aisle width	aisle_wid	Aisle width	Number - integer	in mm	Aisle width >= 1000 mm (AS1428.1-93, Fig. 36, p. 45)
Stage accessibility	wc_stage	Stage access	Boolean	Y/N	Y-accessible, N - inaccessible. Stage, podium, rostrum or like should be accessible to wheelchair user (RD 97/01, cl D3.2). Access should include a ramp (AS1428.2-92, cl 26.2a, p. 36)
Height to operable parts	Oheight	Oper height	Number - integer	in mm	Operable height should be between 500 - 1200 mm, (AS1428.2-92, cl 22.4, p. 32).
Podium: width	wctsp_wid	Podium width	Number - integer	in mm	360 degrees turn requires width >= 2250 mm (AS1428.2-92, cl 26.2b, p. 36).

KNOWLEDGE DISCOVERY PHASE AND COMPUTER-MEDIATED ON-LINE AUDITING PROCESS

Large scale auditing usually means that in order to accomplish an audit project in a timely way, it is usually necessary to put together teams of auditors (Preiser, Rabinowitz & White. 1988). For instance to accomplish the audit of 160 buildings across two campuses within three months, it was necessary to put together an audit team comprising 33 occupational therapy students who volunteered to assist with the accessibility audit as part of their undergraduate professional training commitment. These students were supervised and trained by one full-time and four part-time occupational therapy practitioners employed specifically for the project. Given the number of auditors, considerable attention had to be paid to ensuring reliability and to verification of incoming data. Reliability refers to the reproducibility of a set of measurements under different auditors and across a range of conditions and situations. Ensuring reliability means reducing measurement error by monitoring the variability found in repeated sampling and the establishment of reasonable confidence limits for acceptability of variance in measurements taken. Here on-line technologies are critical to appropriately illustrating and annotating training materials needed to insure reliability of survey procedures.

Primarily auditor or human error, situation-induced error and actual instrument or tool error all cause errors in reliability. Common auditor error relates to low information handling rates (forgetting information), variability in individual performance when problem solving (logical and deductive procedures), variations in force measurements due to differences in strength and fatigue levels, and impairment of accuracy due to changing levels of alertness, fatigue and stress.

Situation-induced error relates to the time of day measurements are taken (i.e., lighting affects accuracy and temperature affects expansion and contraction of materials), the number of people about (i.e., increased stress or distraction) and the weather (i.e., high wind in outdoor locations can affect the accuracy of clinometer readings). Auditor-incurred and situation-induced reliability variance can be corrected in part by development of protocols, cross checks, education and structured opportunities to get feedback on performance.

Therefore, basic training of auditors involved collecting data from a sample of building features, which had already been evaluated by practitioners. This type of 'circuit training' was helpful in assisting students to apply standards, practice measurement protocols, utilize checklists and enter data into the database. Students having completed the entire circuit were then encouraged to compare results and to clarify any outstanding issues relating to measurement, data entry or ambiguity in a group forum conducted after the trial.

In addition, throughout the audit period, weekly meetings were facilitated so students could share, clarify and resolve any measurement issues arising, for example, what should be recorded when horizontal clearance is adequate but an overhanging tree branch obstructs vertical access in a path of travel, etc. Students conducted building audits in self-selected teams of two to three persons with one person having the measurement role and the other the recording role. This team approach provided greater reliability by ensured auditor safety, while encouraging cross checking of data and facilitating peer learning.

Computer-Mediated On-Line Auditing

The scenarios described above illustrate the level of complexity involved in coordination and training necessary for a large-scale auditing project. Computer-mediation of team activities can facilitate and substantially increase the efficiency of auditing activities in these scenarios. The concept of virtual design studios (Maher, Simoff and Cicognani, 1999) addresses the issues of similar scenarios in collaborative design projects. Therefore, we present in detail a number of ways for arranging and organizing the underlying technology relevant for such projects that can be supplemented by on-line methodologies. Project setup is a major criterion in the selection of technological scenarios. As shown earlier, an audit access project comprises several teams, which work in parallel on different parts of the project, thus there is no competition between them. On the other hand, the large amount of collected data requires careful versioning and updating. Current experience is related to manual handling of this type of data.

Internet technologies can be utilized both during the access audit project and in post-

Figure 6: Web-Mediated Team Access Audit Environment.

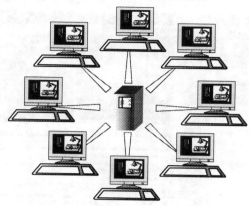

| | TeamWave Client | | TeamWave Server | | Local workplace |

project information dissemination. During the actual access audit procedure the Web may be used as medium for communication and information sharing. The information design is defined by the project structure and collaboration modes. Access audit projects are a combination of different types of collaboration, which leads to different organization of computer-mediated workspaces. The access audit Web mediation can be organized by analogy with the centralized virtual design studio model (Maher, Simoff and Cicognani, 1999, Chapter 7). Figure 6 illustrates one possible way for doing this. The idea is to combine individual and shared workspaces used by the audit team. In this scenario data collection is realized on the spot using mobile personal computers, shown in the figure as separate nodes. Collected data is sorted, cleaned and verified locally, i.e., in the local workspace on each computer. Further data sharing and collaborative analysis is done in the shared workspace supported by groupware technology. A primary issue to be addressed in combining these workspaces is the transition between individual and group work. During an audit process team members shift regularly between individual and group activities, in other words between asynchronous and synchronous collaboration. However, data analysis tools are usually single-user applications. Collaborative activities are usually held in a multi-user groupware environment. Thus, the smoothness of transition between individual and collaborative work in computer-mediated environments is connected with decreasing the gap between the workspaces, ideally having the same workspace both for individual and collective work.

One way to approach this issue is to use the combined metaphor of a desktop for tools arrangement and a room metaphor for information structuring (Greenberg and Roseman, 1998). TeamWave[7] client/server suite is an environment that offers underlying technology suitable for just such an approach. The information space on the server can be organized as a set of rooms, according to some criteria, for example, the division of audited areas to a local work team. The workspace in Figure 6 includes a TeamWave client, which provides the access to the shared workspace and the applications from the local workplace—data analysis, documentation and image processing tools. Figure 7 shows an example of a shared workspace for access auditing. There are five rooms, which correspond to the major auditing

Figure 7: Shared Workspace for a Access Auditing Procedure Based on TeamWave.

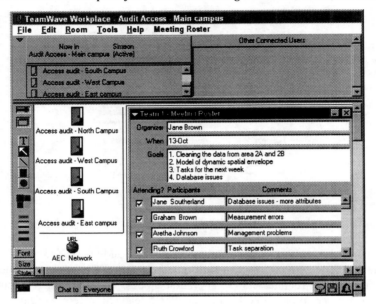

areas—Main, North, West, East and South campuses. Each room accommodates activities and information related to the corresponding campus. The topology of the workplace is defined by the links between related rooms.

Rooms can store a variety of tools which support project scheduling and management, decision making, meetings, file exchange, resource storing, on-line collaboration over text and image data files. Figure 7 illustrates part of the room for the auditing group of the Main campus. It includes a meeting roster with the agenda and participants list for a weekly meeting and also provides Web resources with additional information relevant to team coordination and training. The rooms of other workgroups are accessible through the doorways.

The shared on-line workspace scenario above provides an illustration of how individual and team workspaces could be combined. The selection of particular groupware software will influence how transition between the individual and collaborative workspaces can be achieved. For example, another lightweight groupware, eRoom, bridges the discontinuity of the workspace in distributed desktop environments by adding communication and meeting features directly to the desktop of the operating system, and thus provides a simple way to work collaboratively on documents. Dragging a document from the personal desktop to the browser, which runs eRoom, makes the document immediately available to everyone participating at the team meeting, so that participants can discuss, edit, modify, search, etc. Heavy weight groupware, like Lotus Smartsuite and Domino Server may lead to significant increase of project maintenance costs.

Data Analysis, Pattern Discovery and Feedback to Data Modeling Stage

The data analysis stage identified some unexpected difficulties in the automation of data analysis. They are the result of the standards-centered development of the information model. The original data model was developed on the basis of relevant Australian standards, Human Rights and Equal Opportunity Commission (HREOC) Building Access Guidelines and proposed Building Code of Australia emendations. The entities and their attributes were identified from the requirements specified in the relevant clauses from these documents. It is necessary to point out that during this process we identified some inconsistent and potentially contradictory dimensional data. For example, in the Standards Australia publication relating to requirements for Access and Mobility (AS1428 Parts One and Two), there exist some similarities between requirements for accessible telephones, drinking fountains and washbasins dimensions. Commonalities stem from the common dimensions of wheelchair reach range data, which implicitly formed the basis for the standards. This hidden source creates potential for redundancy, discrepancies, contradictions, misinterpretations and misreferences.

The standards do not provide a functional rationale for understanding and decision making based on disability requirements. Thus, it was difficult to develop data clusters, which form the basis of the queries for audit reporting and interpretation.

For example, in the initial model of the service type "Handrail" we have included the following attributes:

- "intrusion"—to indicate if a handrail obstructs the available circulation space;
- "continue" —to indicate the continuation of a handrail where the handrail adjoins a level landing. This measurement is important in assisting people with visual and balance disabilities in regaining a stable centre balance because climbing stairs requires dynamic gait and it is common for people to trip at the end of a stair;
- "tindic"—to indicate the presence of tactile indicator to inform people with visual disabilities that the handrail finishes;
- "ends"— to indicate that the end of a handrail is turned away the path of travel in order to prevent injuries should someone fall, be pushed or bumped into the handrail end.

In the original model these attributes were of Boolean type. However, during the access audit procedure, implicit relations between these attributes were identified and verification of accuracy was impossible without measurable data as input. For instance, if "continue" is flawed then this will impact on "tindic," but one cannot check data entry reliability on the basis of yes/no response alone.

As a result of these inconsistencies, some attributes were temporarily excluded from the analysis of the building summaries.

Some entities have not been modeled adequately following only the structural constraints from the standards. The problem in this case is not in the standards. The development of simple queries such as compliance with door leaf width is not very helpful in itself, because this attribute is insufficient in determining adequate circulation space for wheel chair users. In order to develop queries that can deal with the complexities of the multiple dimensions it was necessary to develop and prioritize a clustering structure. For example, when considering the dimensions and fixation of a handrail the following query sequence was developed:

- ◆ Is handrail circular with diameter 30-50 mm (inclusive)?
- IF "No" THEN "it does not comply" and "the handrail fails"
- IF "Yes" THEN "it complies to AS 1428.1 for 'crossdiam'

◆ IF "it complies to AS 1428.1" THEN "is the radius of the edges/corners is non-less than 5 mm?

• IF "No" THEN "it does not comply" and "the handrail fails"

• IF "Yes" THEN "it complies to AS 1428.1 for 'exprad'

◆ IF "it complies to AS 1428.1" THEN "is handrail securely fixed and rigid?"

• IF "No" THEN "it does not comply" and "the handrail fails"

• IF "Yes" THEN "the handrail complies for 'rigidfix'

In terms of the database query, for every handrail it is necessary to perform the following queries:

"crossdiam" $\Rightarrow\ \geq 30$ and ≤ 50

"exprad" $\Rightarrow\ \geq 5$

"rigidfix $\Rightarrow$ 'Y'

The process of developing query clusters could not be done *a priori* to the gathering of actual data. Developing query structures happened alongside data collection as reflection on incoming data-assisted prioritization. Although the initial database design has been oriented towards data collection, the information model as originally developed allowed extensions and modifications without affecting collected data.

The development of on-line computational queries was beyond the scope of the audit project as contracted, however, it is an intrinsic part of the development of a Web-mediated on-line auditing tool. As we have shown earlier, the queries are based on the idea of matching disability activities and their spatial requirements against existing space data. Our strategy is based on the Activity/Space model (Maher, Simoff and Mitchell, 1997). The idea is illustrated in Figure 8.

Each disability activity is decomposed into basic activities with their corresponding spatial envelopes and other attributes, like equipment, performer, services and environment (for more details see Section 3 in Maher, Simoff and Mitchell, 1997). On the one hand, activity parameters provide meaningful aggregation of spatial requirements. On the other

Figure 8: On-line Queries Relate Activity Requirements to Standards and Actual Measurements (adapted from De Chiara & Callender, 1990).

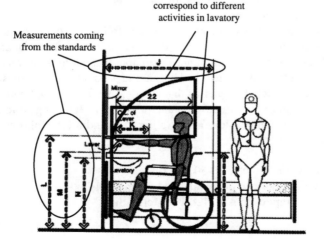

Figure 9. Dynamic Spatial Envelopes for On-line Queries

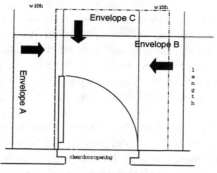

Envelope A: Hinge side approach-door opens
towards the person in a wheelchair

Envelope B: Latch-side approach-door opens
towards the person in a wheelchair

Envelope C: Front approach-door opens
towards the person in a wheelchair

hand, the structure of queries based on activity requirements is clearly separated from their content based on existing standards or measurements, which may change in time. An activity-based approach also allows linking complex queries to the related object. For example, Figure 9 illustrates the concept of a dynamic spatial envelope, which corresponds to a particular conditional activity. The conditional activity determines the relevant spatial envelope, which correspond to the same action under different preconditions. For example, if a person in a wheelchair approaches a door opening from the hinge side of the door leaf, more clear circulation space is required than in a latch-side or frontal approach. The extra space permits the repositioning required to operate the door latch, prior to passing through into the adjacent space.

KNOWLEDGE SHARING: EMPLOYING DATABASE-DRIVEN WEB TECHNOLOGY FOR AUDIT AND ACCESS

Facility Evaluation and Report Generation

Despite not being developed yet to the level of automated query generation and reporting, the database was essential in informing the generation of the final audit report. The database provided a structure that was capable of aggregating elements so data could be clustered and interpreted at a number of levels of abstraction. The basic process used to analyse data was as follows:

1. cluster relevant accessible building elements;
2. aggregate relevant clusters of accessible building elements by levels within a building;
3. aggregate relevant clusters of accessible building elements by building;
4. aggregate relevant clusters of accessible building elements by zone;
5. aggregate relevant clusters of accessible building elements by zone themes.

Using this technique, a summary of each building's performance was generated by manual extraction of data in relation to agreed query clusters. Grouping of data by clusters allowed themes and percentage of compliance to be graphed, reported on and then commented on. Zone summaries were generated in the same way. Zone summaries included reporting on overall building performance for that zone i.e., aggregation of building elements within the zone, which was then combined with summaries of data relating to external links and car parking. Summaries and suggestions for improvements were then generated on this basis for buildings, zones and the facility as a whole. On-line facility evaluation and report generation can be implemented as a set of queries, in a way similar to the information dissemination and management, discussed in the next section.

Information Dissemination and Management

The attribute grouping in our data model provides the flexibility to employ the same data model during the data acquisition stage, the analysis and audit process, and to use the results directly in an on-line Web-based information system. The idea is illustrated in Figure 10. The example shows the use of the data collected for the links. The common part of each entity (see Figure 5) holds the information necessary for answering queries about the degree of accessibility. The answer can span from simple Boolean type "Accessible/Non-accessible" to a certain level of accessibility. To speed up system response the necessary information is pre-computed for each entity (link in the example in Figure 10, space in Figure 5)—the details captured by the specific portion of the entity attributes are analyzed according to access audit evaluation criteria. The "yes/no" answer and degree of accessibility are retrieved from the "Criteria satisfied" field in Figure 10. Formatted information is presented as a Web page. The 'Map database' provides the segments of the map related to the region, covered by the query. The 'CAD database' provides the floor plans of all related buildings. The 'Link geometry' section includes information about actual visualization of the trajectory—line type, color and geometrical parameters. An example of such visualization is shown in Figure 11. When a link is not accessible then it is crossed by a "X", as shown in Figure 10 on the CAD drawing in the building section. Color codes can also be used for labeling different degrees of accessibility.

Taking into account that people with disabilities are part of our target user group, it is also important to consider any additional information that might need to be incorporated to meet users disability requirements. Below we discuss the major disability types that have to be taken into consideration and the corresponding computer support required for enabling Web access to the stored information.

1. *Vision disabilities.* These impairments are supported in computer access by the following basic techniques:
   - screen readers, which provide synthesized speech and, in conjunction with software, produce audio output of information displayed on a computer screen;
   - Braille displays, which provide access to computers, using a special notation of raised dots;
   - screen magnification techniques, which include a magnification lens placed in front of the monitor providing 2-3 times magnification; software programs allowing the user to magnify the screen output up to 8 times; hardware and software solutions which provide multiple larger variations in size of magnification.
2. *Hearing disabilities.* These impairments in the pre-multimedia era of computing have caused fewer problems due to the minimal use of sound. In general, if sound is used to indicate or reinforce a user action, then a visual indication on the screen is required.

Figure 10: Database-Driven Web Information System

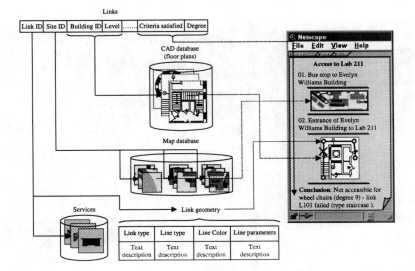

3. *Cognitive disabilities.* These impairments share many of the same characteristics and access issues inherent with low vision and physical disabilities, putting an emphasis to aid comprehension techniques. These may result in extended display times, additional textual descriptions and simplification of the selected set of signs used for navigation.

To provide support for people with visual disabilities the content of the 'Link geometry' database also includes text descriptions of every element presented on the access map. Figure 10 illustrates some of the required fields for a 'Link geometry database'. Developers of Web information systems often rely heavily on graphical modes of communication, such as site plan maps and CAD drawings (as shown in Figure 10 and Figure 11), because they allow the display of complex abstract information in compact formats. This benefits most, but not all users. The users most disadvantaged are people with severe visual impairments who rely on enhanced text-based or auditory communication formats (i.e., screen readers). The incorporation of 'Link geometry' data allows the parallel generation of text descriptions of the accessibility of any potential path of travel. Complying with these issues avoids the situation described below:

"When blind people use the Internet and come across unfriendly sites, we aren't surfing, we are crawling... Imagine hearing pages that say, "Welcome to ... [image].' 'This is the home of ... [image].' 'Link, link, link.' It is like trying to use Netscape with your monitor off and the mouse unplugged. See how far you will get."[8]

Specific challenges of this universally accessible on-line approach include dealing with issues of composing dictionaries, which allow converting graphics into alternative text descriptions so that automatically generated meaningful descriptions correspond to the graphical representation. The on-line interface has to use metaphors compatible with internal cognitive mapping of users. For instance, for visually disabled users a textual navigational path needs to provide considerably more detail than just link numbers. For

Figure 11: Visualization of the Results of an Access Query

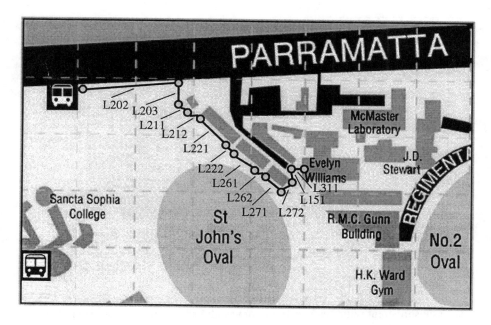

example, a Web page with the following description of the path in Figure 11 will hardly assist a person with visual disability.

> You are at the University drop-off point Camperdown campus Main gate. To go to Evelyn Williams building, you have to follow link L202, then link 203, then link 211, then link 212, then link 221, then link ....

On the Web page the text description of a link should connect spatial references to both

Table 3. Examples of textual alternatives to graphic illustration

Graphic label	Textual description
AP 200	This path starts at Parramatta Road Busstop - University drop off point, Camperdown campus, Main gate. This busstop is situated 20 metres to the north of the main gate. Link 201 is to the north and link 202 is to the south.
Link 202	This runs along the north-south axis and connects the Parramatta Road busstop to the main gate and link 203 .
Link 203	This runs along an east-west axis and connects link 202 and 211.
Link 211	This runs in a west-south direction and connects link 203 and 212.

familiar place names, providing both directional and connection data. Such a requirement adds an additional layer to the backend database. In the simplest case this is a table of attribute-value pairs, where the attribute is the label of the element, and the value is the whole text of the descriptions that goes as a sentence or paragraph on the Web page that displays the result of the query. For instance, in order for the graphical information displayed in Figure 11 to be fully accessible the original database must also contain relevant textual alternatives which can be retrieved with the selection of a start point and a destination or stop point. Table 3 presents an example of such a solution.

The illustration provided in Figure 11 has the Paramatta Road north-west bus stop as a start point and the connecting link (i.e. link 202) needs to be traversed in a southerly direction prior to making a right-hand turn at the intersection of link 203 into the University proper. In other words, entity relations and reference point information using familiar reference point terminology must be included in order to provide any reasonable textual alternative. Note that this is in addition to the text descriptions of the links and other elements presented in Figure 10.

More efficient and sophisticated solutions require the creation of dictionary descriptions where each entry corresponds to a field in the description of an entity in the data model. Such approach will result in extension of entity descriptions (see Table 2), generation of more elaborated and adequate text presentations on the Web pages, from knowledge representations, more compact than the attribute-value representation, shown in Table 3.

The benefit of this approach, if data is captured as a part of the actual audit, is that there is no additional cost in retrospectively collecting data or in complying with anti-discrimination requirements for both facilities and software. Moreover, on-line technologies developed using these principles can be truly inclusive and facilitate planning, problem solving, orientation, and way finding in and about premises not just for the average user but for all users in a nondiscriminatory manner.

BENEFITS AND FURTHER DEVELOPMENT

The development of a methodology for computer-assisted evaluation of the built environment and a database to support data collection and analysis during the physical audit has assisted in ensuring audit validity. Validity was improved by provision of a structure that was logical, extensible and contained measurable elements based on relevant standards and access guidelines. The database demonstrated robustness and was able to accommodate variance in values. Utilization of the database assisted reliable data input by provision of simple online help and provided a means of analyzing the raw data at a level of detail that has previously been impracticable.

All existing physical access checklists and databases reviewed to date contain Boolean data usually in the form of auditor judgements about compliance. Our database is based on actual measurable input, which means that queries can be written to cross check the raw data for data entry error or incompleteness. Moreover, the database development allowed sorting, clustering and aggregation of elements in a time-efficient manner that would have been extremely difficult using the more standard paper-based audit checklists on such a large scale audit. For example, in excess of 3000 hinged door faces were measured, attributes were clustered and then analyzed for compliance. The sheer size of the audit and corresponding amount of paper handling, data extraction and data transcription required would have impacted severely on the resources and data analysis outcomes. Paper-based checklists are cumbersome, inflexible and difficult to check for completeness or reliability of data input.

No existing databases or paper-based checklists consistently link elements to the most recent standards, legislation and specific clauses; without this information it is impossible to cross check elements for validity, accuracy or completeness. Moreover, standards and legislation are socially fixed and are thus liable to change over time as societal values change. Our database separates data collection from analysis and should standards or legislation change, all that will be required is new values for the queries.

The conceptual model that underpins the database makes it possible for the first time to do dynamic searches to determine if an accessible path of travel exists between two points. This requires the development of a query structure to abstract connected links between two points and check for link accessibility. An inaccessible link would indicate a break in the path of travel. More importantly the recording of link lengths permits calculation of distances and thus allows checks on distances overall. Overall distance between access points, drop-off points or car parking can have significant impact on persons with cardiopulmonary impairments and or endurance limitations.

Further development of the database is possible in three major areas, The first and most important would extend and automate the existing manual query structures and would examine the potential to integrate our database with the Standards Australia or other similar databases. Integration of the two databases would permit automatic updating of query values and provide for greater flexibility over the long term. Extension and query integration would significantly extend the capability of the database for any future auditing such as those planned on other university campuses.

The second major improvement would be the compilation of the experience and understanding of the subject gathered during the project so that context-sensitive help could be developed and integrated into both the data-collection forms and the report and query generator.

The third step is the development of the Web-based information system, which utilizes the data model presented in the backend database with distributed access both for submission and retrieval of information. The Web interface, discussed earlier, should be a combination of a graphical (CAD-based) interface similar to ARCHIBUS and readable text descriptions. This combination would make possible the generation of dynamic scaled plans of zones, buildings, levels and spaces, suitable for planning and better accommodating individual students with disabilities. For instance such a development could make the job of the university disability officer much easier when assisting individuals with disabilities in course selection, enrollment, and subject completion. It would permit anticipation of difficulties and would assist in appropriate scheduling of accessible spaces for staff and students.

A full-scale, database-driven Web access audit and information management system can be implemented as a centralized or distributed architecture, or a combination of both architectures. The centralized architecture has the advantage of keeping the data in one place, with the consequences of consistent versioning and technically easier update management. The potential host is the Facilities Management Department. The alternative is to implement the system as a distributed architecture (Colouris, Dollimore and Kindberg, 1994). In this case, the data can be split between different divisions within the organisation. Databases in the divisions are managed independently. The advantage of this approach is

Figure 12. Distributed Web-based access information management

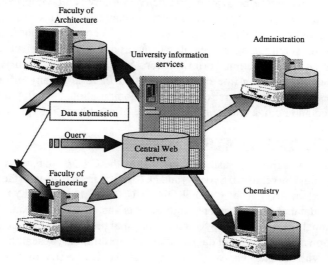

the parallelism during the data acquisition stage - each server is on its own IP address, thus each backend database can be accessed asynchronously. A distributed approach is illustrated in Figure 12. In this case the data submission goes directly to the "regional" servers, when the query is still submitted to the central server which composes the respond collecting data from the "regional" servers.

The strategic planning of accessibility auditing, on-line database development and Web dissemination involves the analysis of the project outcomes and expected functionality with key stakeholders such as therapists and facilities managers (Tan, 1995, Chapter 10). Perspectives on functionality are likely to be substantially different between these users because of differences in values, training and experience with both auditing and on-line computational methodologies. Facilities managers are most likely to be concerned about cost-containment and meeting regulatory compliance criteria at minimum levels, whereas therapists will be most concerned about maximizing functionality for all potential users (i.e., both software and building users). Bridging this divide can be tricky but incorporating both viewpoints will lead to more robust and transparent systems, which will be of the greatest long-term benefit.

CONCLUSION

The results of our preliminary work implies that creating on-line accessibility auditing is indeed possible and likely to make a major contribution to reducing risk and liability for owners and facility managers, while improving and maintaining health and well-being outcomes across acute care and community settings. Inferring from the results of our preliminary work, creating on-line Web-accessible environmental auditing tools is both feasible and likely to be increasingly cost effective for facility managers, auditors and educators. Cost and time efficiencies result from the incorporation of appropriate conceptual data models, object-orientated databases, more flexible search and data mining capability and in-built hyperlinks. Together these new tools make training, collaboration and customization easier. However, there is a need for more research, particularly in the area of predictive validity and prioritization. Predictive validity can be improved by development of performance models that allow greater customization of user needs and profiles. Arbitrary standards are limited in producing reasonable accommodations from a functional perspective. Moreover, tracking and seamlessly incorporating users' perspectives is critical in any ethical process of situational prioritization. As others have previously pointed out it is critical to remember in on-line development that there are many different potential variations in responses to built environments, and computational development needs to be both open ended and humanistic in approach to be of most benefit to practice.

ACKNOWLEDGMENTS

We thank P. Esdaile, M. Saad, and the rest of the CAD/Database group (Office of Facilities Planning, University of Sydney) and D. Crisford from FM~interface (the facilities management system division of CADGROUP AUSTRALIA Pty Ltd.) for briefing and feedback about database development requirements and S. Whybrow and P. Williamson (both occupational therapists employed on the original project) for assistance with advice about automation and clustering of data queries. This preliminary research would have not been possible without the generous assistance of the University of Sydney, the body responsible for contracting and initiating the original database development and accessibility auditing consultancy.

ENDNOTES

1 School of Occupation and Leisure Sciences, Faculty of Health Sciences, University of Sydney, C.Bridge@cchs.usyd.edu.au.

2 Department of Architectural and Design Science, Faculty of Architecture, University of Sydney simeon@arch.usyd.edu.au

3 Both authors were staff members of the University of Sydney at the time of the initial research project.

4 We also use the notion "Room" interchangeably with "Space" where possible. "Room" is accepted term in Structure-Function models.

5 Open Data Base Connectivity, a standard database access method, implemented as a mediator (database driver) between an application and the database management system. If the application is "ODBC-compliant," i. e., produces queries that are understood by the ODBC driver, then the driver translates the application's data queries and requests into commands that particular database management system can interpret.

6 These space types do not have separate tables and are fully covered by the attributes in the Space_Common table.

7 http://www.teamwave.com

8 *New York Times Cybertimes*, 12/1/96, http://www.nytimes.com/library/cyber/week/1202blind.html.

REFERENCES

Americans with Disabilities Act: Accessibility Guidelines. (1991, July 26) Federal Register.

Campbell, L. & Wadell, C. (1997, June) *Electronic Curbcuts: How to build an accessible Web site.* [on-line paper] Available: http://www.jsrd.or.jp/dinf_us/ilf/ecc.htm (Friday, 21st May 1999).

Colouris, G., Dollimore, J. & Kindberg, T. (1994). *Distributed Systems: Concepts and Design.* Addison-Wesley Publishing Co., Reading, MA.

De Chiara, J. & Callender, J. (1990). *Time-Saver Standards for Building Types,* McGraw-Hill, N.Y.

Fox, P. (1995). Environmental modifications in the homes of elderly Canadians with disabilities. *Disabilities and Rehabilitation,* 17, 43-49.

Gero, J. S. (1990). Design prototypes: A knowledge representation schema for design, *AI Magazine,* 11(4), 26-36.

Goldsmith, S. (1997). *Designing for the Disabled: The new paradigm* (4th Ed.). London: RIBA Publications.

Government of Western Australia. (1996). *Access resource kit: With checklists to improve access for people with disabilities.* Perth, Australia: Access Improvements Branch, Disability Services Commission.

Greenberg, S. & Roseman, M. (1998). *Using a Room Metaphor to Ease Transitions in Groupware.* Research report 98/611/02, Department of computer science, University of Calgary, Calgary, Alberta, Canada, January.

Human Rights & Equal Opportunity Commission. (1997). Annual report of the Human Rights and Equal Opportunity Commission. Canberra, Australia.

Iwarsson, S. & Isacsson, A. (1998) ADL dependence in the elderly population living in the community: The influence of functional limitations and physical environmental demand. *Occupational Therapy International,* 5(3) 173-193.

Kelly, B., Deshan, J., Jones, R., & Fisher, K. (1996). *Disability Discrimination Act 1992: Priding equity in access to tertiary institutions.* Brisbane, Australia: Property and Facilities Division, The University of Queensland.

Linn, R. L. (1988). *Educational Measurement* (3rd Ed.) New York. USA: Macmillian.

Martin, E. (1997). *Access to heritage buildings for people with disabilities.* Canberra, Australia: Cox Architects and Planners.

Maher, M. L., Simoff, S. J. & Cicognani, A. (1999). *Understanding Virtual Design Studios,* Springer, London.

Maher, M. L., Simoff, S. J. & Mitchell, J. (1997). Formalising building requirements using an Activity/Space model, *Automation in Construction,* 6, 77-95.

McAuley, H. (1994). Legislation: One step ahead down under. *Access by design,* Sept(65). 8-11.

Preiser, W., Rabinowitz, H. & White, E. (1988). *Post-occupancy evaluation.* Van Nostrand, New York.

Steinfeld, E. & Danford, G. (1997) Environment as a mediating factor in functional assessment. In Dittner S. and Gresham G. (Eds.). *Functional assessment and outcome measures for the rehabilitation professional.* MA: Aspen.

Tan, J. K. H. (1995). *Health management information systems: theories, methods, and applications.* Aspen Publishers, Gaithersburg, MD.

About the Authors

ABOUT THE EDITOR:

Lauren B. Eder received her Ph.D. in Management Information Systems and an MBA from Drexel University, and a B.S. in Business Education from Boston University. She is currently Assistant Professor of Computer Information Systems at Rider University. Previously she was employed for 10 years in various marketing and technical consulting roles with IBM, Digital Equipment Corporation, and Motorola. Dr. Eder's research interests include the adoption and diffusion of information technology in healthcare, and the infusion process of electronic commerce technology. Her research has been published or accepted for publication in *Communications of the ACM, Computer Personnel* and *Information Resources Management Journal*, among other journals, and has also appeared in many national and international conference proceedings. E-mail: eder@rider.edu

CHAPTER AUTHORS:

Monica Adya is Assistant Professor of Information Systems at the University of Maryland Baltimore County (UMBC). She received her PhD from Case Western Reserve University. Her research interests are in decision making and artificial intelligence, with an application area of forecasting. In particular, Dr. Adya has been working on using expert systems for forecasting. She has published papers in *Information Systems Research* and the *Journal of Forecasting*, and she is on the editorial board of the *International Journal of Forecasting* and is serving as the section editor of Research on Forecasting for that journal. Dr. Adya can be reached at adya@umbc7.umbc.edu.

Daniel K. Anderson, M.D., has a consultative clinical internal medicine practice in Grinnell, Iowa, dealing primarily with cardiovascular and renal disease and difficult or complex hypertensive patients. He recently served as assistant professor of internal medicine for Southern Illinois University School of Medicine, where he was also Director of the Springfield Health Information Network and involved in the medical informatics curriculum. He received his M.D. from SIU in 1988 and trained in internal medicine and nephrology, hypertension & electrolyte metabolism at the University of Iowa Hospitals and Clinics in Iowa City, Iowa from 1988-1993. His interest in medical computing is long-standing, and his current practice incorporates a number of database and decision support tools.

James G. Anderson, Ph.D. is Professor and Director, Social Research Institute, Purdue University, West Lafayette, Indiana. He is the associate vice president for Simulation in Health Care Society for Computer Simulation. He is a member of the editorial board of the *JAMIA* and a member of the scientific program committee of the AMIA Annual Symposium, 1999. He has made numerous academic and service contributions to AMIA, the Simulation in Health Care Society for Computer Simulation and the International Institute of Informatics and Systemics.

Malin Brännback has a D.Sc. (Econ. & Bus.Adm.) and a B.Sc. (Pharmacy) from the Åbo Akademi University in Turku. She currently serves as a research director of Innomarket, research which concentrates on new and innovative products and services in the high technology industry. She has served as an associate professor in international marketing at the Åbo Akademi University and as a professor of information systems at the University of Turku. She has taught courses in strategic management, industrial marketing, electronic commerce, and group decision support systems. Her current research activities focus on knowledge-based strategic management, IT-enabled knowledge creation, electronic commerce, drug industry, and healthcare.

Catherine E. Bridge is a tenured Lecturer in the School of Occupation and Leisure Sciences at the University of Sydney. Ms Bridge is passionate about understanding and improving human-design interactions and is currently completing a Ph.D. on redesign for people with disabilities at the University of Sydney, in the Faculty of Architecture where she is an acknowledged expert in the area of environmental assessment and redesign. Her primary research and consultative activities both as a clinician and as an academic have centered on the role of environmental interventions in functional adaptation for people with disabilities. Ms Bridge has authored a number of reports and co-authored a number of other publications including a book chapter in an international undergraduate text.

Angela S. Carillo, M.A. is Assistant Director of the Division of Continuing Medical Education at the University of Alabama School of Medicine at Birmingham, Alabama. She has participated in funds development and evaluation of web courses at UAB.

Linda Casebeer, Ph.D. is Assistant Professor at the University of Alabama at Birmingham School of Medicine in Birmingham Alabama. She also serves as the Associate Director of the Division of Continuing Medical Education at UAB. Her research concerns educational interventions which facilitate changes in physician performance and evaluation of medical informatics interventions.

Walter Fierz studied medicine at the University of Zurich (Switzerland) where he graduated as a medical doctor in 1973. After some clinical experience, he specialized in clinical immunology and was working in experimental clinical immunology in London (England), Würzburg (Germany) and Zurich. Since 1992 he is heading the clinical immunology section of the Institute for Clinical Microbiology and Immunology (IKMI) in St. Gallen (Switzerland). His year-long interest in medical informatics led in 1997 to a collaboration with the Institute for Media and Communication Management (MCM) aimed at the application of the concepts and techniques of knowledge management in the healthcare sector.

Guisseppi A. Forgionne is Professor of Information Systems at the University of Maryland Baltimore County (UMBC). Professor Forgionne holds a B.S. in Commerce and Finance, an M. A. in Econometrics, an M. B. A., and a Ph. D. in Management Science and

Econometrics. He has published 24 books and approximately 125 research articles and consulted for a variety of public and private organizations on decision support systems theory and applications. Dr. Forgionne also has served as department chair at UMBC, Mount Vernon College, and Cal Poly Pomona. He has received several national and international awards for his work.

David W. Forslund, a fellow of the American Physical Society, is a theoretical and computational plasma physicist who has worked in a broad range of plasma physics, from space plasma physics, to magnetic fusion to laser fusion and, more recently, in computer science. He discovered the existence of heat conduction instabilities in the solar wind, co-developed the first consistent model of collisionless shocks with reflected ions, and wrote one of the first codes to numerically evaluate the full electromagnetic dispersion relation for a magnetized plasma. He first emphasized the importance of stimulated Brillouin scattering and stimulated Raman scattering in laser fusion, and first developed a model to explain intense visible harmonics of laser light observed in CO_2 laser-produced plasmas. He published the first accurate calculations of resonance absorption of laser light in arbitrary plasma density profiles. He has developed and maintained the international laser fusion plasma simulation code, WAVE, on a multitude of operating systems and machine architectures. He co-developed the first implicit electromagnetic plasma simulation code (VENUS) and used it to discover the intense surface magnetic fields which have explained a variety of phenomena in the interaction of intense light with plasmas. He has also worked in the area of developing better computational tools in improving the human-computer interface, including the first demonstration of the Network extensible Window System (NeWS™) operating in a useful way between a scientific workstation and a supercomputer. His research has also resulted in the development a distributed particle simulation code in C++ that runs on a network of heterogeneous workstations. As deputy director of the Advanced Computing Laboratory, he helped guide the installation and operation of one of the largest massively parallel supercomputers in the world and led a research project in the practical applications of distributed computing. He has over 60 publications in refereed scientific journals and has given numerous invited talks in plasma physics, computer science, and health informatics. He was principal investigator of a major research project aimed at developing integrated technologies for the National Information Infrastructure. This includes developing a fully functional, distributed graphical patient record system used by radiologists at the National Jewish Center for Immunology and Respiratory Medicine in Denver, Colorado. This first use of truly distributed object technology in healthcare was demonstrated at the Health Information Management Systems Society in 1995. He was principal investigator a project designed to enable portable massively parallel scientific applications. He is the project leader for the TeleMed project funded by the US Medical Research and Materiel Command. He is the technical leader for the Northern New Mexico Rural Telemedicine project funded by the Department of Commerce and has assisted numerous local, state and national organizations in the adoption of advanced information technology. As a member of the Object Management Group, he has worked closely on many of the standard specifications being developed by the CORBAmed healthcare taskforce, including the development and testing of prototypes of those standards. He is engaged by the Government Computerized Patient Record project in the evaluation of the architectural design of a distributed person identification system (EMPI) for linking numerous government health information systems.

Aryya Gangopadhyay is an Assistant Professor of Information Systems at the University of Maryland Baltimore County. His research interests include electronic commerce, multimedia databases, data warehousing and mining, and geographic information systems. He has authored and co-authored two books, numerous papers in journals such as *IEEE Computer, IEEE Transactions on Knowledge and Data Engineering, Journal of Management Information Systems,* and *ACM Journal on Multimedia Systems,* as well as presented papers in many national and international conferences. He can be reached at gangopad@umbc.edu.

Rolf Grütter, lic. oec. HSG, is a scientific project manager and lecturer at the Media and Communications Management Institute (chair Professor Dr. Beat Schmid) of the University of St. Gallen, Switzerland. His research interest concerns the academic discipline of medical informatics in general and the development of medical knowledge media in particular. Rolf studied veterinary medicine at the University of Zurich, Switzerland. In 1983 he accomplished his final exams, in 1990 his doctorate in the field of endocrinology of metabolism at the University of Berne, Switzerland. He studied information management at the University of St. Gallen, completing his licentiate in 1997. Rolf is an active member of the Swiss Society for Medical Informatics (SSMI). He is vitally involved in the establishment of a Swiss Curriculum in Medical and Health Informatics.

Ray Hackney is Director of Business Information Technology Research within the Manchester Metropolitan University. He holds a Cert. Ed, BSc (Hons), MA and Ph.D from leading universities and has contributed to research in the field of information systems with publications in numerous national and international conferences and journals. He has taught on a number of MBA programmes including MMU, Manchester Business School and the Open University. He leads the organising committee for the annual BIT and BITWorld Conference series and is a member of the Strategic Management Society and Association of Information Systems. Dr Hackney has served on the Board of the UK Academy for Information Systems since 1997. He is the Vice President Research for IRMA (USA), Associate Editor of the JGIM, Journal of EUC and ACITM. He is also a reviewer for a number of publishers, journals and conferences and is currently an Associate Editor for ICIS'99. His research interests are the strategic management of information systems within a variety of organisational context.

Christian Heine is research assistant at the Technical University Ilmenau, Germany. He holds a first degree in information systems from the Technical University of Ilmenau. The degree dissertation was on controlling concepts in hospitals. He aspires to be awarded doctor's degree and is studying for his doctorate under Professor Stefan Kirn. The main field of his dissertation is the telemedicine special teleradiology. He took part in several research projects of the public healthcare sector.

Grace J. Johnson is a doctoral student in the Department of Marketing at Southern Illinois University at Carbondale. Her academic background includes an undergraduate degree in psychology and a master's in business, with specialization in marketing. She worked in the pharmaceutical industry and in international business for several years before beginning to pursue her Ph.D. in business. Her academic and work backgrounds have paved the way for her research interests, which include consumer behavior, e-business, and e-medicine.

David Kilman has been working in the computer science side of healthcare for many years. He has built automatic reasoning software in healtcare and contributed significantly to the HL7 and CORBAmed standards for Patient Identification. He was the originator of the concept of workshops held in 1996 to encourage the adoption of open, object-oriented standards for a master patient index. The Person Identification Service standard from the Object Management Group is a direct result of that initiative.

Stefan Kirn heads a chair in information systems at the Technical University Ilmenau, Germany. He holds a Ph.D. in artificial intelligence from University of Hagen (Germany), an M. Sc. in computer science and an M.Sc. in management. Stefan Kirn has published more than 50 papers in peer-reviewed international journals, and at internationally recognized conferences. He is editor-in-chief of the bookseries "Agent Technology" of Addison Wesley Longan (Germany) and the coordinator of a 6-years priority research program on Intelligent Agents in Business Applications in Germany, running from 1999-2006.

Steven P. Klein is an instructor at Southern Illinois University at Edwardsville. He has an M.S. in Computing and Information Systems from SIUE. He also has a B.A. in English from Oklahoma State University. His research interests include Web technologies, expert systems, and simulation.

Robert Klepper is a Professor in the Computer Management and Information Systems Department of the School of Business at Southern Illinois University - Edwardsville. He is author of "Outsourcing Information Technology, Systems, and Services." His research interests include information systems outsourcing, organizational culture and information systems development and use, and electronic commerce.

Rajiv Kohli is the Project Leader - Decision Support Services at the corporate office of Holy Cross Health System. He is also an adjunct Assistant Professor at the University of Notre Dame. He has also taught at the University of Maryland, University College where he was awarded the Teaching Recognition Award. Dr. Kohli received his PhD in 1994 from the University of Maryland, Baltimore County campus. Dr. Kohli's research has or is being published in *Journal of Management Information Systems*, *Decision Support Systems*, *Information Processing & Management*, *International Transactions in Operational Research*, *Topics in Health Information Management*, and *Healthcare Information Management* among other journals. Dr. Kohli's research interests include organizational impacts of information systems, process innovation, and enhanced decision support systems.

Mikko Korpela received his Doctor of Technology degree in 1994 in Information Systems Research. Since 1984 he has been a Senior Researcher at the Computing Centre, University of Kuopio, Finland. He was involved in developing the FileMan/Kernel-based 'MUSTI' hospital information systems in Finland in the mid-1980s, and has been leading the 'FixIT' project to modernize these systems since 1995. In 1989 he was Visiting Research Fellow at the Obafemi Awolowo University, Nigeria. Since 1997 Dr. Korpela has also been a Docent (Associate Professor) in Healthcare Information Systems at the Department of

Computer Science and Applied Mathematics, University of Kuopio.

Robert Kristofco, M.S.W., is Associate Professor of the University of Alabama at Birmingham School of Medicine in Birmingham Alabama. He also serves as the Director of the Division of Continuing Medical Education at UAB. He is a board member and officer of the Alliance for Continuing Medical Education. He has directed medical informatics initiatives including web course development at UAB.

Anand Kumar is an Assistant Professor of Marketing at Southern Illinois University at Carbondale. He holds a PhD in Business from Indiana University, Bloomington. His teaching and research are focused on the general area of consumer behavior. His specific research interests include customer delight, customer value, managerial and consumer decision making, affect, memory, and consumer retention.

Hans Lehmann, Austrian by birth, is a management professional with some 25 years of business experience with information technology. After a career in data processing line management in Austria he worked as an information technology manager in the manufacturing and banking sector in South Africa. After completing an MBA, he joined Deloitte's and worked for some ten years in their international management consultancy firm in Zimbabwe, London and New Zealand. Hans' work experience spans continental Europe, Africa, the United Kingdom, North America and Australasia. He specialised in the development and implementation management of international information systems for a number of blue-chip multi-national companies in the financial and manufacturing sectors. In 1991 Hans changed careers and joined the University of Auckland, New Zealand, where his research focuses on the strategic management of international information systems.

Michèle L. Lemaire, M.D., M.A. is a neuropsychiatrist and a sociologist. She is the co-founder of Anabase International Corp., a global healthcare organization. Anabase provides strategic integrated project planning and management services to optimize drug and medical device research and development. Anabase develops user friendly, Web-based information systems, technology and methodologies to support global clinical research. Under development are Web-based computer-aided chronic disease and patient self-management systems aimed at improving healthcare through empowering both patients and their physician.

Neil McBride is a Principal Lecturer in Information Systems at De Montfort University. Before joining De Montfort University in 1990, he worked as a programmer, analyst and systems development consultant carrying out analysis, development, quality assurance and training. He was involved in the the development and implementation of systems within hospitals. His research interests include object technology, information systems failure, information systems strategy in the public sector, and business strategy for the Internet. He has published papers in European Management Journal, Information Systems Journal and the International Journal of Public Sector Management. His work has applied post-modernism, chaos theory and actor-network theory to understanding information systems problems.

Juha Mykkänen graduated with a master's degree in Computer Science from the

University of Kuopio in 1998, on the architectures of healthcare information systems based on the web browser technology. He has been working in the 'FixIT' project of the University of Kuopio, Computing Centre, since 1997, being in charge of developing the Delphi-FixIT toolkit. His further research interests include the distributed component approach to encapsulating the business logic of healthcare applications.

Joe Noone is a currently undertaking a PhD in the Health Informatics Research Group at the Levels Campus of the University of South Australia. His work centres on the effectiveness and suitability of clinical practice guidelines for health practitioners for the care of the chronically ill. He holds an undergraduate degree of a Bachelor of Health Sciences with Honours.

Arkalgud Ramaprasad is a Professor in the Department of Management at Southern Illinois University at Carbondale and Director of the Pontikes Center Management of Information. He teaches and conducts research in strategic management and management of information, and promotes industry-university cooperation in education and research related to management of information. He obtained his PhD from the University of Pittsburgh in 1980. Prior to that he obtained his MBA from Indian Institute of Management, Ahmedabad, India, and BE (Electrical) from the University of Mysore. He has published in *Behavioral Science, Management Science, Academy of Management Review, Omega, Decision Sciences* and other journals. He has received research grants from major corporations such as Comdisco, Chrysler, IBM and Bozell Worldwide.

Mika Räsänen graduated with a master's degree in Computer Science from the University of Kuopio in 1999, on the application integration architectures of healthcare information systems, with emphasis on the distributed objects technology. His study was part of the 'FixIT' project of the University of Kuopio, Computing Centre.

Madhusudhan Reddy is an MBA student at Southern Illinois University at Carbondale.

Pekka Reijonen received his M.Soc.Sc. in Psychology from the University of Turku. He is a researcher at the Information Systems Laboratory Laboris at the University of Turku. His research interests are usability and deployment issues of information systems in organizations and he currently is working on a project defining end-users' skills and knowledge requirements and their evaluation.

Hellevi Ruonamaa received her master's degree in mathematics from the University of Helsinki in 1985. She has been working in the University of Kuopio, Computing Centre, since 1989, being in charge of the FileMan/Kernel technology and coordinating the technological development in the 'FixIT' project since 1995.

Simeon J. Simoff has an original interdisciplinary way in design computing, combining in his teaching and research the elegant and structured approach of mathematics, visual attractiveness and beauty of multimedia computing, and dynamics of computer-mediated communication. He has published numerous papers in journals and books in data analysis, artificial intelligence and design science, and co-authored a book about virtual design studios. Currently Dr Simoff is a Research Fellow at the Key Centre of Design Computing and Cognition, University of Sydney. His teaching and research work is connected with data mining and analysis for knowledge discovery in digital media, distributed information systems, multimedia communication and flexible learning environments.

Riitta Söderlund has a DDS (Specialist in Healthcare) and a M.Sc. (Computer Science) from the University of Turku. She currently serves as a researcher of Innomarket, the research of which concentrates on new and innovative products and services in the high technology industry. She has served as an assistant in the Department of Computer Science at the University of Turku and as a dentist in the Health Center of Turku. Her current research activities focus on information technology used in healthcare, especially on the issue of whether it is possible to make activities of healthcare more efficient and effective using new IT solutions.

Marko Sormunen graduated with a master's degree in Computer Science from the University of Kuopio in 1998, on converting a client/server systems development toolkit to the Java applet technology. He has been working in the 'FixIT' project of the University of Kuopio, Computing Centre, since 1997, being in charge of developing the Web-FixIT toolkit.

Katarina Stanoevska-Slabeva studied business administration at the Faculty of Economics of the University "Kiril and Metodij" in Skopje, Macedonia, and accomplished her doctorate at the University of St. Gallen, Switzerland, in 1997 in the field of knowledge management and business process redesign (http://www.netacademy.org/netacademy/register.nsf/homepages/kstanoevska-slabeva). She is currently working as a senior lecturer and as a scientific project manager of the research area "Media Platforms and Management" at the Institute for Media and Communications Management at the University St. Gallen. Her research interests are knowledge media platforms, ontologies, concepts for management of knowledge management platforms and reference models for component-based knowledge management.

Jeanine W. Turner received her Ph.D. from the Ohio State University. Her research explores the human factors and management issues involved in the introduction of new communication technologies within organizations and the development of virtual organizations. Specifically, she has studied the implementation of telemedicine technology as a means of augmenting the delivery of healthcare services, use of computer-mediated bulletin boards as a form of social support, and use of videoconferencing technology and the internet for distance education. Turner is an assistant professor in The McDonough School of Business at Georgetown University and holds a joint appointment with the Georgetown University School of Medicine.

Jim Warren is Director of the Health Informatics Research Group and Senior Lecturer in Computer and Information Science at the University of South Australia. He is interested in the nexus of human-computer interaction and decision support, especially as it applies to the health sector. Much of his work focuses on technology for the future computing workstation of the general practitioner. He is also interested in on-line learning environments. He holds the PhD in Information Systems and B.S. in Computer Science from the University of Maryland Baltimore Country (UMBC).

Bernard M. Waxman is an associate professor ast Southern Illinois University at Edwardsville since 1989. He has an M.A. degree in mathematics from the University of Illinois at Urbana-Champaign and a Doctoral degree in computer science from Washington University in St. Louis. His research interests include computer networks and algorithms with an emphasis on approximation algorithms and multicast routing. Prior to receiving his degree in computer science, Dr. Waxman served as the president of a professional photoprocessing laboratory and taught high school mathematics.

Terence Wee, a postgraduate student at the University of Auckland, is currently on a year's work-experience in Singapore.

Jerry B. Weinberg is an Assistant Professor in the Department of Computer Science of the School of Engineering at Southern Illinois University – Edwardsville. He received the B.S. degree in nursing from Indiana State University, Terre Haute, the B.S. degree in computer science from the University of South Carolina, Columbia, and the M.S. and Ph.D. degree in computer science from Vanderbilt University, Nashville, TN. His research interests include abductive reasoning, inductive learning, medical diagnosis, and the application of conceptual clustering and concept formation to database mining and knowledge discovery. Dr. Weinberg is a member of AAAI, IEEE, and ACM.

Xudong William Yu is an Assistant Professor in the Computer Science Department at Southern Illinois University-Edwardsville. He received his Ph.D. in computer science from Vanderbilt University in 1992. His research interests include model-based reasoning and diagnosis, hybrid systems for diagnosis, knowledge-based systems, modeling and analysis of complex systems, and machine learning.

David Ziege is the manager of financial analysis at the corporate office of Holy Cross Health System. He has worked at the corporate office for nine years, the last four years as project leader for the cost function. He received his MS in administration from the University of Notre Dame in 1996 and his BS in accounting from Ball State University in 1986. Mr. Ziege's work has recently been published in *Topics of Health Information Management.* His professional interests involve incorporating cost and DSS information into managing operations.

Index

A

access 227
access point 246
accessibility auditing 240
Active Server Pages 194
ActiveX Database Objects 197
Actor-Network Theory 17
artificial intelligence 146
asynchronous 253

B

benefits expected from teleradiology 47
breast cancer 141
Breast Cancer Analysis System (BCAS) 144
British National Health Services 230

C

cancer 141
cancers 222
cardiovascular diseases 222
Center for Information Technology 127
central database system 125
chronic hypertension 189
client/server architecture 92, 115
client/server networks 172
clinical decision-making 172, 173
clinical practice 182
clustering techniques 142
cognitive disabilities. 258
communication flows 34
communication tools 222
components 92
computational queries 256
computer decision support systems 233

D

computer-assisted access evaluation, 239
computer-based clinical decision support systems 181
computer-mediated communication 15
computer-mediated network 15
computer-mediated workspaces 252
conceptualizations of the teleradiology network 47
CORBA 5
CORBAmed 7
cost accounting methodology 110
cost allocation system 119
cost information systems 109, 111
cost of distributing 181
cost-containment imperatives 222

data analysis 144
Data integrity 79
data mining 148
Data verification 79
data warehousing 144
Database Group 127
decision support 144, 191
decision support system 144
Department of Veterans Affairs 92
development tools 88
diabetes 206
diabetes care and management 206
diabetic 206
Dicom 46
direct-to-consumer advertising 33
discrimination complaint 240
disease management program 40
disease prevention 222